Pharmaceutical Bioequivalence

DRUGS AND THE PHARMACEUTICAL SCIENCES

A Series of Textbooks and Monographs

edited by

James Swarbrick
AAI, Inc.
Wilmington, North Carolina

1. Pharmacokinetics, *Milo Gibaldi and Donald Perrier*
2. Good Manufacturing Practices for Pharmaceuticals: A Plan for Total Quality Control, *Sidney H. Willig, Murray M. Tuckerman, and William S. Hitchings IV*
3. Microencapsulation, *edited by J. R. Nixon*
4. Drug Metabolism: Chemical and Biochemical Aspects, *Bernard Testa and Peter Jenner*
5. New Drugs: Discovery and Development, *edited by Alan A. Rubin*
6. Sustained and Controlled Release Drug Delivery Systems, *edited by Joseph R. Robinson*
7. Modern Pharmaceutics, *edited by Gilbert S. Banker and Christopher T. Rhodes*
8. Prescription Drugs in Short Supply: Case Histories, *Michael A. Schwartz*
9. Activated Charcoal: Antidotal and Other Medical Uses, *David O. Cooney*
10. Concepts in Drug Metabolism (in two parts), *edited by Peter Jenner and Bernard Testa*
11. Pharmaceutical Analysis: Modern Methods (in two parts), *edited by James W. Munson*
12. Techniques of Solubilization of Drugs, *edited by Samuel H. Yalkowsky*
13. Orphan Drugs, *edited by Fred E. Karch*
14. Novel Drug Delivery Systems: Fundamentals, Developmental Concepts, Biomedical Assessments, *Yie W. Chien*
15. Pharmacokinetics: Second Edition, Revised and Expanded, *Milo Gibaldi and Donald Perrier*
16. Good Manufacturing Practices for Pharmaceuticals: A Plan for Total Quality Control, Second Edition, Revised and Expanded, *Sidney H. Willig, Murray M. Tuckerman, and William S. Hitchings IV*
17. Formulation of Veterinary Dosage Forms, *edited by Jack Blodinger*
18. Dermatological Formulations: Percutaneous Absorption, *Brian W. Barry*
19. The Clinical Research Process in the Pharmaceutical Industry, *edited by Gary M. Matoren*

20. Microencapsulation and Related Drug Processes, *Patrick B. Deasy*
21. Drugs and Nutrients: The Interactive Effects, *edited by Daphne A. Roe and T. Colin Campbell*
22. Biotechnology of Industrial Antibiotics, *Erick J. Vandamme*
23. Pharmaceutical Process Validation, *edited by Bernard T. Loftus and Robert A. Nash*
24. Anticancer and Interferon Agents: Synthesis and Properties, *edited by Raphael M. Ottenbrite and George B. Butler*
25. Pharmaceutical Statistics: Practical and Clinical Applications, *Sanford Bolton*
26. Drug Dynamics for Analytical, Clinical, and Biological Chemists, *Benjamin J. Gudzinowicz, Burrows T. Younkin, Jr., and Michael J. Gudzinowicz*
27. Modern Analysis of Antibiotics, *edited by Adjoran Aszalos*
28. Solubility and Related Properties, *Kenneth C. James*
29. Controlled Drug Delivery: Fundamentals and Applications, Second Edition, Revised and Expanded, *edited by Joseph R. Robinson and Vincent H. Lee*
30. New Drug Approval Process: Clinical and Regulatory Management, *edited by Richard A. Guarino*
31. Transdermal Controlled Systemic Medications, *edited by Yie W. Chien*
32. Drug Delivery Devices: Fundamentals and Applications, *edited by Praveen Tyle*
33. Pharmacokinetics: Regulatory · Industrial · Academic Perspectives, *edited by Peter G. Welling and Francis L. S. Tse*
34. Clinical Drug Trials and Tribulations, *edited by Allen E. Cato*
35. Transdermal Drug Delivery: Developmental Issues and Research Initiatives, *edited by Jonathan Hadgraft and Richard H. Guy*
36. Aqueous Polymeric Coatings for Pharmaceutical Dosage Forms, *edited by James W. McGinity*
37. Pharmaceutical Pelletization Technology, *edited by Isaac Ghebre-Sellassie*
38. Good Laboratory Practice Regulations, *edited by Allen F. Hirsch*
39. Nasal Systemic Drug Delivery, *Yie W. Chien, Kenneth S. E. Su, and Shyi-Feu Chang*
40. Modern Pharmaceutics: Second Edition, Revised and Expanded, *edited by Gilbert S. Banker and Christopher T. Rhodes*
41. Specialized Drug Delivery Systems: Manufacturing and Production Technology, *edited by Praveen Tyle*
42. Topical Drug Delivery Formulations, *edited by David W. Osborne and Anton H. Amann*
43. Drug Stability: Principles and Practices, *Jens T. Carstensen*
44. Pharmaceutical Statistics: Practical and Clinical Applications, Second Edition, Revised and Expanded, *Sanford Bolton*
45. Biodegradable Polymers as Drug Delivery Systems, *edited by Mark Chasin and Robert Langer*

46. Preclinical Drug Disposition: A Laboratory Handbook, *Francis L. S. Tse and James J. Jaffe*
47. HPLC in the Pharmaceutical Industry, *edited by Godwin W. Fong and Stanley K. Lam*
48. Pharmaceutical Bioequivalence, *edited by Peter G. Welling, Francis L. S. Tse, and Shrikant V. Dinghe*
49. Pharmaceutical Dissolution Testing, *Umesh V. Banakar*
50. Novel Drug Delivery Systems: Second Edition, Revised and Expanded, *Yie W. Chien*
51. Managing the Clinical Drug Development Process, *David M. Cocchetto and Ronald V. Nardi*
52. Good Manufacturing Practices for Pharmaceuticals: A Plan for Total Quality Control, Third Edition, *edited by Sidney H. Willig and James R. Stoker*
53. Prodrugs: Topical and Ocular Drug Delivery, *edited by Kenneth B. Sloan*
54. Pharmaceutical Inhalation Aerosol Technology, *edited by Anthony J. Hickey*
55. Radiopharmaceuticals: Chemistry and Pharmacology, *edited by Adrian D. Nunn*
56. New Drug Approval Process: Second Edition, Revised and Expanded, *edited by Richard A. Guarino*
57. Pharmaceutical Process Validation: Second Edition, Revised and Expanded, *edited by Ira R. Berry and Robert A. Nash*
58. Ophthalmic Drug Delivery Systems, *edited by Ashim K. Mitra*
59. Pharmaceutical Skin Penetration Enhancement, *edited by Kenneth A. Walters and Jonathan Hadgraft*
60. Colonic Drug Absorption and Metabolism, *edited by Peter R. Bieck*
61. Pharmaceutical Particulate Carriers: Therapeutic Applications, *edited by Alain Rolland*
62. Drug Permeation Enhancement: Theory and Applications, *edited by Dean S. Hsieh*
63. Glycopeptide Antibiotics, *edited by Ramakrishnan Nagarajan*
64. Achieving Sterility in Medical and Pharmaceutical Products, *Nigel A. Halls*
65. Multiparticulate Oral Drug Delivery, *edited by Isaac Ghebre-Sellassie*
66. Colloidal Drug Delivery Systems, *edited by Jörg Kreuter*
67. Pharmacokinetics: Regulatory · Industrial · Academic Perspectives, Second Edition, *edited by Peter G. Welling and Francis L. S. Tse*
68. Drug Stability: Principles and Practices, Second Edition, Revised and Expanded, *Jens T. Carstensen*
69. Good Laboratory Practice Regulations: Second Edition, Revised and Expanded, *edited by Sandy Weinberg*
70. Physical Characterization of Pharmaceutical Solids, *edited by Harry G. Brittain*

ADDITIONAL VOLUMES IN PREPARATION

Modern Pharmaceutics: Third Edition, Revised and Expanded, *edited by Gilbert S. Banker and Christopher T. Rhodes*

Pharmaceutical Powder Compaction Technology, *edited by Christer Nyström and Göran Alderborn*

Pharmaceutical Bioequivalence

edited by

Peter G. Welling
Parke-Davis Pharmaceutical Research Division
Warner-Lambert Company
Ann Arbor, Michigan

Francis L. S. Tse
Sandoz Research Institute
East Hanover, New Jersey

Shrikant V. Dighe
Center for Drug Evaluation and Research
Food and Drug Administration
Rockville, Maryland

informa
healthcare

First published in 1991 by Marcel Dekker Inc, 270 Madison Avenue, New York, NY 10016.

This edition published in 2010 by Informa Healthcare, Telephone House, 69-77 Paul Street, London EC2A 4LQ, UK.

Simultaneously published in the USA by Informa Healthcare, 52 Vanderbilt Avenue, 7th Floor, New York, NY 10017, USA.

Informa Healthcare is a trading division of Informa UK Ltd. Registered Office: 37–41 Mortimer Street, London W1T 3JH, UK. Registered in England and Wales number 1072954.

©2010 Informa Healthcare, except as otherwise indicated
Printed and bound in India by Replika Press Pvt. Ltd.

No claim to original U.S. Government works

Reprinted material is quoted with permission. Although every effort has been made to ensure that all owners of copyright material have been acknowledged in this publication, we would be glad to acknowledge in subsequent reprints or editions any omissions brought to our attention.

All rights reserved. No part of this publication may be reproduced, stored in a retrieval system, or transmitted, in any form or by any means, electronic, mechanical, photocopying, recording, or otherwise, unless with the prior written permission of the publisher or in accordance with the provisions of the Copyright, Designs and Patents Act 1988 or under the terms of any licence permitting limited copying issued by the Copyright Licensing Agency, 90 Tottenham Court Road, London W1P 0LP, UK, or the Copyright Clearance Center, Inc., 222 Rosewood Drive, Danvers, MA 01923, USA (http://www.copyright.com/ or telephone 978-750-8400).

Product or corporate names may be trademarks or registered trademarks, and are used only for identification and explanation without intent to infringe.

This book contains information from reputable sources and although reasonable efforts have been made to publish accurate information, the publisher makes no warranties (either express or implied) as to the accuracy or fitness for a particular purpose of the information or advice contained herein. The publisher wishes to make it clear that any views or opinions expressed in this book by individual authors or contributors are their personal views and opinions and do not necessarily reflect the views/opinions of the publisher. Any information or guidance contained in this book is intended for use solely by medical professionals strictly as a supplement to the medical professional's own judgement, knowledge of the patient's medical history, relevant manufacturer's instructions and the appropriate best practice guidelines. Because of the rapid advances in medical science, any information or advice on dosages, procedures, or diagnoses should be independently verified. This book does not indicate whether a particular treatment is appropriate or suitable for a particular individual. Ultimately it is the sole responsibility of the medical professional to make his or her own professional judgements, so as appropriately to advise and treat patients. Save for death or personal injury caused by the publisher's negligence and to the fullest extent otherwise permitted by law, neither the publisher nor any person engaged or employed by the publisher shall be responsible or liable for any loss, injury or damage caused to any person or property arising in any way from the use of this book.

A CIP record for this book is available from the British Library.

Library of Congress Cataloging-in-Publication Data available on application

ISBN-13: 9780824784843

Orders may be sent to: Informa Healthcare, Sheepen Place, Colchester, Essex CO3 3LP, UK
Telephone: +44 (0)20 7017 5540
Email: CSDhealthcarebooks@informa.com
Website: http://informahealthcarebooks.com/

For corporate sales please contact: CorporateBooksIHC@informa.com
For foreign rights please contact: RightsIHC@informa.com
For reprint permissions please contact: PermissionsIHC@informa.com

Preface

A systemically acting drug must be absorbed from the site of administration to an extent and at a rate that will elicit a required therapeutic effect for a desired period of time. The rate and extent of drug absorption are a function of many factors, including the site of administration, the physicochemical characteristics of the compound, and the dosage form. If two or more different dosage forms are intended to exert an identical therapeutic effect, it is essential that they have the same bioavailability.

These statements regarding bioequivalence and bioavailability, while appearing to be exquisitely simple and straightforward, have given rise to heated controversy in pharmaceutical and clinical circles for many years. Compounding the issues of bioequivalence and bioavailability are those of therapeutic efficacy and equivalence as well as the underpinnings of economic factors. These have created a jumble of rules, interpretations, and opinions from which we have not yet extricated ourselves.

In order to help resolve the many controversies and misunderstandings currently surrounding bioequivalence and bioavailability, we invited a number of scientists from academia, industry, and regulatory agencies to contribute to this book. Our intention was to present informed opinions from those actively involved in addressing problems associated with the many aspects of drug bioequivalence and bioavailability as well as those involved in "setting the ground rules" from regulatory bodies worldwide. The response to our invitation was extremely gratifying and reflects not only the dedicated enthusiasm of the authors but also the urgency of the topic.

This book consists of 16 chapters and is divided into three major sections. Part One addresses major concerns including bioequivalence and therapeutic equivalence, study design for bioavailability and bioequivalence assessment, statistical criteria, disease state, mechanisms of absorption, luminal gut wall metabolism, bioequivalence of oral versus parenteral formulations, and in vitro–in vivo relationships. Part Two addresses species differences in physiology and pharmacokinetics affecting drug absorption and pharmacodynamic models. Part Three collectively presents the current opinions of regulatory agencies in the United States, Canada, Europe, Scandinavia, and Australia. This book thus presents a broad spectrum of information and opinions from a variety of perspectives on this controversial and fascinating topic.

If presenting this wealth of current material in a single book helps to provide greater understanding of the problems associated with bioequivalence and bioavailability monitoring, resolves misconceptions regarding bioequivalence and therapeutic equivalence, and provides direction in the design and interpretation of bioequivalence and bioavailability studies, then we have achieved our goal.

We are indebted to many of our colleagues for their kind advice in the design of this book. We gratefully acknowledge the authors for giving up so much of their valuable time to contribute to this endeavor. We must also thank Executive Secretaries Christine Cavanna and Rosemary Valentino for their continued help and support, and for keeping the whole thing straight.

Peter G. Welling
Francis L. S. Tse
Shrikant V. Dighe

Contents

Preface   *iii*
Contributors   *vii*

Part One
Bioequivalence and Its Determination

1. Bioequivalence and Therapeutic Equivalence   1
   Roger L. Williams

2. Study Design for the Assessment of Bioavailability
   and Bioequivalence   17
   Francis L. S. Tse, William T. Robinson, and Miles G. Choc

3. Statistical Criteria   35
   Carl M. Metzler

4. Influence of Disease on Bioavailability   67
   Wolfgang A. Ritschel and Donald D. Denson

5. Factors Influencing Bioavailability and
   Bioequivalence   117
   Arzu Selen

6. The Role of Intestinal Metabolism on Bioavailability 149
   William H. Barr

7. Bioavailability of Transdermal and Topical Dosage Forms 169
   Marvin C. Meyer

8. In Vitro Methods to Determine Bioavailability:
   In Vitro–In Vivo Correlations 223
   Peter G. Welling

Part Two
Species Differences, Pharmacodynamic Models

9. Animal Models for Oral Drug Absorption 235
   Jennifer B. Dressman and Kenji Yamada

10. Interspecies Scaling in Pharmacokinetics 267
    Patrick J. McNamara

11. Pharmacodynamic Models in Bioequivalence 301
    S. Thomas Forgue and Wayne A. Colburn

Part Three
Perspectives of Regulatory Agencies, Worldwide, on Bioequivalence Testing

12. Bioequivalence: A United States Regulatory Perspective 347
    Shrikant V. Dighe and Wallace P. Adams

13. Bioequivalence: A Canadian Regulatory Perspective 381
    Iain J. McGilveray

14. Bioequivalence: A European Community Regulatory Perspective 419
    A. G. Rauws

15. Bioavailability and Bioequivalence: An Australian Perspective 443
    Susan Walters and Rodney Charles Hall

16. Bioequivalence: A Nordic Perspective 453
    Tomas Salmonson, Hans Melander, and Anders Rane

Index 463

Contributors

Wallace P. Adams, Ph.D.   Division of Bioequivalence, Center for Drug Evaluation and Research, Food and Drug Administration, Rockville, Maryland

William H. Barr, Pharm D., Ph.D.   Professor and Chairman, Department of Pharmacy and Pharmaceutics, Medical College of Virginia, Virginia Commonwealth University, Richmond, Virginia

Miles G. Choc, Ph.D.* Department of Drug Metabolism, Sandoz Research Institute, East Hanover, New Jersey

Wayne A. Colburn, Ph.D.   Vice President, Clinical Development Division, Harris Laboratories, Inc., Scottsdale, Arizona

Donald D. Denson, Ph.D.   Associate Professor of Anesthesia, College of Medicine, and Associate Professor of Pharmacy, Director of Research, Division of Anesthesia, University of Cincinnati Medical Center, Cincinnati, Ohio

---

**Current affiliation*: Vice President and Scientific Director, Biodecision Laboratories, Pittsburgh, Pennsylvania

Shrikant V. Dighe, Ph.D.   Director, Division of Bioequivalence, Center for Drug Evaluation and Research, Food and Drug Administration, Rockville, Maryland

Jennifer B. Dressman, Ph.D.   Associate Professor of Pharmaceutics, College of Pharmacy, The University of Michigan, Ann Arbor, Michigan

S. Thomas Forgue, Ph.D.   Senior Research Associate, Pharmacokinetics/Drug Metabolism, Parke-Davis Pharmaceutical Research Division, Warner-Lambert Company, Ann Arbor, Michigan

Rodney Charles Hall, Ph.D.   Medical Director, Merck Sharp & Dohme (Australia) Pty. Ltd., South Granville, New South Wales, Australia

Iain J. McGilveray, Ph.D.   Head, Biopharmaceutics Section, Drug Toxicology Division, Health Protection Branch, Bureau of Drug Research, Ottawa, Ontario, Canada

Patrick J. McNamara, Ph.D.   Associate Professor, College of Pharmacy, University of Kentucky, Lexington, Kentucky

Hans Melander, M.Sc.   Head of Biostatistics, Division of Pharmacotherapeutics, Medical Products Agency, Uppsala, Sweden

Carl M. Metzler, Ph.D.   Distinguished Scientist, Research Biostatistics, The Upjohn Company, Kalamazoo, Michigan

Marvin C. Meyer, Ph.D.   Professor and Associate Dean for Research and Research Training, College of Pharmacy, University of Tennessee, Memphis, Tennessee

Anders Rane, M.D.   Professor, Division of Clinical Pharmacology, University Hospital, and Medical Products Agency, Uppsala, Sweden

A. G. Rauws, Dr. Biochem.   Pharmacokinetic Consultant, Staff Bureau Sector of Pharmacology and Toxicology, National Institute of Public Health and Environmental Protection, Bilthoven, The Netherlands

Wolfgang A. Ritschel, Ph.D., M.D.   Professor and Chairman, Division of Pharmaceutics and Drug Delivery Systems, University of Cincinnati Medical Center, Cincinnati, Ohio

William T. Robinson, Ph.D.   Director, Department of Drug Metabolism, Sandoz Research Institute, East Hanover, New Jersey

Contributors

Tomas Salmonson, Ph.D. Head of Pharmacokinetics, Division of Pharmacotherapeutics, Medical Products Agency, Uppsala, Sweden

Arzu Selen, Ph.D. Research Associate, Pharmacokinetics/Drug Metabolism Department, Parke-Davis Pharmaceutical Research Division, Warner-Lambert Company, Ann Arbor, Michigan

Francis L. S. Tse, Ph.D. Assistant Director, Drug Metabolism Department, Sandoz Research Institute, East Hanover, New Jersey

Susan Walters, Ph.D. Drug Evaluation Branch, Therapeutic Goods Administration, Canberra, Australia

Peter G. Welling, Ph.D., D.Sc. Vice President, Pharmacokinetics and Drug Metabolism, Parke-Davis Pharmaceutical Research Division, Warner-Lambert Company, Ann Arbor, Michigan

Roger L. Williams, M.D. Director, Office of Generic Drugs, Center for Drug Evaluation and Research, Food and Drug Administration, Rockville, Maryland

Kenji Yamada, Ph.D. Department of Drug Metabolism, Taisho Pharmaceutical Company, Saitama, Japan

Pharmaceutical Bioequivalence

Part One
Bioequivalence and Its Determination

Part One
Bioequivalence and Its Determination

1
Bioequivalence and Therapeutic Equivalence

Roger L. Williams
Center for Drug Evaluation and Research
Food and Drug Administration
Rockville, Maryland

INTRODUCTION

The health professional today is often confronted with a bewildering array of medications for a single indication. Different classes of agents are available to treat a single condition, and within each class many different agents may be available that exhibit, more or less, the same beneficial and adverse effects [1]. For a single agent, different salt forms may be available. Finally, a specific drug salt may be prepared as a capsule or tablet, each with different excipients, coatings, and coloring agents, which may affect the release rate of the drug from the formulation. The bulk of prescription drug products fall into this final category; of the approximately 10,000 prescription drugs available in 1990, over 80% are available from more than one source [2]. It is a remarkable practitioner who can select one agent knowledgeably from this potentially large group of comparable products and administer it rationally in a therapeutic setting. In many instances, specific labeling claims will distinguish between different drugs that are prescribed for the same indication. When the same tablet or capsule is available from different sources, with only excipient, color, and coating differences, the labeling can be similar or identical. The availability of drug formulations from different sources with similar or identical labeling is an increasingly common occurrence in clinical practice: one example is the introduction of a generic formulation for a marketed product that has lost patent protection; a second example is substitution of one formulation of a patent-protected drug for another as a result of manufacturing changes; and a third example is the introduction of a new formulation intended for sale to replace the clinical trial drug product used in the New Drug Application (NDA) process. Issues surrounding the substitution of one formulation for another are thus not "generic-innovator" or "new-old" issues, but rather, are a part of the development of many, if not most, drug products.

Marketing of different formulations of the same drug substance, given in the same strength, the same dosage form, by the same route, and according to the same labeling has posed a special challenge to health care professionals, regulatory agencies and pharmaceutical scientists. In part, this challenge arises from economic issues and issues over who controls drug prescribing. Substitution of one product for another can now occur, with little input from, and perhaps even lack of awareness of, the practitioner—although practitioners throughout the United States retain authority to prevent substitution. In part, the challenge arises from the regulatory and scientific task of developing a set of criteria to judge whether one formulation can be substituted for another without a labeling change and in the absence of clinical trials. This judgement is now based on several factors, perhaps the most important of which is the in vivo bioequivalence study. This chapter will explore theoretical and observational aspects of the clinical bioequivalence study as a determinant of therapeutic equivalence and substitution, in the absence of labeling changes. In bioequivalence studies, usually an unapproved formulation is compared with the original brand name (innovator's) formulation. In the following discussion, the approved formulation is termed the *reference formulation*, and the brand name formulation is termed the *test formulation*. The chapter will focus on the determination of equivalence of orally administered capsules and tablets, with the expectation that concepts in this setting can usually be generalized to formulations intended for other routes of administration.

BACKGROUND

In the United States, the Food, Drug and Cosmetic (FD&C) Act of 1938 and the Kefauver-Harris Amendment to this act in 1962 require that safety and efficacy data be generated to support claims for active ingredients in a drug product before approval for sale. In the last several decades, societal judgments in the United States, translated into scientific standards by the Food and Drug Administration (FDA) and presented publicly in several formats, have allowed the substitution of one formulation for another, without a requirement to repeat expensive and time-consuming clinical safety and efficacy studies. The scientific rationale for these judgments is that a set of biopharmaceutic, pharmacokinetic, and statistical standards can be established to document that a test formulation is therapeutically interchangeable with a reference formulation in the absence of clinical trials. A test formulation that meets these criteria is termed *bioequivalent* to, and therapeutically interchangeable with, the reference formulation. Since the early 1970s, in the United States [3,4], these criteria have been embodied in regulatory policies of the FDA to allow marketing of generic drug formulations. Summaries of the criteria, the regulatory history underlying their creation, and exceptions to general provisions have recently been published [5]. These criteria are also generally applicable when a marketed product is reformulated for manufacturing or marketing reasons. The mechanism by which a generic product can be marketed in the United States is through submission and approval of an Abbreviated New Drug Application (ANDA). For reformulation of a patent-protected product, a supplement to the New Drug Application (NDA) is usually required. Before 1984, generic formulations were allowed primarily for innovator products that were approved for sale before 1962, providing acceptable marketing conditions for the primary drug product has been developed during the Drug Efficacy Study Implementation [5]. Although never absolute, this partial barrier to generic substitution for drugs approved after 1962 was removed in 1984, with passage of the Drug Price Competition and Patent Term Restoration Act, which allows marketing of any off-patent drug, provided specific ANDA criteria are met. Details of the history and regulation of generic drug development and substitution have been recently reviewed [6,7].

Criteria by which one formulation can be deemed equivalent to another in part focus on product and manufacturing documentation of similarity. The product documentation criteria require that the new formulation contains the same active ingredients in the same dose form and strength, is intended for the same route of administration, and is labeled comparably with the formulation it is designed to replace. The manufacturing documentation criteria relate to manufacturing processes to ensure that drug products exhibit known and consistent stability, purity, and potency. A final requirement for a determination of equivalence between one formulation and another is usually an in vivo human bioequivalence study to confirm that levels of drug or metabolite in selected biological fluids are comparable after administration of each formulation. Currently, in the United States, certain existing drug formulations do not require in vivo bioequivalence studies, but virtually all new tablet or capsule formulations from which measurable amounts of drug or metabolites are absorbed into the systemic circulation require a human bioequivalence study for approval. Although continually evolving, clinical trial methodology and pharmacokinetic and statistical criteria to document bioequivalence have become relatively standardized in the last two decades. More recently, attempts have been made to extend these principles to allow marketing approval of a controlled-release formulation for an immediate-release formulation without a requirement for clinical trials [8].

Inherent in the demonstration that one formulation is bioequivalent to another is the expectation that formulations deemed bioequivalent will be therapeutically interchangeable. Products that are judged bioequivalent according to current pharmacokinetic and statistical guidelines can thus be used interchangeably, with the understanding that risk and efficacy after either formulation should be similar. This is an important conclusion that must be convincing not only to the pharmaceutical sponsor and the FDA, but to the constituency who will use the new formulation, namely, patients and health care professionals. Historically, development of bioequivalence regulations and guidelines has focused on pharmacokinetic and statistical practices as a means of defining bioequivalence [9]. This emphasis arose from clear evidence of bioinequivalence between formulations that were nominally identical [10-12]. More recently, and perhaps coincident with the development of better ways to assess drug pharmacologic effects, the focus has shifted somewhat to an examination of the assumption that bioequivalence and therapeutic equivalence are one and the same. Surprisingly, relatively few studies have been performed to assess this assumption. Although many critiques of generic and other forms of substitution have been advanced [13-19], specific challenges to bioequivalence judgments as a means of predicting therapeutic equivalence frequently focus on (1) the criteria used to establish or refute equivalence in a clinical bioequivalence study and (2) the performance of the standard clinical study in a young healthy male population.

IN VIVO BIOEQUIVALENCE: CRITERIA AND ISSUES

Specific national regulatory requirements to document bioequivalence are reviewed in other chapters. Common to all these requirements is an in vivo bioequivalence study in which the test and reference formulations are usually administered to the same individuals on separate occasions, with collection of blood or urine samples, or both, for a specified period after each dose. Assays of these biological samples yield plasma or urine concentration-time curves for drug and metabolite(s) from which pharmacokinetic variables are calculated and compared by standard statistical tests. The resulting pharmacokinetic data and associated statistical analyses are examined according to a set of predetermined criteria, to confirm or refute the judgment that drug delivery and disposition are equivalent after administration of the test and reference formulations. At its simplest, an in vivo bioequivalence study involves administration of the test and reference formulations, each as a single dose, to healthy male volunteers in an open-label crossover fashion, with randomization for treatment sequence and allowance for adequate washout between the two doses. The time selected for washout is usually a minimum of 10 half-lives of the active moiety with the longest half-life. Healthy male volunteers are generally selected for the study to assure a homogeneous study population and to spare patients the rigors of a clinical investigation. Homogeneity in the study population permits focus on formulation, rather than between- and within-individual factors that affect drug absorption and disposition. Variations to this general approach are determined usually by specific characteristics of the drug. Pending regulatory approval, in vivo bioequivalence studies in animals have been proposed as a means of establishing bioequivalence for drugs not suitable for administration to healthy volunteers. Dosing to steady state may be required for drugs that exhibit nonlinear absorption or disposition characteristics. Irrespective of specific design criteria, the in vivo human bioequivalence study is the sine qua non to document bioequivalence and, by implication, therapeutic equivalence and substitutability. Issues of therapeutic equivalence versus bioequivalence will necessarily focus on the design and execution of the human in vivo bioequivalence study.

Pharmacokinetic Criteria

Pharmacokinetic parameters derived from blood or urine concentration–time curves generated in a clinical bioequivalence study generate information about the rate and extent of drug absorption for each formulation tested. Rate of absorption is frequently the more difficult determination, relying as it does on assumptions of the process by which a drug is absorbed and eliminated. Compartmental models, graphical procedures, and observational methods are used to compare drug absorption between two formulations. Compartmental models assume that absorption occurs by a specific rate process (e.g., first-order, zero-order kinetics). Graphical methods (Wagner–Nelson for drugs exhibiting one-compartment characteristics and Loo–Riegelman for drugs exhibiting multicompartmental characteristics) relate percentage drug absorbed versus time and can be used to compare test and reference formulations. Neither method assesses the extent of absorption, and both require information about drug disposition following an intravenous dose to ensure adequate description of the elimination rate constant(s) [20]. Observational methods assess rate of absorption directly from a comparison of peak drug or metabolite concentration and time of this concentration after administration of the test and reference formulations. Currently, and perhaps for reasons that relate more to ease of application than to a specific scientific rationale, the most frequently applied methodology is observational, namely, determination of peak concentration (C_{max}) and the time of its occurrence.

The extent of drug absorption is measured by area under the plasma concentration–time curve either after a single dose with extrapolation to infinity (AUC) or over an interdose interval ($AUC_{INTERDOSE}$) after administration of the test and reference formulations at constant rate and dosing intervals to steady state. Determination of bioavailability (F) requires administration of an intravenous dose. Because intravenous dosing is usually not performed in bioequivalence studies, only relative bioavailability is determined. In the past, an oral solution was sometimes included in a bioequivalence study to assess drug absorption in the absence of formulation factors, but, generally, this is neither now recommended nor performed. Although problems can arise in the determination of AUC or $AUC_{INTERDOSE}$ when sampling or assay limitations lead to a relatively large fraction of total AUC in the extrapolated area, the determination of extent of absorption is generally more straightforward than determination of rate of absorption. Reliance on AUC from two different dosing periods in a bioequivalence study assumes that clearance is the same during each dosing period. Analysis for sequence effects can sometimes indicate whether there is systematic deviation from this assumption in a specific study.

Statistical Criteria

The further analysis of pharmacokinetic data from a bioequivalence study involves the determination of whether the test and reference formulations differ within a predefined level of statistical significance. A commonly applied test in this determination is analysis of variance to assess treatment, period, and sequence effects. Interpretation can be difficult when a large difference in a particular parameter is not accompanied by a demonstration of a statistically significant difference, and the converse, when a small difference is found to be statistically significant. Additional tests are employed to assess the power and significance of the primary statistical observation. Power analysis evaluates the likelihood of falsely rejecting (type I error) or accepting (type II error) the null hypothesis that no difference exists between pharmacokinetic variables of the test and reference formulations. Power analysis and other statistical tests, such as confidence interval analysis [21] and the two one-sided tests [22], are necessary to judge the significance of a primary statistical observation. Just as the primary statistical test requires judgment of the significance of a given probability, these additional tests require a judgment of what difference is considered important. Historically, a difference of 20% in a pharmacokinetic variable has been defined as an important, as opposed to a statistically significant, difference. This 20% allowance is embodied in power analyses and in both the two one-sided and confidence interval tests. In a modified form, it is an integral part of the "75-125 rule," which is now less frequently applied.

One challenge to the in vivo bioequivalence study to document therapeutic equivalence is based on the assumption that the 20% guideline allows a difference of 20% in the means of pharmacokinetic variables (e.g., C_{max} and AUC) measured after administration of the test and reference formulations [23]. In fact, the current tests for bioequivalence are usually based on an analysis of mean ± the standard deviation (SD) of the individual formulation-associated *differences* in observed values for a specific pharmacokinetic variable. If two formulations behaved identically in vivo, this difference would be zero, with a standard deviation of zero. Current FDA rulings suggest that the mean difference and the 90% confidence interval (CI) of the difference ($\pm$ 2 SD) should be within a range of $\pm$ 20% about zero. This criterion is not the same as allowing the means of pharmacokinetic variables from two formulations to differ by 20%. A difference of this magnitude would almost certainly not meet current criteria for bioequivalence on the basis of confidence interval testing. Historically, differences between AUC means after test and reference formulations generally differ by 5% or less [24].

Pharmacokinetic Issues

Despite the rarity of mean differences greater than 5% in pharmacokinetic variables in an in vivo bioequivalence study, a specific pharmacokinetic variable in a single individual can frequently show differences of 20% and more from the group mean. Although differences of this magnitude are almost certainly attributable to within-individual, rather than formulation, factors, it is useful to consider the variation in pharmacokinetic variables that are required to produce $\pm 20\%$ differences in C_{max} and AUC. Simulated plasma concentration–time curves after an oral dose of a drug that exhibits first-order absorption and disposition according to a one-compartment model are shown in Figures 1–3. The middle baseline curve in Figures 1 and 2 was generated using the following parameters: (1) oral dose, 500 mg; (2) plasma clearance (CL), 5 L/hr; (3) plasma volume of distribution (V), 50 L; (4) rate constant of absorption (k_a), 0.70 hr^{-1}; (5) rate constant of elimination (k), 0.10 hr^{-1}; and (6) bioavailability (F), 0.5. These absorption

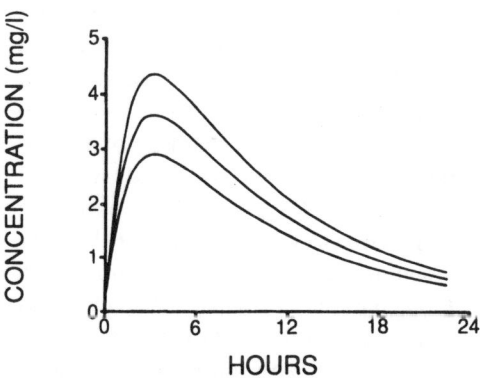

Figure 1 Simulated curves denoting a $\pm 20\%$ variation in extent of absorption; F varies from 0.4 (lower curve), to 0.5 (middle curve), to 0.6 (upper curve). See text for pharmacokinetic parameters used in the simulations.

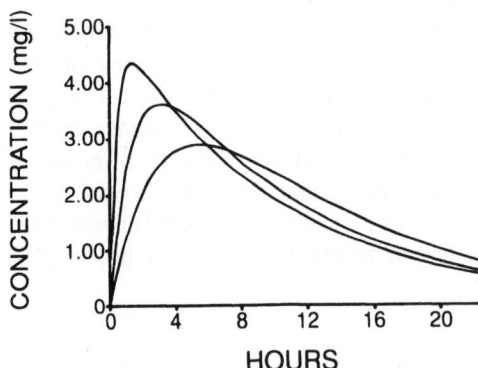

Figure 2 Simulated curves denoting a ±20% variation in C_{peak}; k_a varies from 0.34 hr^{-1} (lower curve), to 0.70 hr$_{-1}$ (middle curve), to 2.3 hr^{-1} (upper curve). See text for pharmacokinetic parameters used in the simulations.

and disposition parameters are characteristic of a drug that is relatively rapidly absorbed, but slowly cleared from the plasma, with an absorption half-life of about 1 hr and an elimination half-life of about 7 hr. The middle baseline curve in Figure 3 was simulated using the following pharmacokinetic parameters: (1) oral dose, 500 mg; (2) CL, 35 L/hr; (3) V, 50 L; (4) k_a, 0.10 hr^{-1}; k, 0.7 hr^{-1}; F, 0.5. These variables are representative of a rapidly cleared drug that exhibits absorption rate-limited kinetics, with an absorption half-life of about 7 hr and an elimination half-life of about 1 hr. The upper and lower curves in Figure 1 reflect a ±20% variation in extent of absorption (F = 0.4 and 0.6) without change in other pharmacokinetic parameters. This variation is directly reflected in ±20% changes in C_{max} and AUC and is true for any drug, irrespective of its absorption and disposition parameters. Because of the exponential character of absorption in the model, however, changes in rate of absorption are not directly reflected in C_{max} changes. To achieve a ±20% variation in C_{max} with only a change in absorption rate constant (see Fig. 2), k_a is required to vary from 0.34 hr^{-1} (lower curve) to 2.3 hr^{-1} (upper curve), representing a change in absorption half-life from about 2 to 0.3 hr. For a drug exhibiting the pharmacokinetic characteristics simulated by the curves in Figure 2, absorption must thus vary over a sevenfold range to produce a ±20% variation in C_{max}. When absorption is rate-limiting (see Fig. 3), the absorption rate constant is require to vary between 0.077 hr^{-1} (lower curve, absorption half-life 9 hr) and 0.13 hr^{-1} (upper curve, absorption half-life 5.3 hr) to produce a ±20% variation in C_{max}—approximately a twofold difference.

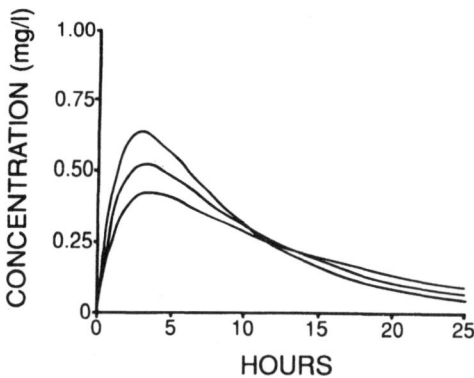

Figure 3 Simulated curves denoting a ±20% variation in C_{peak} for a drug with absorption rate-limited disposition; k_a varies from 0.077 hr^{-1} (lower curve), to 0.10 hr^{-1} (middle curve), to 0.13 hr^{-1} (upper curve). See text for pharmacokinetic parameters used in the simulations.

The simulations in Figures 2 and 3 demonstrate that substantial changes in the rate of absorption are sometimes necessary to produce ±20% changes in C_{max}. Depending on the relationship between the absorption and elimination rate constant, it may not be possible to achieve a 20% increment in C_{max}. This limit is indicated in Figure 4, which presents a comparison between the percentage change in absorption rate constant required to produce a 20% increment in C_{max} (ordinate) and the ratio of absorption and elimination rate constants (k_a/k) (abscissa). As an example, when k_a is approximately tenfold greater than k, k_a must increase by more than 500% to produce a 20% increment in C_{max}. The value of k_a approaches infinity when the k_a/k ratio approaches a limiting value of approximately 17. The relationships displayed in Figure 4 suggest that C_{max} is not a sensitive indicator of absorptive processes, particularly when absorption is rapid relative to elimination. In a sense, this observation may be encouraging because it suggests that marked differences in absorption rate for rapidly absorbed drugs can occur, without a corresponding increment in C_{max}. However, the consequences of not detecting manyfold differences in rate constants in standard bioequivalence studies for certain drugs and in specific patient populations remain to be explored. When saturable first-pass metabolism exists, differences in absorption rate may produce marked differences in C_{max} and AUC. It is thus possible that absorption rate differences may be exaggerated in special patient populations with greater saturation of absorptive processes. Martis and Levy [25] and Rubin and Tozer [26] have emphasized the importance of absorption rate in assessing bioequivalence in the presence of saturable metabolism.

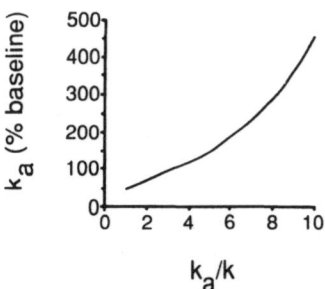

Figure 4 Percentage change in k_a required to produce a 20% increment in C_{peak} relative to the ratio of absorption and elimination rate constants (k_a/k) for a drug exhibiting linear and monoexponential absorption and elimination.

Pharmacodynamic Issues

The judgment of therapeutic equivalence relative to bioequivalence is closely related to the relationship between drug concentration and pharmacologic effect. Most drugs produce their beneficial and toxic pharmacologic effects as a consequence of interaction with one or more receptors. It is generally assumed that unbound drug at the receptor site equilibrates with unbound drug in other tissues and fluids of the body, including the intravascular space. This assumption underlies the construction of pharmacokinetic and pharmacodynamic models that relate total or unbound drug concentrations in plasma or blood at a given time to a pharmacologic effect of interest. Although several models of drug effect versus concentration have been proposed (linear, log-linear), one that is now most commonly used is the E_{max} model [27]. In this model, drug effect (E) is initially linearly related to concentration, but approaches a limit (E_{max}). The concentration at which effect is half maximal is termed the EC_{50}. This relationship is defined in the following equation:

$$\text{Effect} = \frac{E_{max} \cdot C}{EC_{50} + C}$$

The shape (sigmoidicity) of the E_{max} concentration–response relationship can be modified by adding an exponent (γ) to C in the above equation, which is useful in modeling variation in the rate of change in pharmacologic effect to concentration. This variation reflects that the concentration–response relationship is steep for some drugs and flat for others. A reasonable therapeutic goal is to administer a drug in the range at which effect is linearly related to concentration.

The E_{max} relationship between drug concentration and effect is pertinent to an assessment of the relationship between bioequivalence and therapeutic equivalence. For drug dosages at concentrations that lie in the linear portion of the concentration–response curve, concentration differences that might occur with substitution of one formulation for another produce equivalent differences in pharmacologic effect. When a drug is administered at concentrations close to E_{max}, differences in concentrations produced by different formulations will be less important. In the simulations in Figure 5, effect is expressed as percentage E_{max} versus time for a drug exhibiting the same primary pharmacokinetics and variation in absorption rate constant as the example depicted in Figure 2. The difference between the two sets of curves in Figure 5 is produced by a priori determination of the concentration at which effect is half-maximal (EC_{50}). In the lower set of curves, EC_{50} was chosen to be 10.8 mg/L, and in the upper set EC_{50} was chosen to be 1.2 mg/L. The lower set of curves thus reflects a linear relationship between concentration and effect, whereas the upper set reflects concentrations approaching E_{max}. Although the shape of the effect curves is the same, irrespective of the EC_{50}, the effect of different rates of absorption on pharmacologic effect expressed as percentage of E_{max} is substantially different. When concentration approaches E_{max} (see upper set of curves, Fig. 5), the percentage change in effect with a $\pm 20\%$ variation in C_{max} changes effect from about 70 to 78% of E_{max}—a fractional increment in response of about 10%. When the concentration attained relative to C_{50} is low (see lower set of curves, Fig. 5), a $\pm 20\%$ change in peak concentration varies effect from about 20 to 28% of E_{max}, a fractional increment of about 40%.

The shape (sigmoidicity) of the E_{max} relationship can also attenuate or magnify formulation differences in absorption. For a drug with a flat concentration–response E_{max} relationship ($\gamma < 1$), the effect of change in absorption rate on pharmacologic effect is small, whereas for a drug with a steep concentration–response curve ($\gamma > 1$), small absorption rate differences can move effect from none to maximal. Olson et al. used simulated data in a pharmacokinetic–pharmacodynamic model to suggest that sigmoidicity was a more important determinant of drug action than a $\pm 20\%$ variation in rate or extent of absorption [28]. This observation is perhaps more pertinent to between-individuals, rather than within-individual, comparisons. Concentration differences produced by different formulations within a single individual, who presumably has a more or less fixed concentration–response relationship, are directly related to pharmacologic response, depending, as noted, on the relationship between concentration, EC_{50}, and the shape of the concentration–response curve.

Although, ideally, a drug should reach a therapeutic response at concentrations well below those at which toxicity appears, many drugs produce some toxicity at or below concentrations associated with the desired pharmacologic effect. Within an individual, several pharmacokinetic and pharmacodynamic relationships can exist that reflect both beneficial and adverse drug actions. Low

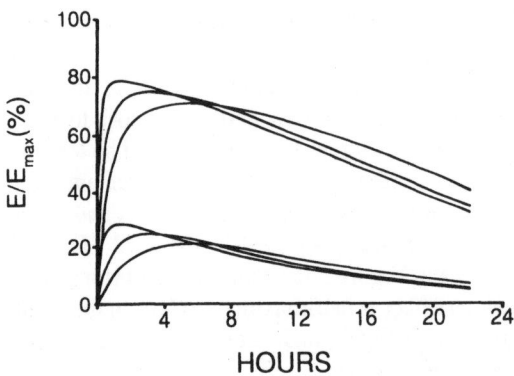

Figure 5 Simulated curves of pharmacologic effect using the E_{max} model for a drug exhibiting the same pharmacokinetic parameters and variation in absorption rate constant as the drug denoted in Figure 2. EC_{50} chosen as 10.8 mg/L (lower set of curves) or 1.2 mg/L (upper set of curves). See text for discussion.

therapeutic index drugs are frequently characterized by steep concentration–response relationships and manifestations of toxicity at or below concentrations at which maximum benefit occurs. For these drugs, efficacy and toxicity are closely related and confined to a narrow concentration range. Drugs with steep concentration–response relationships and manifestations of toxicity at or below concentrations at which maximum benefit occurs are strong candidates for inclusion on lists of narrow therapeutic range drugs. It has been argued that bioequivalence requirements for these drugs should be more stringent, and for certain drugs (e.g., warfarin) these more stringent requirements have, in fact, been applied. Pharmacokinetic and pharmacodynamic information required to identify the therapeutic window of a drug is frequently lacking. The information is difficult to obtain and, in any event, varies from patient to patient. More stringent restrictions on bioavailability requirements for these drugs would not obviate the requirement on the part of the health care professional to monitor the clinical status of the patient.

IN VIVO BIOEQUIVALENCE: CLINICAL STUDIES

Studies in Healthy Men

A frequent criticism of bioequivalence testing as a predictor of therapeutic equivalence is the decision to perform in vivo studies in healthy male volunteers. A principal argument for the use of this population is that the focus of a bioequivalence study should be on formulation factors and not on inter- or intraindividual factors (e.g., age, race, gender, diet, disease state, smoking history) that are known to affect drug absorption and disposition under certain conditions of use. Additional factors supporting this decision are the desire to avoid unnecessary drug administration to elderly or diseased populations or to pregnant women.

The argument in favor of performing bioequivalence studies in specific patient populations is generally based on the well-established argument that drug disposition in these populations frequently differs from that in healthy subjects. Following drug absorption into the systemic circulation, this argument is not compelling. Once a drug enters the systemic circulation, distribution and elimination should be consistent in a given individual, regardless of the formulation from which it was derived, barring some postabsorptive interaction between drug and excipients that at this time is generally hypothetical [29].

Certainly within-individual factors, such as age, race, gender, diet, and smoking history are known to affect drug pharmacokinetics and pharmacodynamics, but assessment of these effects generally does not lie in the province of a bioequivalence study. Before entry into the systemic circulation, however, a drug traverses an impressive array of barriers in the gut lumen, gut wall, portal vascular system, and liver before entry into the systemic circulation. At any point in this sequence, degradation can occur, with or without production of a active metabolite, as can interactions between drug, metabolite(s) and excipients. Within-individual factors, such as age and disease state, can disturb the barriers that a drug must transit to gain access to the systemic circulation. For example, alterations in gastric pH and emptying time, intestinal blood flow, and mucosal absorptive area, all have been reported to change in the elderly and in many diseased states. It is also known that formulation excipients can alter both the rate and extent of drug absorption. What seems much less well studied is whether these drug-absorption and drug-excipient interactions can somehow combine to produce alterations in drug absorption that would be detectable primarily in a patient population. In this event, bioavailability studies in healthy men might not adequately test comparability between two formulations under actual conditions of use.

Methods to Document Bioequivalence and Therapeutic Equivalence

Questions on the integrity of an in vivo bioequivalence study as a predictor of therapeutic equivalence could be assessed in several ways. One way involves the performance of specific clinical studies to confirm that a product determined to be bioequivalent in healthy subjects is also bioequivalent in the patient populations for which the drug was intended. A second way would be through postmarketing surveys of blood concentrations or therapeutic responses produced by different formulations of the same drug under actual conditions of use. A third method relies on anecdotal reports from the clinic. None of these methods has been systematically employed to confirm current bioequivalence methodology.

Despite decades of use of many different formulations of the same drug, anecdotal confirmation of therapeutic inequivalence in formulations determined to be bioequivalent has been rare [J. Morrison, personal communication]. When therapeutic failure can be attributable to a drug product, as opposed to drug or disease factors, failure is more readily attributable to manufacturing and quality control issues than to putative errors arising from bioequivalence testing. In the setting of wide within- and between-individual variation in pharmacokinetic parameters and pharmacodynamic response, contributions from formulation differences should usually be negligible. Although the long, and generally successful, history of substitution of one formulation for another that is based on current bioequivalence methodology in healthy men argues that the standard methodology is sound, underlying assumptions and methodology could be readily confirmed, either through specific prospective studies or through some form of postmarketing surveillance.

SUMMARY

Substitution of one drug formulation for another is now a common practice in clinical drug development and clinical medicine. General methods have been established to document that the in vivo absorption and disposition of the new formulation will be comparable with the one it is designed to replace or to compete with. A primary element of these methods is the in vivo bioequivalence study that is generally performed in healthy men. Criteria have been established to allow the assertion that when one formulation is bioequivalent, it is also therapeutically equivalent to another. In certain instances, these criteria are not especially sensitive and suggest that documentation of bioequivalence should be extended to specific patient populations. In addition, some underlying principles remain to be validated in specific scientific studies. Despite these caveats, the long history of successful substitution of one formulation for another—and the likelihood that drug and patient, rather than formulation factors are more likely to influence drug kinetics and response—argue that current methods of establishing bioequivalence will also result in therapeutic equivalence.

ACKNOWLEDGMENT

The author gratefully acknowledges the assistance of Thomas N. Tozer in the preparation of this manuscript.

REFERENCES

1. American College of Physicians. *Ann. Int. Med. 113*:160 (1990).
2. *Food Drug Lett. 365*:2 (1990).
3. *Fed. Reg. 34*:2673 (1969).
4. *Fed. Reg. 35*:6574 (1970).
5. *Fed. Reg. 54*:28873 (1989).
6. B. L. Strom. *N. Engl. J. Med. 316*:1456 (1987).
7. S. L. Nightingale and J. C. Morrison. *JAMA 258*:1200 (1987).
8. J. P. Skelly, et al. *Pharm. Res. 4*:75 (1987).
9. Drug Bioequivalance Study Panel Report. *Drug Bioequivalence.* Office of Technology Assessment (July 15, 1974).
10. W. L. Chiou. *J. Clin. Pharmacol. 12*:296 (1972).
11. J. Lindenbaum, et al. *N. Engl. J. Med. 285*:1344 (1971).
12. H. MacDonald, F. Pisano, J. Burger, A. Dornbush, and E. Pelcak. *Clin. Med.* 30 (1969).
13. H. R. Dettelbach. *J. Clin. Pharmacol. 26*:307 (1986).
14. R. Spector. *Iowa Med.* p. 24, (Jan. 1986).
15. P. P. Lamy. *J. Clin. Pharmacol. 26*:309 (1986).
16. J. L. Colaizzi and D. T. Lowenthal. *Clin. Ther. 8*:370 (1986).
17. L. A. Gottschalk. *J. Clin. Psychiatry 47*:3 (1986).
18. G. L. Klein. *Ann. Allergy 58*:350 (1987).
19. B. L. Diamond and J. W. Albrecht. *Psychopathology 20*:92 (1987).
20. M. Gibaldi and D. Perrier. *Pharmacokinetics.* Marcel Dekker, New York, 1982.
21. W. J. Westlake. *Current Concepts in the Pharmaceutical Sciences, Dosage Form Design and Bioavailability.* Lea & Febiger, Philadelphia, pp. 149–179 (1973).
22. D. J. Schuirmann. *J. Pharmacokinet. Biopharm. 15*:657 (1987).
23. American Association of Family Physicians, Committee on Public Policy. Appendix A. *Drugs Devices* p. 525 (1989).
24. *FDA Drug Bull. 16*:14 (1986).
25. L. Martis and R. H. Levy. *J. Pharmacokinet. Biopharm. 1*:283 (1973).
26. T. N. Tozer and G. M. Rubin. *Saturable Kinetics and Bioavailability Determination.* pp. 473–513.
27. N. H. G. Holford and L. B. Sheiner. *Clin. Pharmacokinet. 6*:429 (1981).
28. S. C. Olson, M. A. Eldon, R. D. Toothaker, J. J. Ferry, and W. A. Colburn. *J. Clin. Pharmacol. 27*:342 (1987).
29. G. A. Faich, J. Morrison, E.V. Dutra, D. B. Hare, P. H. Rheinstein. *N. Engl. J. Med. 316*:1473 (1987).

2
Study Design for the Assessment of Bioavailability and Bioequivalence

Francis L. S. Tse, William T. Robinson, and Miles G. Choc*
*Sandoz Research Institute
East Hanover, New Jersey*

INTRODUCTION

The term *bioavailability* was originally used to indicate the rate and relative amount of the administered drug that reaches the general circulation intact [1]. Over the years, it has been expanded to include the systemic availability of all active metabolites, particularly those with a pharmacologic activity similar to that of the parent drug [2]. Two drug products are generally considered to be *bioequivalent* if they yield comparable bioavailability when administered to the same individuals under similar dosage conditions. This simple definition, however, has led to controversy over its proper interpretation and evaluation. Several decades after the emergence of the concept of bioavailability and bioequivalence, regulatory authorities have not established a single set of requirements concerning the need, design, conduct, and interpretation of studies to determine product bioavailability and bioequivalence that would be universally acceptable. This phenomenon reflects, at least in part, the continued progress made in the various scientific arenas, for example, improvements in analytical methodology yielding lower limits of detection, discovery of active metabolites, new drugs with unique pharmacokinetic

---

*Current affiliation: Biodecision Laboratories, Pittsburgh, Pennsylvania.

characteristics, novel and controlled drug delivery systems, increased understanding of pharmacokinetic–pharmacodynamic relationships, as well as rational application of statistical methods to drug product evaluation. The present chapter reviews the various factors influencing the design of bioavailability and bioequivalence studies, and discusses the contemporary approaches to study design using specific examples based on work performed at Sandoz Research Institute on the phenothiazine analogue thioridazine and the new antipsychotic agent clozapine.

During the course of drug discovery and development, different bioavailability and bioequivalence studies are conducted for different objectives that, in turn, govern the design of these studies. The most common types of bioavailability and bioequivalence studies are described below.

TYPES OF BIOAVAILABILITY-BIOEQUIVALENCE STUDIES

1. *Study to evaluate the absolute bioavailability* of an oral, topical, intramuscular, or any other dosage form. Ideally, the test dosage form should be compared with an intravenous reference dose. In reality, however, a suitable intravenous form may not be readily available, and the test dosage form is usually compared, instead, with an oral solution or suspension to determine if the former would be adequate for subsequent clinical studies. Normally, the study is conducted in 6–12 subjects using a single-dose crossover design.
2. *Dose proportionality study* to determine if bioavailability parameters [i.e., peak concentration (C_{max}) and area under concentration–time curve (AUC)] are linear over the proposed dose range to be used in medical practice. Oral doses usually are given as a solution or suspension covering the therapeutic range for a single dose and tested using a three-way crossover design (low, mid, and high dose) in 12–18 subjects.
3. *Intra/intersubject variability study* to determine what the variability of bioavailability parameters are at any one dose level. Oral doses at one dose level are usually given as a solution or suspension in a mock three-way crossover design.
4. *Dosage form(s) study* to determine if that used during clinical trials is bioequivalent to that proposed for marketing. This is normally a single-dose crossover study evaluating the highest strength of the proposed marketed dosage form. The number of subjects to be used is dependent on available information on dose proportionality and inter- and intrasubject variability.
5. *Dosage form proportionality study* to determine if equipotent drug treatments administered as different dose strengths of the market form produce equivalent drug bioavailability. Normally, multiple strengths are evaluated by bracketing (i.e., studying the lowest and highest strengths at the same dose level in a

single-dose crossover design). The number of subjects again is based on dose proportionality and inter- and intrasubject variability of the drug.
6. *Effect of various types of intervention studies* to examine the effects of, for example, food and concomitant medication on bioavailability parameters. These are normally single- or multiple-dose studies conducted using the dosage form proposed for marketing.
7. *Bioequivalence study* needed as a result of changes in the formulation or manufacturing process (i.e., to show that the old and the new product are bioequivalent).
8. *ANDA bioequivalence studies* conducted for the purpose of filing an abbreviated new drug application (ANDA). The goal is to show that a generic drug is bioequivalent to the innovator's product in order to make claims of therapeutic equivalence.

FACTORS INFLUENCING THE DESIGN OF BIOAVAILABILITY–BIOEQUIVALENCE STUDIES

Intersubject and Intrasubject Variability

Since no two persons are identical in the way their bodies handle and respond to drugs, the question of intersubject variability is well recognized in bioavailability and bioequivalence studies. The use of a crossover design is but one attempt to address this issue. For some drugs, variation in pharmacokinetic parameters can occur over time, even within the same subject, caused primarily by changes in clearance because of variations in enzyme levels, inhibitors, inducers, urinary pH, and so forth. The magnitude of intrasubject variability has considerable impact on the design of bioequivalence studies and, therefore, should be determined when the drug is in its early phase of development.

The bioavailability of orally administered drugs depends, in part, on the extent of first-pass metabolism. For drugs subject to a high hepatic (perfusion-limited) clearance, changes in intrinsic clearance could result in altered bioavailability (F), without a significant effect on the subsequent disposition rate. Examples of such drugs include alprenolol [3], propranolol [4], and lidocaine [5]. In contrast, when the hepatic extraction ratio is low, such as for antipyrine [6] and theophylline [7], variation in intrinsic clearance is often reflected by altered clearance (CL) and half-life, instead of absolute bioavailability, which generally remains high. Thus, a drug with a high first-pass effect would tend to show greater variability in bioavailability secondary to variation in hepatic intrinsic clearance, compared with one with a low hepatic extraction ratio. However, it is interesting to note that the degree of variability in the commonly used bioavailability parameters [i.e., AUC after a single dose and average steady-state blood concentration ($\bar{C}_{ss}$)

during chronic dosing] is inherently no different between high- and low-clearance drugs [8]. As shown in Eq. (1) and (2),

$$\text{AUC} = \frac{F \cdot \text{dose}}{\text{CL}} \quad (1)$$

$$\bar{C}_{ss} = \frac{F \cdot \text{dose}}{\text{CL} \cdot \tau} \quad (2)$$

where CL is the total body clearance of drug and τ is the dosing interval, AUC and $\bar{C}_{ss}$ are functions of both F and CL. Therefore, variability in AUC or $\bar{C}_{ss}$ reflects variability in the intrinsic clearance of drugs of both high and low hepatic clearance, albeit through F in the former case and through CL in the latter.

Michaelis-Menten Kinetics

From Eqs. (1) and (2), it is clear that the use of AUC or $\bar{C}_{ss}$ in determining bioavailability is based on the premise that the overall clearance is the same for both the test drug product and the reference. Therefore, differences in bioavailability are usually attributed to differences in absorption. However, for drugs following Michaelis-Menten or other forms of nonlinear elimination kinetics, differences in bioavailability can occur, even when the degree of absorption is equivalent [9]. Drugs absorbed from the gastrointestinal tract are normally transferred through the portal circulation to the liver, where the enzymes responsible for most metabolic reactions are located. Thus, the absorbed drug can be partially or entirely metabolized before reaching systemic circulation. In the presence of Michaelis-Menten kinetics, the degree of this first-pass effect is a function of the drug concentration in portal blood, and this concentration is influenced by both the dose level as well as by the rate of absorption. Continued presentation of low blood levels of drug to the liver may not saturate the metabolic pathways; however, rapid presentation of the same dose could saturate the metabolic pathway(s). Various methods have been proposed for the determination of bioavailability of drugs demonstrating Michaelis-Menten kinetics [10-16]. The advantages and limitations of these methods were discussed in a recent review [17].

Bioavailability of Metabolite(s)

In principle, one metabolic pathway may take over when another becomes saturated. Therefore, two products from which similar amounts of the same drug are absorbed at different rates could yield comparable bioavailability of the parent compound, yet show different quantitative blood profiles of the multiple metabolites. This is of particular concern if the metabolites in question are pharmacologically active. The logical solution to this problem would be to make bioavailability assessments that are based on the blood concentrations of unchanged drug as well as all active metabolites. In practice, however, it is sometimes difficult to elucidate the structure and the pharmacologic activity of all the metabolites, and the issue of metabolite bioavailability should be addressed on a case-by-case basis. Normally, this becomes an important consideration only for drugs with a high first-pass metabolism or with metabolites present in large quantities or contributing significantly to therapeutic activity. For example, for the phenothiazine analogue thioridazine, the FDA requires that its two major active metabolites mesoridazine and sulforidazine be assayed together with the parent drug in all ANDA-type bioequivalence studies [18].

Conventional versus Controlled-Release Dosage Forms

In contrast with the conventional immediate-release dosage form, controlled-release products basically are designed to provide long-acting therapy. This can be accomplished through a number of ways, as illustrated in Figure 1. Oral delayed-release products generally consist of the immediate-release drug form, albeit enteric-coated for release in the intestines. Repeated-action products

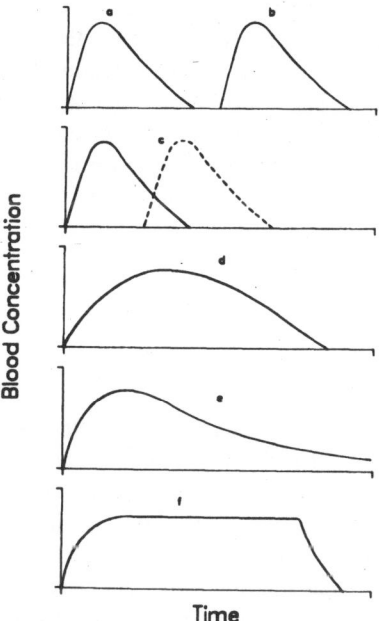

Figure 1 Various types of dosage forms (a) immediate release, (b) delayed release, (c) repeated action, (d) prolonged release, (e) sustained release, and (f) controlled release. (From Ref. 19.)

generally contain two doses of the drug, the first for immediate release and the second enteric-coated for (also rapid) release at a later time. Prolonged-release products deliver the drug slowly and are useful when an immediate therapeutic effect is not required. Sustained-release products often contain an immediate-release loading dose intended to rapidly establish therapeutic drug concentrations in blood and a slow-release drug component intended to maintain these concentrations for a prolonged period. Controlled-release products are sustained-release products that are capable of maintaining a constant and predictable blood level of drug for a predetermined period.

In addition to demonstrating equivalent steady-state performance to a currently marketed immediate-release or controlled-release drug product that contains the same active ingredient, a controlled-release dosage form must prove the controlled-release characteristic claimed. Furthermore, its plasma concentration profile should rule out the possibility of any uncontrolled or rapid release of product.

Blood Concentration–Pharmacologic Response Relationship

Usually there is some relationship between drug concentration in blood or plasma and that at the site of action. Therefore, two bioequivalent drug products should deliver the active ingredient to its site of action at the same rate and extent, thereby ensuring therapeutic equivalence. However, a difference in bioavailability between two drug products may result in a large or small difference in therapeutic response, depending on the nature of the blood concentration–pharmacologic response relationship. This is illustrated in Figure 2 [20]. Normally, drugs with a higher therapeutic index or a relatively flat dose–response curve are less likely to be subject to bioavailability-related alterations of clinical effect [21].

COMMON CONSIDERATIONS IN STUDY DESIGN

Single Versus Multiple Dosing

For drugs intended for long-term use, it would seem obvious that a multiple-dose study design is preferred to a single-dose design, since the former more accurately reflects the recommended use of the drug. Steinijans et al. [22] compared the conclusions drawn from single- and multiple-dose studies of theophylline in the same subjects and found that, although both single- and multiple-dose AUC data yielded similar estimates of the extent of bioavailability, the peak–trough characteristics (and, hence, the absorption rate) at steady-state cannot be predicted, based on the single-dose results (also refer to later Case Study II). Other advantages of using a multiple-dose regimen in bioavailability–bioequivalence studies include

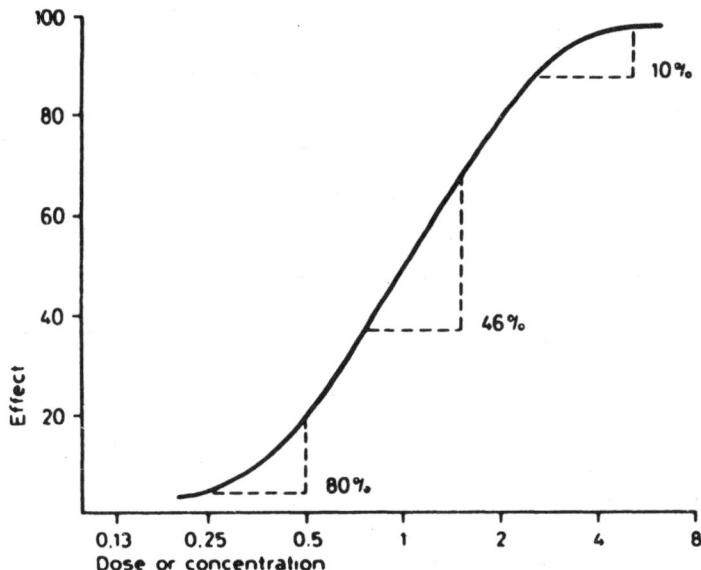

Figure 2 Effect of a 50% decrease in bioavailability on pharmacologic effect. (From Ref. 20.)

1. Multiple-dosing studies can be conducted in patients. This would allow the use of higher doses that, in turn, could yield higher drug concentrations in blood. Not only are these higher drug concentrations more easily determined, but also, in using a steady-state study design, drug concentrations need be measured only over a dosing interval, avoiding the need to measure lower concentrations during a disposition phase. In contrast, single-dose studies are usually performed in normal subjects. Use of this population avoids ethical issues of drug "holidays," concomitant medication, and disease-related effects, and provides pharmacokinetic data in a stable group of subjects with whom other groups may be compared. However, single-dose studies are more taxing from an analytical point of view.
2. Because of potential intraindividual variability, it is desirable to minimize the duration of the overall study. This goal is accomplished in multiple-dosing studies by eliminating long washout periods between doses. Therefore, the washout period and the dosing to steady-state period can be one and the same.
3. Usually a smaller intersubject variability is observed in steady-state studies, which may permit the use of fewer subjects.

4. Saturable pharmacokinetics, if present, can be more readily detected at steady-state following multiple dosing.

On the other hand, multiple-dosing studies may be ethically undesirable in some respects. Healthy subjects should not be dosed with any drug for an extended time. In patients, the disease state may introduce variability, reducing the statistical power of the study. Multiple-dosing studies, in general, are also more difficult to conduct, particularly in terms of controlling subject compliance with dietary and dosing restrictions.

Normal Subjects Versus Patients

Since patients represent the target population for which the drug is intended, they have the potential of providing results that would most accurately reflect the performance of the drug product during therapeutic use. However, as previously stated, patients are typically used only in multiple-dosing studies. Additionally, they tend to be more difficult to control (see foregoing) than normal subjects, often resulting in greater variability in the data.

Monitoring Parent Drug Alone Versus Drug and Metabolites

Significant advances have been made in recent years in the use of in vitro methodology for studying drug metabolism; for example, qualitative information (metabolite pattern) can be obtained from cell preparations of different organs from animals and humans, structure elucidation by techniques such as liquid chromatography–mass spectrometry (LC-MS/MS) and diode array detection, and estimation of hepatic clearance with liver microsomes [23]. Consequently, it has become increasingly possible to identify, synthesize, and pharmacologically characterize potential human metabolites of a compound during its early (preclinical) stage of development. This would afford time for assay development for active metabolites so that they can subsequently be monitored in human samples, including those obtained from the bioavailability and bioequivalence studies. Especially for drugs subject to an extensive first-pass effect, claims of bioequivalence should be based on circulating levels of the parent drug as well as active metabolites to represent therapeutic equivalence.

Statistical Concerns

In bioavailability and bioequivalence studies, it is normally assumed that each subject remains biologically constant throughout the study. Since this is rarely true, and since no two subjects are identical, it becomes critically important that the experimental data be analyzed by an appropriate statistical test. The intended statistical analysis should dictate the study design so that design constraints do not compromise study objectives. Some commonly encountered statistical issues in bioavailability-bioequivalence studies have been summarized in a recent article by Metzler [24].

CASE STUDY I: THIORIDAZINE

A compound that has potential bioequivalence problems encompassing virtually all of the complicating factors outlined in the foregoing is thioridazine, a phenothiazine product which is an anxiolytic agent at low doses but at medium and high doses is effective in controlling severe symptoms of psychotic and nonpsychotic mental disorders. The drug is subject to presystemic metabolism and exhibits considerable intersubject variability. It is biotransformed to two active principal metabolites (mesoridazine and sulforidazine) and has been shown to follow saturable pharmacokinetics [25]. The U. S. Food and Drug Administration (FDA) presently accepts single-dose studies for up to 100 mg thioridazine, but requires multiple-dose studies for 150- or 200-mg tablet strengths. It is also required that the parent drug and the metabolites, mesoridazine and sulforidazine, be monitored in these studies.

Thioridazine (Mellaril) is currently administered on a two- to four-times-a-day regimen. Since it is administered over an extended time to psychiatric patients, often in an institutionalized setting, development of a sustained-release form for once-a-day dosing was desired to increase patient compliance and reduce institutional care costs. Because of the complex characteristics of thioridazine disposition and the need for multiple-dose strengths, several of the factors discussed earlier (influencing study design) had to be considered in the developmental program for such a dosage form(s).

Mechanistic Study

Preliminary studies with the dosage form demonstrated sustained release of drug, but with an overall reduction in bioavailability ($\sim 25\%$). This prompted a mechanistic study to examine the effect of site of absorption on bioavailability and extent of absorption. A protocol for the gastrointestinal intubation of radiolabeled (^{14}C) drug was developed [26]. Study data were obtained from eight individuals. Before dosing, the intestinal feeding tubes were positioned and their location confirmed by fluoroscopy. Three individuals were positioned with intubation into the proximal region (beyond the ligament of Treitz and into the proximal jejunum), and five were positioned with intubation into the distal region (distal jejunum or below). Subjects were administered a 50-mg dose on two occasions, once as a bolus drink solution and once as a 4-hour infusion through their respective intestinal feeding tubes. Plasma and urine samples were collected at intervals for up to 120 hr after dosing.

On the basis of the radioactivity in urine ($\sim 30\%$ of the dose), the absorption in both intubation groups (proximal and distal) was identical with the oral bolus treatment. However, bioavailability was reduced in both intubation groups relative to the bolus group (~30%) for the principal plasma components, thioridazine, mesoridazine, and sulforidazine. No distinctions were evident between the two intubation groups, with both being significantly different from the oral bolus dose. These results suggested that development of any sustained-release form of this drug that releases drug in transit through the gastrointestinal tract would provide suboptimal bioavailability relative to an oral bolus dose.

Bioavailability Relationship: Sustained-Release Versus Immediate-Release Forms

The results from the mechanistic study were in concert with the preliminary observations of reduced bioavailability for the sustained-release (SR) form relative to the immediate-release (IR) forms and suggested an additional study to confirm the interchangeability of SR and IR in terms of extent of bioavailability. A single-dose study in normal volunteers was designed that addressed this issue, with the additional objective, to compare the intrasubject plasma level variability of the SR and IR forms. To address the interchangeability question, a single dose of 100 mg with the SR tablet was compared to a 75-mg dose with the IR tablets; variability of the dosage forms was addressed by repeated dosing in each individual (randomized, double-switchback crossover design, IR: SR: IR: SR or SR: IR: SR: IR). Within-subject variability was estimated using the ratio (SR/IR) of the intrasubject coefficients of variation (CV; defined as the intrasubject standard error divided by the subject's mean).

Data from 27 male subjects completing the study indicated that 100-mg SR was interchangeable with 75-mg IR in terms of extent of bioavailability. Differences in extent of bioavailability were less than 15% in all comparisons, and equivalence between treatments was supported by the two one-sided tests [27] and Westlake's symmetric 95% confidence intervals [28]. A pilot study (n = 6) in patients comparing the two higher strengths (2 × 200 mg and 1 × 400 mg) to Mellaril IR (300 mg) also confirmed the proportional difference in bioavailability. For dosage form variability, the comparison of intrasubject CVs showed that the within-subject plasma variations were comparable for the two forms (SR and IR). Therefore, substitution of the SR for the IR form resulted in comparable plasma concentration variability.

Effect of Food

A normal part of any SR development program is the study to examine the effect of concomitant food administration. Twenty-four male volunteers completed this two-period crossover study in which each subject received a single 100-mg (SR) dose either fasted or in conjunction with a standard breakfast (two eggs, two slices bread with butter, two strips of bacon, 8 oz orange juice, and 8 oz whole milk). Four hours after the morning dose, a standard lunch (cold-cut sandwiches and 8 oz whole milk) was given in both treatment periods. Assessments were based upon statistical comparison of the mean bioavailability parameters (AUC, C_{max}, t_{max}) and examination of individual plasma concentration–time curves for evidence of "dose-dumping" (i.e., immediate release of the medication from the SR form as a result of food interaction).

The mean plasma concentrations (Fig. 3) and statistical analysis for all three components demonstrated the lack of any significant global food interaction. Plasma profiles for thioridazine, mesoridazine, and sulforidazine were essentially superimposable for the two treatments, with the exception of a slight delay (1–4 hr) in appearance in plasma when the drug was administered with food. Examination of the individual thioridazine data showed that the majority of individuals had comparable plasma levels in both treatments (i.e., C_{max} was essentially the same). The observed plasma level variability was typical of variations observed with the IR form [29].

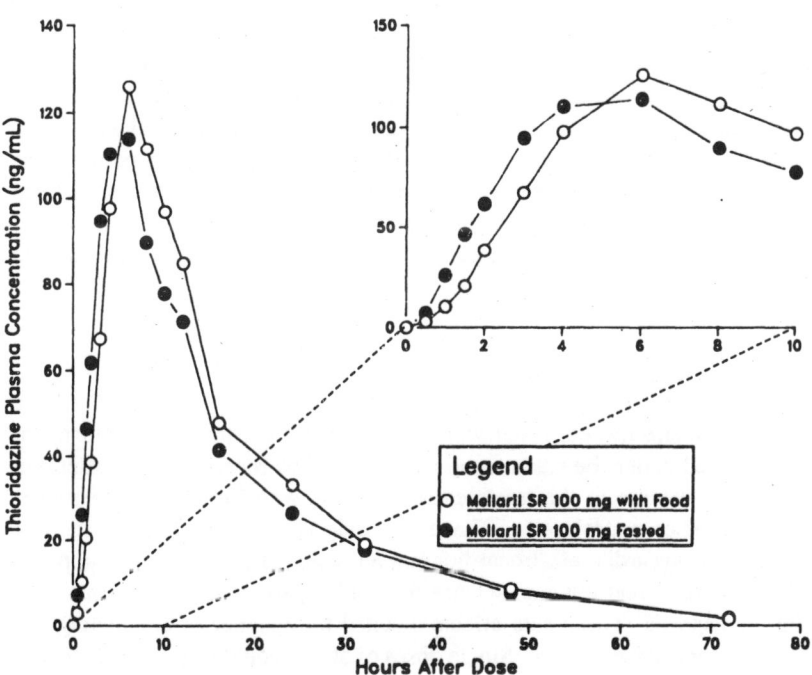

Figure 3 The effect of a high-fat meal on the bioavailability of a Mellaril 100-mg modified-release formulation given to normal volunteers.

Dosage-Form Proportionality

Because of the broad therapeutic range that exists for thioridazine, and other drugs in this class, there is a need for multiple-dose strengths. For the Mellaril SR tablet, four different dose strengths (50, 100, 200, 400 mg) were developed. For ethical reasons, the two higher dose strengths were tested in patient populations, since normal volunteers could not tolerate doses of this magnitude without a potential safety problem (i.e., orthostatic hypotension). As noted earlier, however, the two lower strengths are well tolerated in normal volunteers. Since the 100-mg strength was used in previous studies, it was used as the reference in two subsequent dosage-form proportionality studies: 2×50 mg versus 1×100 mg conducted as a single-dose study in normal volunteers; and 2×200 mg and 1×400 mg versus 4×100 mg conducted as a steady-state study in patients.

The results of these two studies demonstrated the proportionality of the various dosage forms, as evidenced by the superimposable plasma concentration profiles (Fig. 4 shows the results for thioridazine from the steady-state study in patients).

Summary

The design of this development program was complicated by the nature of the drug (high variability, first-pass, active metabolites, necessity to dose in patients) and the dosage form (sustained-release tablet). Particular deviations from a "normal" program were the mechanistic study performed to rationalize the observed decreased bioavailability (SR vs IR) and the subsequent study to confirm the equivalence of unequal dose strengths (SR vs IR). The comparison of dosage form variability is also important when developing novel dosage form replacements. Our example shows how to combine two of these objectives into one study to conserve development time.

CASE STUDY II: CLOZAPINE

Clozapine, a dibenzodiazepine derivative, is a broad-spectrum neuroleptic agent that is marketed under the trade name Clozaril. It has received much attention because of its success in the treatment of patients with histories of treatment resistance to other neuroleptics. The major side effects of this drug include hypotension, tachycardia, electrocardiogram ST segment depression, leukopenia or agranulocytosis, and lowered seizure threshold, particularly in patients who may be predisposed. These side effects dictated the manner of conducting the biopharmaceutical development. Single doses of 50 mg could be tolerated by normal young healthy male volunteers; however, even at these doses, severe hypotension was a high risk. Since the dosage forms developed included strengths above 50 mg, the bioavailability studies had to be conducted in a patient population.

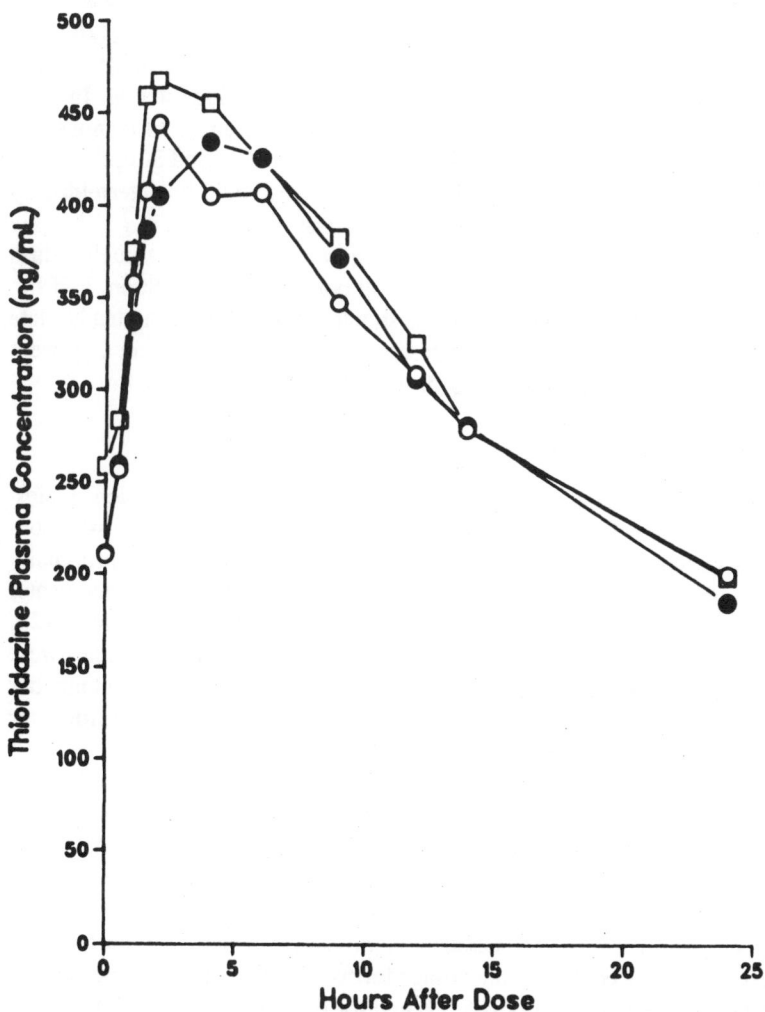

Figure 4 Steady-state plasma concentrations of thioridazine in patients given once-a-day 4 × 100-mg, 2 × 200-mg, or 1 × 400-mg tablets of a modified-release formulation of Mellaril.

Dose Proportionality

In a two-center study, 11 patients with diagnosed schizophrenia completed this three-period open-label sequential design study [30]. Each patient was brought up in dose slowly (37.5 mg hs for 6 days) before stabilization at 37.5 mg bid q12h (7 am, 7 pm). After 1 week of stabilization, this same regimen was maintained for 1 week at each of three dose levels, 37.5, 75, 150 mg bid q12h using an oral solution as the formulation. On day 7 of each period, sufficient plasma samples were collected to define one complete daytime dosing interval. In addition, several trough values were collected on days 5, 6, and 7 to demonstrate attainment of steady state. After the last morning dose of period 3, each patient had a drug holiday so that individual patient half-lives could be determined by collecting plasma samples for 148 hr after this last dose.

The results of the study are shown in Figure 5. Individual trough values demonstrated achievement of steady state at all dose levels. In addition, half-life ($t_{1/2}$) data suggested that each individual should have achieved a steady state (99%) within 7 days of dosing. The increases in AUC_{0-12}^{SS}, C_{max}^{SS}, and C_{min}^{SS} were directly and proportionally related to dose. The mean $t_{1/2}$ was 17 hr.

Bioavailability Assessment

To establish the bioavailability of the marketed 25- and 100-mg tablets against a solution and clinical research capsule, a four-way crossover study was conducted in a patient population using a design similar to the dose proportionality study (unpublished data). Thirty patients successfully completed this three-center study. Dosing for each cell of the study was for 14 days at 100 mg bid q12h, and there was no washout period between periods. Several plasma samples were collected at trough to establish attainment of steady state, and a sufficient number were collected on day 14 of each period to define the plasma level profile over the daytime-dosing interval.

Since half-lives of up to 33 hr were observed in the earlier dose–proportionality study, a more conservative 14-day treatment period was selected for this pivotal study. Trough values indicated that all subjects attained a steady state. All major bioavailability parameters, with the exception of the parameter "time to peak," showed differences, in pair-wise comparison of means, of less than 20%. Some of these comparisons achieved statistical significance, which was the result of small variances in the content of the dosage forms. For example, the true percentage of label for the solution was 105.3% and for the 100-mg tablet 97.1%. This difference of 8.2 percentage units was sufficient to show statistical significance. An adjustment of bioavailability parameters by the percentage of label for content provided comparisons indicative of bioequivalent products.

Single-Dose Versus Multiple-Dose Kinetics

The half-life data for the two foregoing studies (mean $t_{1/2}$ of 15–17 hr) differed from single-dose data. An earlier ADME study in normal male volunteers, not described here, indicated a $t_{1/2}$ of about 8 hr, and this was calculated using data over three half-lives. This difference could not be rationalized in terms of nonlinear

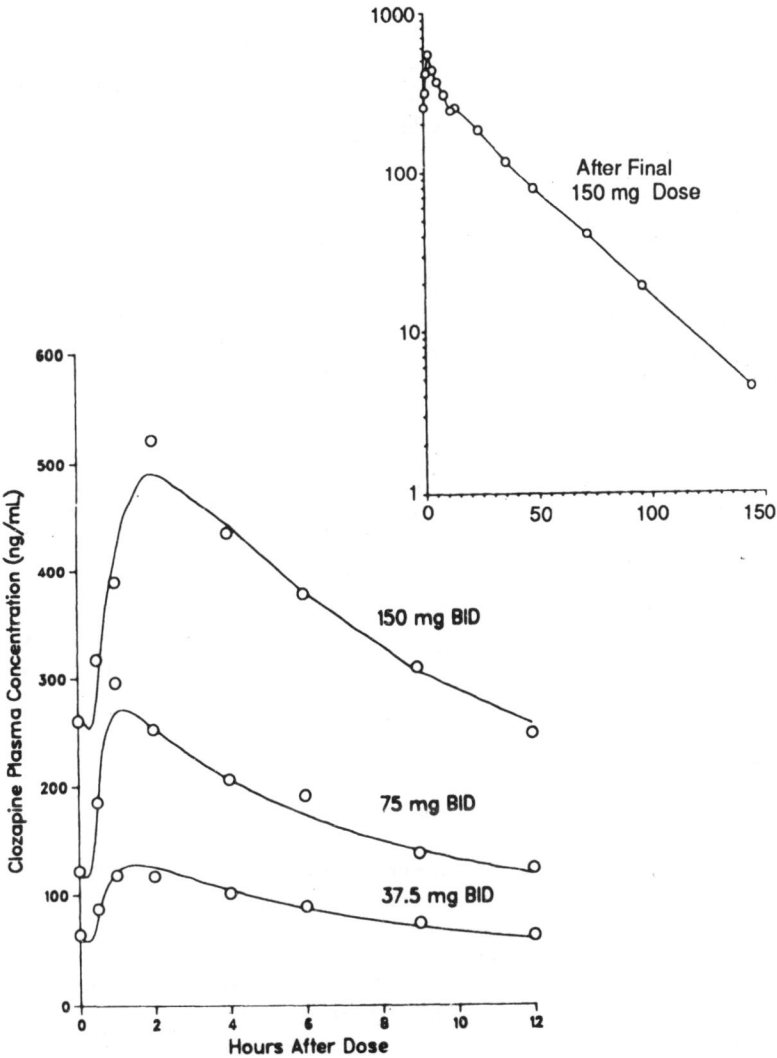

Figure 5 Steady-state plasma concentration of clozapine in patients given 37.5 mg, 75 mg, and 150 mg (bid) of an oral solution.

kinetics in light of the linear dose–response data collected at steady state. In addition, there appeared to be no relationship to demographic data. Potential reasons for the difference could have been: patient (drug history) versus normal volunteer; or single- versus multiple-dose kinetics. We chose to investigate the latter by dosing

16 patients, after an appropriate washout, with 75 mg of clozapine single-dose, followed by a multiple-dose phase for 7 days, followed by another 75-mg dose after an appropriate washout period [31]. In addition, the effect of food on clozapine bioavailability was woven into the single-dose cells by using a crossover design. Sufficient plasma samples to define half-lives were collected after each single dose and after the last dose of the multiple-dosing period.

Analysis of all data showed that there was no food effect on the bioavailability of clozapine. In addition, the apparent half-life after each single dose was confirmed to be about 8 hr. After multiple dosing, the apparent $t_{1/2}$ was 14 hr. Therefore, the differences in apparent half-lives across various studies was determined to be directly related to the dose regimen; single-dose kinetics were not predictive of the steady state.

Summary

The development program for clozapine was complicated by the need to use steady-state study designs in a patient population. Even though the drug had apparent linear kinetics at steady state, single-dose kinetics were not predictive of the steady state. Through careful study design that used drug holidays to collect half-life data and by incorporating secondary objectives, such as food effects, the overall kinetics and bioavailability of clozapine were well described with three studies.

REFERENCES

1. The Editors. Pharmacokinetics and biopharmaceutics: A definition of terms. *J. Pharmacokinet. Biopharm.* 1:3–4 (1973).
2. C. T. Viswanathan and J. P. Skelly. Role of metabolite in drug development—FDA point of view. In *Program and Abstracts of the 37th National Meeting of the American Pharmaceutical Association Academy of Pharmaceutical Sciences*. American Pharmaceutical Association, Philadelphia, p. 152 (1984).
3. G. Alván, K. Piafsky, M. Lind, and C. von Bahr. Effect of pentobarbital on the disposition of alprenolol. *Clin. Pharmacol. Ther.* 22:316–321 (1977).
4. D. M. Kornhauser, A. J. J. Wood, R. E. Vestal, G. R. Wilkinson, R. A. Branch, and D. G. Shand. Biological determinants of propranolol disposition in man. *Clin. Pharmacol. Ther.* 23:165–174 (1978).
5. P. N. Bennett, L. J. Aarons, M. R. Bending, J. A. Steiner, and M. Rowland. Pharmacokinetics of lidocaine and its de-ethylated metabolite: Dose and time dependency studies in man. *J. Pharmacokinet. Biopharm.* 10:265–281 (1982).
6. R. A. Branch, D. G. Shand, G. R. Wilkinson, and A. S. Nies. Increased clearance of antipyrine and d-propranolol after phenobarbital treatment in the monkey. *J. Clin. Invest.* 53:1101–1107 (1974).
7. R. A. Upton, J. F. Thiercelin, T. W. Guentert, S. M. Wallace, J. R. Powell, L. Sansom, and S. Riegelman. Intraindividual variability in theophylline pharmacokinetics:

Statistical verification in 39 of 60 healthy young volunteers. *J. Pharmacokinet. Biopharm. 10*:123-134 (1982).
8. M. Rowland. Models to identify sources of pharmacokinetic variability. In *Variability in Drug Therapy: Description, Estimation, and Control* (M. Rowland, L. B. Sheiner, and J.-L. Steimer, eds.) Raven Press, New York, p. 19 (1985).
9. W. Jusko, J. Koup, and G. Alván. Nonlinear assessment of phenytoin bioavailability. *J. Pharmacokinet. Biopharm. 4*:327-336 (1976).
10. G. M. Rubin and T. N. Tozer. Theoretical considerations in the calculation of bioavailability of drugs exhibiting Michaelis Menten elimination kinetics. *J. Pharmacokinet. Biopharm. 12*:437-450 (1984).
11. L. Martis and R. Levy. Bioavailability calculations for drugs showing simultaneous first-order and capacity-limited elimination kinetics. *J. Pharmacokinet. Biopharm. 1*:283-294 (1973).
12. F. Keller and J. Scholle. First-pass effect: Nonlinear concept comprising an explicit solution of integrated Michaelis-Menten equation. *J. Pharm. Sci. 70*:195-198 (1981).
13. P. Veng-Pederson. Novel method of calculating absolute bioavailability in nonlinear pharmacokinetics. *J. Pharm. Sci. 74*:90-93 (1985).
14. J. A. Waschek, G. M. Rubin, T. N. Tozer, R. M. Fielding, W. R. Couet, D. J. Effeney, and S. M. Pond. Dose-dependent bioavailability and metabolism of salicylamide in dogs. *J. Pharmacol. Exp. Ther. 230*:89-93 (1984).
15. Y. Kasuya, K. Mamada, S. Baba, and M. Matsukura. Stable-isotope methodology for the bioavailability study of phenytoin during multiple-dosing regimens. *J. Pharm. Sci. 74*:503-507 (1985).
16. G. M. Rubin, J. A. Waschek, S. M. Pond, D. J. Effeney, and T. N. Tozer. Concurrent intravenous administration of a labeled tracer to determine the oral bioavailability of a drug exhibiting Michaelis-Menten metabolism. *J. Pharmacokinet. Biopharm. 15*:615-631 (1987).
17. T. N. Tozer and G. M. Rubin. Saturable kinetics and bioavailability determination. In *Pharmacokinetics: Regulatory-Industrial-Academic Perspectives* (P. G. Welling and F. L. S. Tse, eds.) Marcel Dekker, New York, pp. 473-513 (1988).
18. S. V. Dighe. Current bioavailability and bioequivalence requirements and regulations. Presented to the Regulatory Affairs Professionals Society, Morristown, New Jersey, August 3, 1983.
19. L. Krówczyński. *Extended-Release Dosage Forms*. CRC Press, Boca Raton, Fl., p. 5 (1987).
20. G. Levy. Bioavailability, clinical effectiveness, and the public interest. *Pharmacology 8*:33-43 (1972).
21. D. L. Azarnoff and D. H. Huffman. Therapeutic implications of bioavailability. *Annu. Rev. Pharmacol. Toxicol. 16*:53-66 (1976).
22. V. W. Steinijans, R. Sauter, J. H. G. Jonkman, H.-U. Schulz, H. Stricker, and H. Blume. Bioequivalence studies: Single vs multiple dose. *Int. J. Clin. Pharmacol. Ther. Toxicol. 27*:261-266 (1989).
23. T. F. Woolf and T. Chang. Recent advances in drug metabolism methodology. In *Pharmacokinetics: Regulatory-Industrial-Academic Perspectives* (P. G. Welling and F. L. S. Tse, eds.) Marcel Dekker, New York, pp. 451-471 (1988).

24. C. M. Metzler. Bioavailability/bioequivalence: Study design and statistical issues. *J. Clin. Pharmacol.* 29:289–292 (1989).
25. R. Axelsson and E. Martensson. The concentration pattern of nonconjugated thioridazine metabolites in serum by thioridazine treatment and its relation to physiological and clinical variables. *Curr. Ther. Res. Clin. Exp.* 21:561–586 (1977).
26. M. G. Choc, F. Hsuan, W. T. Robinson, and W. H. Barr. Comparison of absorption and bioavailability of thioridazine after GI intubation in normal male volunteers. *Pharm. Res.* 5:S172 (1988).
27. D. J. Schuirmann. A comparison of the two one-sided tests procedure and the power approach for assessing the equivalence of average bioavailability. *J. Pharmacokinet. Biopharm.* 15:657–680 (1987).
28. W. J. Westlake. Response to T. B. L. Kirkwood: Bioequivalence testing—a need to rethink. *Biometrics* 37:589–594 (1981).
29. M. G. Choc, H. M. Proskin, J. H. Gogerty, and H. J. Schwarz. Variability of thioridazine and metabolite plasma concentrations after administration of identical tablets on three occasions. *Pharm. Res.* 4:S97 (1987).
30. M. G. Choc, R. G. Lehr, F. Hsuan, G. Honigfeld, H. T. Smith, R. Borison, and J. Volavka. Multiple-dose pharmacokinetics of clozapine in patients. *Pharm. Res.* 4:402–405 (1987).
31. M. G. Choc, F. Hsuan, G. Honigfeld, W. T. Robinson, L. Ereshefsky, M. L. Crismon, S. R. Saklad, J. Hirschowitz, and R. Wagner. Single- vs multiple-dose pharmacokinetics of clozapine in psychiatric patients. *Pharm. Res.* 7:347–351 (1990).

3
Statistical Criteria

Carl M. Metzler
The Upjohn Company
Kalamazoo, Michigan

INTRODUCTION

Scope of the Chapter

This chapter will discuss some of the statistical concepts useful in the estimation of bioavailability and in the evaluation of bioequivalence. No attempt is made at a complete statistical treatment. For example, it is assumed that the reader is familiar with the concept of sampling from populations. In bioavailability trials, or experiments, of a formulation, we assume that the tablets or capsules we observe are sampled from the total production (or population) of the product. Distinctions between items in a sample (e.g., tablets) and measurements of the items in the sample (AUCs of the tablets) will be made only when necessary for clarity. No attempt is made at rigor; we will say for example, "The mean of the formulation is. . ." when we really mean "The mean of the population (or distribution) of the areas under the concentration–time curves (AUCs) of the formulation is. . ." (Actually, of course, we do not sample from a population of AUCs. We choose, in some way, a sample of individuals, and from each of these individuals we observe an AUC. We call these AUCs "a sample of AUCs.") As long as there is little chance of misunderstanding, we feel that an attempt at rigor in this context would lead to poorer, not better, communication.

An attempt will be made to distinguish between populations and samples, for this is crucial to understanding much of the material. Common statistical notation and conventions will be used. Greek letters will be used for population parameters; the "hat," ^ , will be placed over them for estimates obtained from a sample. Thus "mu," μ, will designate the mean of a population, and "mu hat" or "X bar," $\hat{\mu} = \bar{X}$ the estimate of μ calculated from a sample. The number of observations in a sample will usually be called N, the "sample size."

Details of statistical methods will be given only when necessary for understanding in the context of this chapter. Computational formulae will usually not be given. Only enough discussion of bioavailability will be given to make the chapter somewhat self-contained. For a more complete discussion of bioavailability-bioequivalence as a statistical problem see Metzler [1]. For a reading of basic statistical concepts and computations the texts by Freedman and coauthors [2] or by Snedecor and Cochran [3] are recommended.

Bioavailability and Bioequivalence

Although bioavailability and bioequivalence are well-defined and thoroughly discussed in other chapters, a definition is given here to be used in this chapter. Quite often after an active drug molecule is shown to be efficacious and safe by clinical trials, the active molecule is formulated into another product. Since clinical trials are expensive (in many types of resources), researchers sought for a way to establish the safety and efficacy of the new product without clinical trials in patients. *Bioequivalence* of formulations was developed as a concept that would permit the new formulation to be considered as not different from the old formulation in efficacy and safety. (In this chapter the terms *reference formulation* and *test formulation* will be used for the old and new formulations.)

Considerations of pharmacology and pharmacokinetics suggest that if both formulations deliver the active ingredient to the circulating blood at the same rate, and to the same extent, then the pharmacologic responses, desired or undesired, should be the same. The rate and extent of the appearance of drug in the blood is the *bioavailability* of the drug product, and is estimated by assaying concentrations of the drug, usually in plasma samples. Other observations of bioavailability, such as drug in urine, or pharmacodynamic effects, are also used. The extent of bioavailability is often estimated by calculating the area under the concentration-time curve (AUC), and the maximum concentration (C_{max}). Rate of availability is estimated by (t_{max}) the time after dosing at which C_{max} is observed or estimated. The relative bioavailability of the two formulations can be used

Statistical Criteria

to determine if the two are bioequivalent. Relative bioavailability can be expressed as either a difference or a ratio.

In this chapter, bioequivalence is defined as

Bioequivalent: In bioequivalence testing a *test formulation* (test) is said to be *bioequivalent* to a *reference formulation* (ref) if

$$A < \Theta < B$$

Where Θ is a measure of relative bioavailability and A and B are limits of acceptable relative bioavailability.

Although, for many drugs, not much is known about the relationships of circulating drug concentrations, efficacy, and side effects, an often-used rule is that the test formulation should be from 80 to 120% as available as the reference formulation. Thus if

$$\Theta = 100 \, (AUC_{test}/AUC_{ref}), \, A = 80\% \text{ and } B = 120\%$$

then the test formulation would be said to be equivalent to the reference formulation if Θ is between 80 and 120%. (Although the methods of this chapter apply to all bioavailability and bioequivalence parameters, for convenience AUC will usually be used to illustrate.)

Sometimes *bioequivalence* is stated as "the difference between the average bioavailabilities should not be greater than 20% of the average of the reference average." Here,

$$A = -20\%, \, B = 20\%, \text{ and } \Theta = 100 \, (AUC_{test} - AUC_{ref})/AUC_{ref}$$

This definition is a statement about the relative bioavailability of the total production of the two formulations; evaluations and decisions about bioequivalence are based on samples, of course. That is the major reason that statistical criteria are of interest.

Sources of Variability

There are many recognized sources of variability in bioavailability studies. Statistics deals with variability in several ways: It identifies and isolates sources of variability; it measures and tests sources of variability for their significance; it provides measures of uncertainty (usually in the form of probability statements) for estimates and decisions that must be made in the presence of variability; and it provides experimental designs that enable variability to be handled in the most efficient manner.

The variability of most interest is due to formulation differences. Most of this chapter is concerned with ways to estimate and evaluate that source of variability as precisely as possible. To do this, other sources of variability must be accounted for. One of the largest sources of variability is subject-to-subject differences. If each subject is used more than once in a study, then, with proper design and analysis, the variability associated with these differences can be isolated from the other sources of variability. Consequently, some type of crossover design is usually the most efficient for bioequivalence comparisons. Other sources of variability that may be identified are due to the periods, sequence, carryover, and groups. All the other variability that is not identified is labeled "error."

Characteristics and Distribution of Bioavailability Data

Many statistical methods are based on the assumption that the random variables involved are normally distributed. Actually, most methods in common use are quite robust, even if this assumption is violated, and work quite well if the random variable is only symmetric about the mean. Thus, skewness of the data, or the presence of a few extreme values, is usually the problem. There have been many suggestions that bioavailability data should be transformed in some way; most often by taking the logarithm of the data before doing any computation.

Care must be taken to understand the nature of the nonmornality of the data and how it will affect the various statistical procedures. For many data sets, such as AUC or C_{max}, it is the subject effect that skews the data. One or two subjects may have exceptionally large (or small) drug concentrations. This skewness may be caused by size, body type, or by polymorphic metabolism. In many cases, the data may be better represented by the mixture of two distributions, with unequal means (and perhaps unequal variances), than by a skewed distribution.

If the data are being summarized by averages or confidence intervals, then skewness of the data will affect the statistics. But if an analysis of variance (AOV) is being computed, with subjects as one of the sources of variance, then the residuals may very well be symmetric, and the analysis valid. In this chapter the attempt will be made to indicate when transforming the data, or using nonparametric methods, are useful, and when transformations may be counterproductive.

The data in Table 1 represents AUCs from two typical two-formulation, two-period bioequivalence trials. They will be used to illustrate the statistical concepts in this chapter. It is possible to get some ideas of the nature of this data even without formal statistical analysis. In addition to subject, period, and formulation identification for each AUC, Table 1 also shows the rank of each AUC within its formulation. Note that subjects with the largest (or smallest) AUC values tend to have the same rank in each formulation. Other subjects have somewhat different ranks in the two formualtions, but only one subject has ranks that differ by more than 3. This suggests the kind of subject effect mentioned earlier, which when removed in an AOV will likely cause the residuals from the statistical model to be more nearly symmetric.

Statistical Criteria

Table 1 AUCs from a Two-Period, Two-Formulation Crossover

Subject	Reference formulation			Test formulation		
	Period	AUC	Rank	Period	AUC	Rank
Data Set A						
1	1	83.97	12	2	76.72	12
2	1	62.67	9	2	47.56	8
3	1	55.31	8	2	40.14	7
4	1	34.10	5	2	33.34	6
5	1	27.75	3	2	27.38	5
6	1	78.03	11	2	74.62	11
7	2	24.47	2	1	23.34	3
8	2	34.91	6	1	26.78	4
9	2	31.33	4	1	13.42	1
10	2	54.23	7	1	48.50	9
11	2	23.17	1	1	13.80	2
12	2	66.76	10	1	50.14	10
Data Set B						
1	1	117.6	16	2	125.8	16
2	1	49.2	6	2	57.9	9
3	1	45.4	5	2	57.8	8
4	1	20.4	1	2	30.2	2
5	1	51.9	7	2	53.4	5
6	1	108.9	15	2	96.8	14
7	1	41.0	4	2	36.5	3
8	1	26.4	2	2	28.2	1
9	2	54.5	8	1	66.4	11
10	2	71.5	12	1	55.3	7
11	2	60.8	10	1	59.3	10
12	2	56.0	9	1	54.0	6
13	2	83.4	13	1	100.3	15
14	2	102.5	14	1	94.8	13
15	2	32.3	3	1	47.5	4
16	2	66.5	11	1	73.4	12

Figure 1 shows normal probability plots of the data. The vertical scale is in units of AUC, and the horizontal scale is standardized normal variables, calculated as though the data were from a normal distribution. If the data are from a normal distribution they will lie on approximately a straight line. The solid lines in the figures are the best fits through the data. Data set A has a good fit, set B has a lot of deviation at the larger AUC values, which *may* suggest some skewness

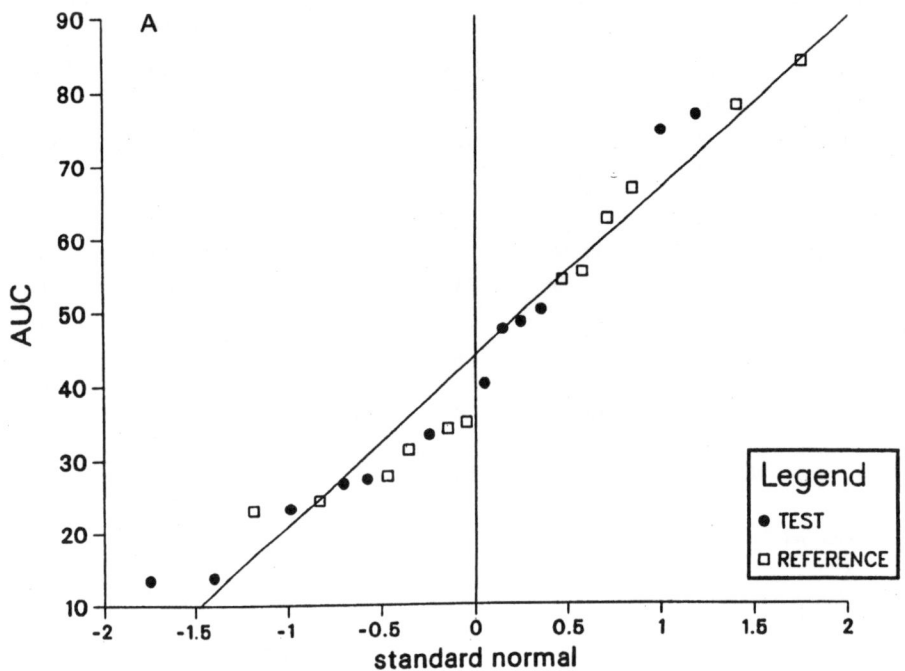

Figure 1 Normal plot of AUCs, set A and set B.

to the right. Additional use of these plots, and the characteristics of these data sets, will be discussed in following sections.

ESTIMATES OF RELATIVE BIOAVAILABILITY

Estimates for a Single Formulation

Estimates of Average Values

The two most commonly used estimates of average value are the mean, often denoted by mu (μ) and the median. For symmetric *populations* these values are equal; in *samples* from such populations they will almost always differ at least a little owing to sampling variation. If the population is skewed or if there are extreme values of outliers, then the population mean and median will differ, and the sample values will also differ.

For a sample of N AUCs, the sample mean, which estimates the population mean, is defined as

Statistical Criteria

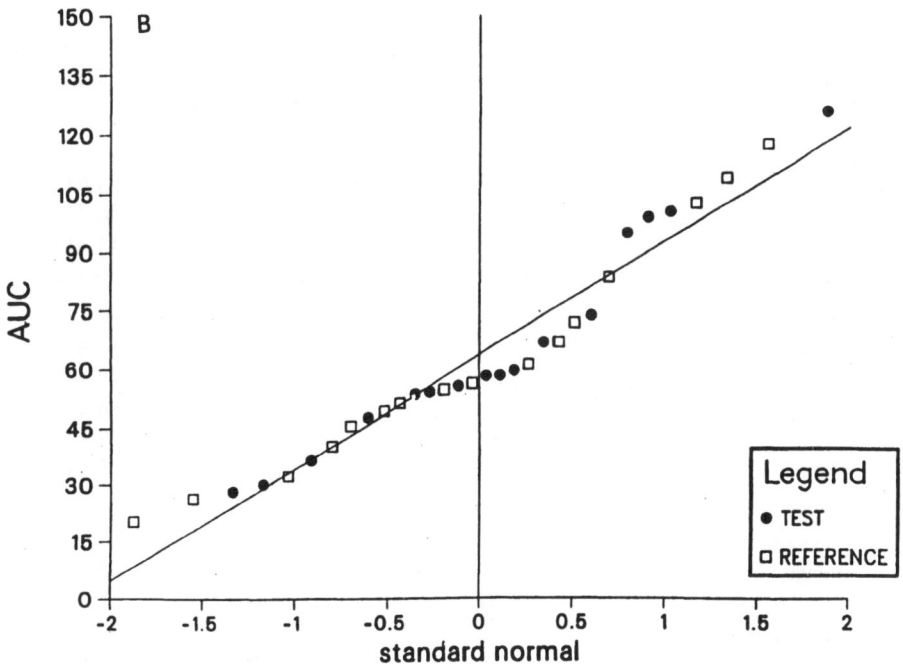

Figure 1 *Continued*

$$\hat{\mu} = \bar{X} = \Sigma \, AUC/N \qquad (1)$$

The median is that value which divides the sample in half, that is, there are as many sample values less than the median as there are sample values greater than the median. If N is odd, then the median is one of the sample values; if N is an even number, then the median is half the sum of the two "middle values" when ranked from smallest to largest. The median is also called the 50th percentile. Other sample percentiles also provide information about the population. In general, the "Pth" percentile is that value such that P percent of the sample is smaller, and (100 − P) percent of the sample is larger. In most cases the percentiles will not be observed values, but will be interpolated between two observed values.

Summary statistics for the AUCs of Table 1 are shown in Table 2. In this table the mean and median provide information, or estimates, only of the average, or *location*, of the formulations from which they are sampled.

In Set A they suggest that the AUCs from the reference formulation are, on

Table 2 Summary Statistics for AUCs of Table 1

Statistic	Total data	Formulation	
		Reference	Test
Data Set A			
N	24	12	12
Mean	43.85	48.06	39.64
Median	37.52	44.57	36.74
Minimum	13.42	23.17	13.42
Maximum	83.97	83.97	76.72
Percentiles			
10th	18.48	23.56	13.53
25th	26.93	28.64	24.20
50th	37.52	44.57	36.74
75th	60.83	65.74	49.73
90th	77.38	82.19	76.09
Variation			
Standard deviation	21.19	21.48	20.95
Range	70.55	60.80	63.30
Quartile range	33.90	37.09	25.53
CV (coefficient of variation)	48.32%	44.71%	52.84%
Data Set B			
N	32	16	16
Mean	63.31	61.77	64.85
Median	56.90	55.25	57.85
Minimum	20.4	20.4	28.2
Maximum	125.8	117.6	125.8
Percentiles			
10th	28.80	24.60	29.60
25th	45.92	42.10	48.98
50th	56.90	55.25	57.85
75th	80.80	80.42	89.45
90th	106.98	111.51	107.95
Variation			
Standard deviation	27.60	28.82	27.18
Range	105.4	97.2	97.6
Quartile range	34.98	38.32	40.48
CV (coefficient of variation)	43.59%	46.65%	41.91%

average, greater than those of the test formulation. This is true at every percentile; thus the reference population is located above, or to the right of, the test population. The opposite is true in population B, for which the test population seems to be to the right of, or greater than, the reference population. These statistics also give some information about the shape of the distributions, and an indication of the variability of the formulation. For both formulations of both data sets the means are larger than the medians, suggesting a skewness to the right. This is a little stronger in set B than in set A (see Fig. 1 again).

Estimates of Variability

In most situations, estimates of the average, or "location," of a population is not sufficient information. Something must usually be known about variability also. The most used measure of variability is the variance, or its square-root, the standard deviation (SD). The standard deviation is in the same units as the observations and the mean. It is usually denoted by sigma (σ). The sample standard deviation,

$$SD = s = \hat{\sigma} = \sqrt{\{\Sigma\ [X - \bar{X}]^2/(N - 1)\}} \quad (2)$$

is the estimate of the population standard deviation. Much of the popularity of the standard deviation as a measure of variability is a result of the unique role it plays in the normal probability distribution. The normal distribution is completely determined by μ and σ, and thus all percentiles can be written as functions of μ and σ. Some of these are

Percentile	
2.5	$\mu - 1.960\sigma$
5.0	$\mu - 1.645\sigma$
10.0	$\mu - 1.282\sigma$
25.0	$\mu - 0.674\sigma$
34.0	$\mu - 1.000\sigma$
50.0	μ
66.0	$\mu + 1.000\sigma$
75.0	$\mu + 0.674\sigma$
90.0	$\mu + 1.282\sigma$
95.0	$\mu + 1.645\sigma$
97.5	$\mu + 1.960\sigma$

The 2.5 and 97.5 percentiles are approximately 2 SD below and above the mean. It is easy to remember that "the mean, plus or minus 2 SD, contains 95% of the population." From the 25th to the 75th percentile (i.e., the *quartile range*)

is about 1.35 SD. The quartile range is a useful nonparametric estimate of the variability of the data. The total range, maximum−minimum, is not so useful, since it can be very much affected by one outlier, an observation either very small or very large.

Estimates of Relative Bioavailability

Ratios and Differences of Point Estimates

The estimates of average bioavailability for each formulation can be used to estimate the *relative bioavailability*. Relative bioavailability may be expressed as the ratio (or percentage) of the test formulation to the reference formulation. Relative bioavailability may also be expressed by comparing the difference of the bioavailabilities with the reference bioavailability. Thus different ways of estimating Θ, relative bioavailability, of the data in Table 1, are:

A1. $\Theta = R_{mean} = 39.64/48.06 = 0.825$ (82.5%)
A2. $\Theta = R_{median} = 36.74/44.57 = 0.824$ (82.4%)
A3. $\Theta = D_{mean} = (39.64 - 48.06)/48.06 = -0.175$ (−17.5%)
A4. $\Theta = D_{median} = (36.74 - 44.57)/44.57 = -0.176$ (−17.6%)
B1. $\Theta = R_{mean} = 64.85/61.77 = 1.050$ (105.0%)
B2. $\Theta = R_{median} = 57.85/55.25 = 1.047$ (104.7%)
B3. $\Theta = D_{mean} = (64.85 - 61.77)/61.77 = 0.050$ (5.0%)
B4. $\Theta = D_{median} = (57.85 - 55.25)/55.25 = 0.047$ (4.7%)

With the use of the ratio of the means, the test formulation of set A is 0.825 as bioavailable as the reference formulation; that is, A1 shows its relative bioavailability to be 82.5%. Item A3 says it in another way; the difference in the bioavailabilities of the test and reference formulations is −17.5% of the reference mean. For this data set the relative bioavailabilities estimated by the medians are very similar to the estimates from the means.

In set B the test formulation is more available than the reference formulation. By B1 its relative bioavailability is 1.05; the difference between the formulations is 5.0% of the reference mean, B3.

Means and Medians of Ratios

Since most bioequivalence studies are crossovers in which each individual is dosed with both formulations, a natural variable is the ratio within each subject. Unfortunately, these are ratios of random variables, and their probability distribution is very difficult to work with. Therefore, it is difficult to estimate the variability or base decision rules on ratios. (More will be said about possible ways to work with individual ratios in the later section: Nonparametric Intervals). They do, however, provide estimates of relative bioavailability.

Table 3 lists the ratios and differences of the AUCs of Table 1. Note that in

Statistical Criteria

Table 3 Ratios and Differences in AUCs from Table 1

Subject	Reference	Test	Ratio	Difference
Data Set A				
1	83.97	76.72	0.914	−7.25
2	62.67	47.56	0.759	−15.11
3	55.31	40.14	0.726	−15.17
4	34.10	33.34	0.978	−0.76
5	27.75	27.38	0.987	−0.37
6	78.03	74.62	0.956	−3.41
7	24.47	23.34	0.954	−1.13
8	34.91	26.78	0.767	−8.13
9	31.33	13.42	0.428	−17.91
10	54.23	48.50	0.894	−5.73
11	23.17	13.80	0.596	−9.37
12	66.76	50.14	0.751	−16.62
Mean			0.809	−8.413
Mediam			0.831	−7.690
Standard deviation			0.172	6.459
Data Set B				
1	117.6	125.8	1.070	8.2
2	49.2	57.9	1.177	8.7
3	45.4	57.8	1.273	12.4
4	20.4	30.2	1.480	9.8
5	51.9	53.4	1.029	1.5
6	108.9	96.8	0.889	−12.1
7	41.0	36.5	0.890	−4.5
8	26.4	28.2	1.068	1.8
9	54.5	66.4	1.218	11.9
10	71.5	55.3	0.773	−16.2
11	60.8	59.3	0.975	−1.5
12	56.0	54.0	0.964	−2.0
13	83.4	100.3	1.203	16.9
14	102.5	94.8	0.925	−7.7
15	32.3	47.5	1.471	15.2
16	66.5	73.4	1.104	6.9
Mean			1.094	3.08
Median			1.069	4.35
Standard deviation			0.201	9.82

set A all the test AUCs are smaller than the reference AUCs, so that all ratios are less than 1 and all differences are negative. This strongly suggests that the test formulation is not as bioavailable as the reference formulation. In set B, six of the test formulation AUCs are less than reference AUCs, but ten are larger. This suggests that perhaps there is no difference; it is only the variability that makes the average values of the test formulation greater than the reference.

Also note that the averages of the ratios are not the same as the ratio of the averages computed in the previous section; nor are the *median differences* the same as the *differences of the medians*. Which is the correct estimate of relative bioavailability? There is no one correct estimate; the various estimates all have their uses.

Confidence Intervals

We know that the estimates of average or location in the foregoing two sections on estimates, being based on sample results, are themselves variable, or uncertain. The estimates of variability of observations, discussed earlier, can be used to construct estimates that show both location and variability. These are called confidence interval estimates. Three classes of confidence intervals often used in bioavailability and bioequivalence are discussed in this chapter.

Classical t-Based Confidence Intervals

The most common confidence intervals are based on the Student's t distribution. (Because of their long history in statistics these will be called "classic.") If the normal distribution, with mean μ and variance σ^2, is a reasonable model for the population being studied, then the mean $\bar{X}$ of a sample of size N also has a normal distribution with mean μ and variance σ^2/N. (The standard deviation of $\bar{X}$, $\sigma/\sqrt{N}$, is often called the *standard error*.) If the population variance σ^2 is known, then the distribution of $\bar{X}$ is known, and statements can be made about its variability. But usually, σ^2 can only be estimated by the sample variance s^2. When s is used in place of σ, rather than using the normal distribution, the distribution of Student's t with $N - 1$ degrees of freedom (df) is used. The percentiles of the t-distribution depend on the sample size, but they can be easily obtained from tables or computer programs.

Confidence intervals are statements about a population parameter, such as the mean. The "90% confidence interval for the mean" is

$$\bar{X} \pm t_{.05}\, s/\sqrt{N} \tag{3}$$

where $-t_{.05}$ is the fifth percentile of the t-distribution with $N - 1$ df, $\bar{X}$ and s are the sample mean and standard deviation, and N is the sample size. (The fifth percentile is used because the interval is symmetric, with 5% of the distribution less than the left end of the interval, and 5% greater than the right end.) Note

Statistical Criteria

that this interval is symmetric about the sample mean. This is an *estimate* of the population mean plus a statement about the *variability* of the estimate. It says that at a confidence level of 90% the population mean is in the interval. The confidence level is not about this particular interval, for it either does, or does not, contain the population mean. The confidence is in the method; if this method is used to construct a large number of confidence intervals from samples, then in 90% of the cases the interval will contain the population mean μ.

For the reference formulation of set A, $\bar{X} = 48.06$, $s = 21.48$, $df = 11$, $t_{.05} = -1.796$ and $\sqrt{12} = 3.464$. Thus the 90% confidence interval (CI) is

$$48.06 \pm (1.796 \times 21.48/3.464) = 48.06 \pm 11.14 \text{ or } (36.92, 59.20)$$

It can be said "At a 90% level of confidence, the mean of the reference population is between 36.92 and 59.20." Interval estimates can be computed for any level of confidence less than 100%; for illustrations in this section the 90% or 95% levels are used.

An interval estimate can also be computed for $\mu_{test} - \mu_{ref}$, the difference between the means of the reference and test AUCs of set A. From Table 3, $\bar{X} = -8.413$ and $s = 6.46$; N and df are the same as above. Again, $t_{.05} = 1.796$, so that the 90% confidence interval for the mean difference (or the difference of the means) is -8.413 ± 3.35, or $(-11.76, -5.06)$. With a 90% confidence the mean difference is negative, since the upper end of the confidence interval is -5.06. When a confidence interval such as this is computed, it is sometimes said

$$\text{Prob } (-11.76 < \mu_{test} - \mu_{ref} < -5.06) = 0.90$$

but as noted earlier, since our confidence is in the method, not the computed interval, this is not a correct probability statement.

For set B the 90% confidence interval for the mean difference is $(-1.224, 7.387)$, so that although the point estimate of the difference is 3.08, at the 90% level of confidence it could be zero or even negative. Although Table 3 gives means and standard deviations for the individual ratios, these cannot be used to construct confidence intervals, since the distribution of the ratios is not a normal distribution.

Westlake's Symmetric Intervals

After noting that the definition of bioequivalence is symmetric about zero for differences, and about 1 for ratios, Westlake [4,5] suggested that, for bioavailability purposes, confidence intervals about zero or 1 would be more useful than the confidence intervals symmetric about the sample value. To construct these intervals two values of t must be found, t_l and t_u, such that the amount of the t-distribution between t_l and t_u is the level of confidence. That is, for a symmetric 90% confidence interval, 90% of the t-distribution must be between t_l and t_u. Westlake had suggested that these values of t can be found by interpolating in tables of the percentiles of the t-distribution. But it is easy to write computer programs to find the correct values; such a program, in the SAS language, is in Metzler [6].

For the mean difference of AUCs of set A, the 90% confidence interval symmetric about zero is $(-11.0, 11.0)$. The two t values used to compute this interval are $t_1 = -1.37$ and $t_u = 10.2$. That is, 90% of the t-distribution with 11 degrees of freedom lies between -1.37 and 10.2.

Figure 2 shows the t-distribution and the two types of confidence intervals for the mean difference of the two sets of AUCs of set A. In Figure 2a values symmetric about $\bar{X}$ are used to mark off the central 90% of the distribution. In Figure 2b values symmetric about a sample mean of zero are used. Because the sample mean, -8.42, is so far from zero (off the figure to the right) almost all of the 90% is below t_1, and t_u is also so far to the right that it is out of the figure. Only 0.13% of the distribution is above t_u. In effect the symmetric about zero interval is obtained by swapping probability from the upper tail to the lower tail until the interval limits are equal distance from zero.

If $\bar{X} = 0$, then the two types of confidence intervals will be exactly the same. Whenever the sample mean is not exactly zero, the symmetric intervals will always be longer than the classic ones. In the example used here, the length of the classic 90% confidence interval is 6.70 AUC units (i.e., from -11.76 to -5.06). The symmetric interval is 22 AUC units in length; 3.3 times as long as the classic interval. As seen in Figure 2b most of this length contains very little probability. Also note that, whereas the classic intervals give an indication both of location and variability, since they are centered on the sample mean, the symmetric intervals give little information about either location or variability.

Confidence Intervals as Percentage

The confidence intervals computed in the previous sections were in the units of the AUCs. Since bioequivalence is often stated as a percentage of the reference mean, it is useful to convert the confidence intervals to percentages. If the population mean were known, the intervals could be converted by dividing their endpoints by the population mean. The first attempts to convert confidence intervals to percentages simply used the sample reference mean, rather than the population mean. With this technique, the 90% confidence intervals computed in the previous section for the mean difference between the two formulations of set A are $(-24.5\%, -10.5\%)$ and $(-22.9\%, 22.9\%)$. Interpreting the classic confidence interval, with a certainty of 90%, the mean difference between the two formulations is between -24.5% and -10.5% of the reference mean.

But, as pointed out by Mandallaz and Mau [7], the reference mean is itself a random variable, and a correction must be made to the confidence interval if the sample mean is used. The correction consists of multiplying s in Eq. (3) by the square root of $\{0.5 + (\bar{X}_{test}/\bar{X}_{ref})^2/2\}$. With this correction the confidence

Statistical Criteria

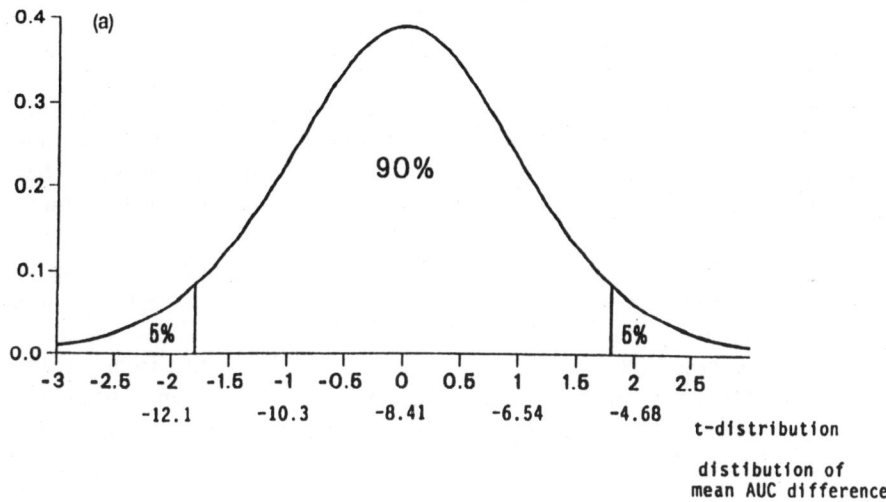

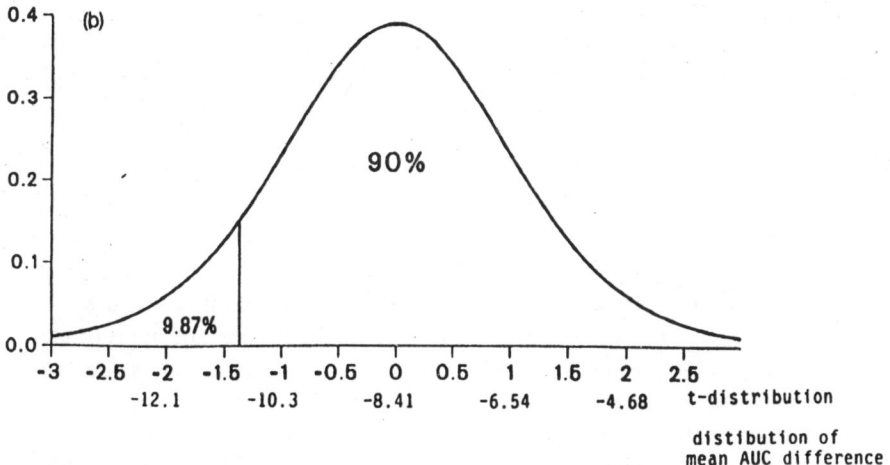

Figure 2 (a) Classic *t*-based confidence interval; (b) symmetric confidence interval.

intervals are (−23.9%, −11.1%) and (−22.4%, 22.4%). Note that these intervals are shorter, but the differences are small. When the mean of the test formulation is larger than the mean of the reference formulation, the correct intervals will be longer. Since the correct intervals are as easy to compute as the approximate ones, they will be used in this chapter.

Nonparametric Intervals

Since some bioavailability data appears to be strongly skewed, proposals have been made to use nonparametric confidence intervals. They are called nonparametric because they do not depend on assumption of the t-distribution. These nonparametric intervals can also be used to compare confidence intervals for individual ratios.

The most common nonparametric intervals are computed by ranking the means of all possible pairs of the data [see Ref. 8]). That is, each data point in a set is paired with every other data point, including itself, and the means computed. These $N(N + 1)/2$ means are ranked, and then, either from prepared tables or by approximation from the normal distribution, ranks from each end of the list are picked to be the ends of the interval. The method is illustrated with the differences of set A from Table 3. The first mean is $(-17.91 - 17.91)/2$, the second mean is $(-17.91 - 16.62)/2$, and so on. The last two means are $(-0.76 - 0.37)/2$ and $(-0.37 - 0.37)/2$. The tables in Hollander and Wolfe [9] indicate that in this list of $(12 \times 13)/2 = 78$ means the 14th and 65th means give a 95% confidence interval. Accordingly, the nonparametric 95% confidence interval is $(-12.56, -3.81)$. This can be converted to percentage by dividing by 44.57, the *median* of the reference formulation. This is an approximation, since there is no correction for using a sample statistic, rather than a population parameter. Dividing by the median of the reference formulation gives a 95% confidence interval in percentages $(-28.2\%, -8.5\%)$.

It can be seen that the nonparametric interval is longer than the t-based interval. This reflects the common inefficiency of nonparametric methods when they are applied to data that are approximately symmetric. Accordingly, the nonparametric interval is used only for very skewed data. It can be used for individual ratios, however, where the t-based intervals are not appropriate. By using the ratios for set A from Table 3, and going through the same procedure of forming 78 means, the 95% confidence interval for the *average ratio* is (0.69, 0.94). Since this is an interval on ratios, multiplying by 100 produces the confidence interval for percentages, (69%, 94%). Subtracting 100% from each endpoint gives the 95% confidence interval on the differences, $(-31\%, -6\%)$.

Another way to use individual ratios is to use the bootstrap methodology to construct confidence intervals. This has not yet been well studied, but in the future, may provide a tool for using this natural variable for relative bioavailability.

ANALYSIS OF VARIANCE

Analysis of variance (AOV) is often used to test the hypothesis that the means of two populations are equal; in bioequivalence studies, AOV has been used to test that the mean AUCs of two formulations are equal. This is not usually the question of interest; thus, many applications of AOV in bioavailability or bioequivalence studies have been a misuse of the method. The AOV does have uses in bioavailability, however, and in this section, the most important use of AOV is discussed and application made to bioavailability.

Identifying Sources of Variation

The most important use of AOV is to identify sources of variation and estimate the size of that variability. In most bioavailability studies there are three readily identified sources of variation: formulation, subjects, and periods. Interest is usually in only the formulations, the others are nuisance variances to be identified and removed.

In the design used in Table 1 there are two sequences of formulation assignment; half the subjects get test, then reference, the other half get reference, then test. These sequences may also be an effect in the statistical model.

An often used statistical model for AUCs is

$$AUC = M + S_j + s_{l(j)} + P_i + F_k + e_{il(j)k} \qquad (4)$$

where M is the overall mean, S_j is sequence effect, $s_{l(j)}$ is the subject in sequence effect, P_i is period effect, F_k is formulation effect, and $e_{il(j)k}$ is the error term. By *error term* is meant all those other sources of variation which are not identified. Subjects are said to be "in sequence" because each subject occurs with only one sequence, whereas each sequence occurs with every formulation and period. Often effects are classifed as "fixed" or "random," with fixed effects those about which inferences are made and the variances of random effects are estimated. But for purposes of removing the variability by AOV this classification is not needed. Furthermore, in the two-period, two-formulation experiment, such as shown in Table 1, all the effects have to be one kind or the other.

The coefficients of variation (CV) in Table 2 are between 42% and 53%; this is quite high. But the variances in those tables include all the variation: subject, period, and, for the total data set, formulation. We now want to divide the total variation into its identifiable parts. Table 4 shows AOV tables for the two data sets. The parts of the table will be identified and interpreted.

Since a mean has to be estimated, the degrees of freedom (*df*) is 1 less then the number in the classification. Thus the *df* for the total sum of squares (SS) is $N - 1$; the *df* for formulation, perids, and sequences is 1. The SS represents the total variation about the mean of that effect. The SS of the total is the number from which the variance of the data set is computed. Note that if the standard

Table 4 Analysis of Variance Tables for AUCs of Table 1

Source of variation	df	Sum of squares	Mean square	F	p
Data Set A					
Total	23	10,328.91			
Sequences	1	2,218.37	2,218.37	2.98	0.115
Subject (sequences)	10	7,456.37	745.64	34.25	<0.001
Formulations	1	424.70	424.70	19.51	0.001
Periods	1	11.79	11.79	0.54	0.479
Error	10	217.68	21.77		
Root mean square error = 4.67 CV = 10.64%					
Data Set B					
Total	31	23,613.23			
Sequences	1	412.00	412.00	0.26	0.620
Subject (sequences)	14	22,401.87	1,600.133	30.97	<0.001
Formulations	1	75.95	75.95	1.47	0.245
Periods	1	0.16	0.16	<0.01	0.956
Error	14	723.15	51.66		
Root mean square error = 7.19 CV = 11.35%					

deviation of set A, 21.19, is squared and then multiplied by 23, the result is 10,328.91, the total SS. The SS of all the effects add up to this total SS. Thus the total SS has been partitioned into the identifiable sources of variation plus the error SS.

The *mean square* (MS) is SS divided by *df* and is the quantity used to compute the F-statistic. For formulation, period and subject (sequences) the error MS is used to compute F. The F-statistic for sequences is obtained by dividing the sequences MS by the subject (sequences) MS. Although we are not interested in testing hypotheses, the F-statistic and its accompanying probability level give some idea of the relative strengths of the effects. As in most bioavailability trials, subjects are a large source of variation for both data sets.

The *root mean square error* is the square root of the error mean square, and is an estimate of the standard deviation of the error term. It can also be used to make probability statements about the formulation means; it will be used for this purpose in the next section. The CV is the error standard deviation divided by the AUC mean. Note how much smaller are the CVs in Table 3 than those in Table 1; this decrease in variability has been obtained by removing the known sources of variation. The standard deviations from the AOV are also smaller, but not by so much, than the standard deviations of the differences given in

Table 3. In taking differences within each subject, the subject effects are removed, but not the other effects.

Uses of Analysis of Variance in Bioavailability Studies

Some of the usefulness of AOV has been suggested in the previous section; it is a way to identify sources of variation and evaluate their relative contribution to the total variability. Periods, for example, are mostly a random effect; they depend on availability of the clinic and other logistic problems. As such they will from time to time reach a level of significance. But if periods are a large part of the total variation, one should probably look for something in the experimental setup that is not as well controlled as it should be. Likewise, subjects are usually assigned to sequences at random, and the sequence effect will occasionally be significant. However, one problem with this simple two-period, two-formulation design is that interactions between the factors cannot be evaluated. (This will be further discussed in the section on experimental designs, in which other designs will be recommended.) The sequence effect is exactly the same as the formulation by period interaction (the statistical term is "completely confounded"). Thus, a large sequence effect may indicate that the difference between the formulations is not the same in both periods. In set A, the sequence effect, although not "statistically significant" is a large part of the total variation. The means for each formulation in each period are the following:

	Period 1	Period 2	Overall
Reference	56.97	39.14	43.85
Test	29.33	49.96	39.64

In period 1 the reference mean AUC is 27.6 units larger than the test mean AUC; in period 2 it is 10.5 units smaller. This is also an indication that something may have gone wrong with the implementation of the study. With this kind of interaction, it is difficult to say much about relative bioavailability.

Normal plots are often useful in evaluating an AOV. Figure 3 shows the residuals (error) from fitting the AOV model. The residuals from set B lie nicely scattered along the line and give no indication of any problem with model. The residuals of set A, however, indicate some problems. There are large, nonrandom deviations from the straight line. To further identify the problem, the deviations have been coded by both formulation and period. The reference residuals are open symbols, the test residuals closed. Residuals from period 1 are circles, from period 2 squares. If the residuals are random normal deviates then they

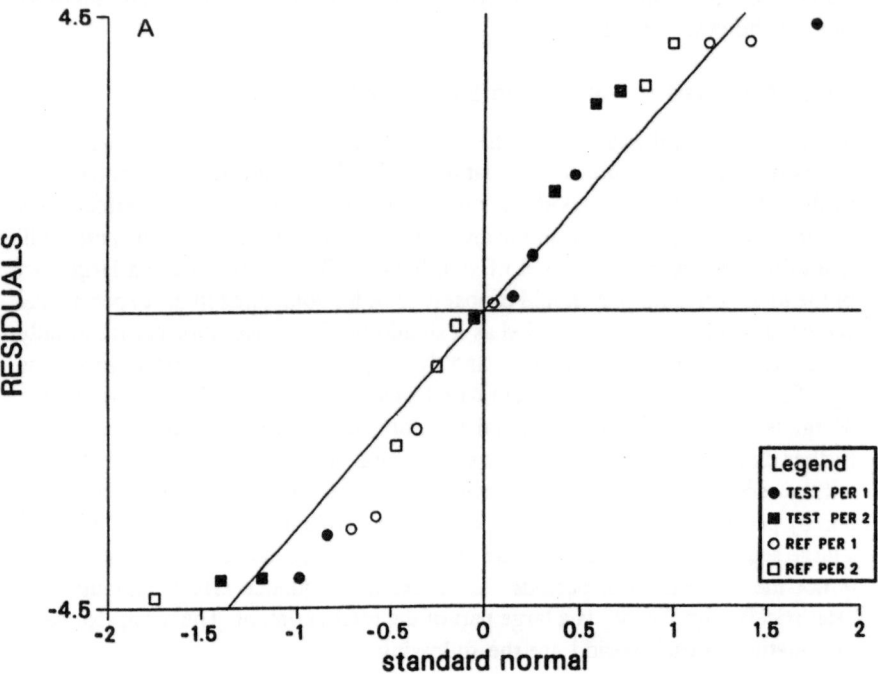

Figure 3 Normal plot of residuals from AOV, set A and set B.

should be randomly distributed along the line. But there is clustering, runs of the same formulation and of the same period. This is further evidence of the possible formulation by period interaction.

The most important use of AOV in bioavailability–bioequivalence studies in estimating the standard deviation of the error. Since all subjects have had both formulations in both periods, the standard deviation for the AOV may be used to compute confidence intervals on the mean differences. The s used in Eq. (3) will be from the AOV tables, rather than from Table 3, the 90% and 95% confidence intervals for the two data sets, expressed as percentages of the reference mean, are

	90% CI	95% CI
Set A	(−24.1%, −10.9%)	(−25.6%, −9.4%)
Set B	(−2.4%, 12.4%)	(−4.0%, 14.0%)

These were computed using the correction proposed by Mandallaz and Mau,

Statistical Criteria

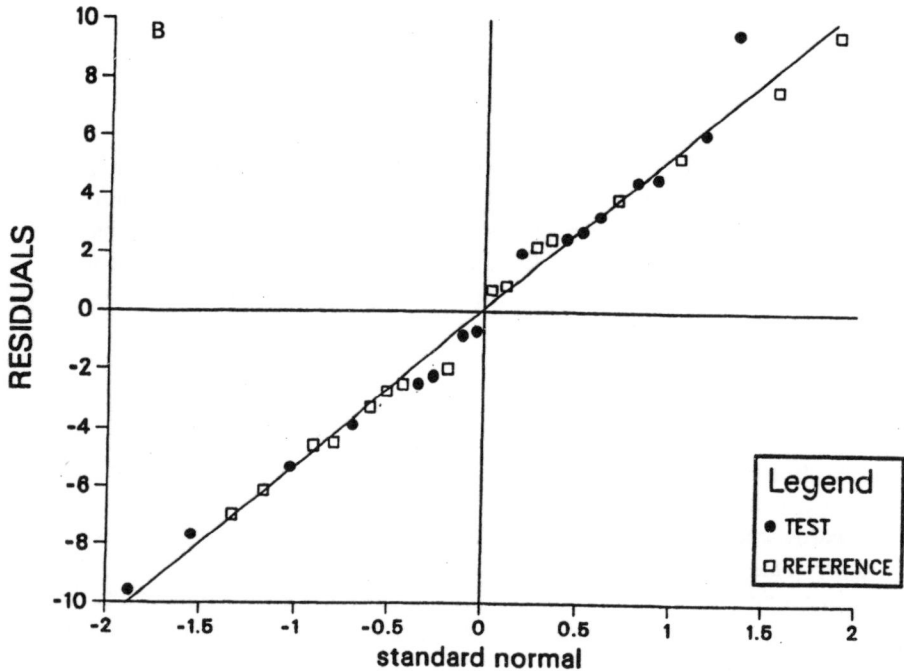

Figure 3 *Continued*

dividing by the reference mean and changing to percentage. These intervals are a little shorter than those computed with s from Table 3.

DECISION RULES FOR BIOEQUIVALANCE

Decisions about bioequivalence are made in many contexts; often a pharmaceutical company will have a series of formulations and for planning drug development must decide if two of the formulations are equivalent. More well know is the situation in which the producer of a drug product makes application to a regulatory agency that two formulations are equivalent. The latter context will be used in this section on decision rules; applications to other contexts are readily made.

Precise Definition of Equivalence

In the previous sections the point and interval estimates of the bioavailability of a single formulation have been discussed, and the application of these to relative bioavailability has also been shown. These have been in terms of AUCs, but they also apply to other measures of bioavailability such as C_{max} and t_{max}. Bioequivalence involves the comparison of the measures of bioavailability of two or more formulations. The same methods of comparison are appropriate for comparing the effects of an intervention, such as meals, on the bioavailability of a single formulation.

Some of the controversy of bioequivalence evaluation has arisen from a lack of a precise statement of the definition of bioequivalence. A precise definition was given in the first section of this chapter. If the interval of acceptable bioequivalence (A and B in the definition) is taken as $\pm 20\%$, then the inequality of that definition can be stated in the following alternate forms:

$0.8\mu_{ref} < \mu_{test} < 1.2\mu_{ref}$

$|\mu_{test} - \mu_{ref}| < .2\mu_{ref}$

$0.8 < \mu_{test}/\mu_{ref} < 1.2$

The decision of bioequivalence is well-defined if the population mean bioavailabilities are known. However, the decision must usually be made based on partial knowledge (i.e., the information contained in samples from the populations). This puts the problem in a statistical context.

In considering decision rules for deciding bioequivalence it is helpful to form a "truth table" which shows the consequences of right and wrong decisions (Figure 4).

In Figure 4 it is assumed that when two formulations are truly bioequivalent and the decision is **bioequivalent**, everyone gains; the consumer because they have a choice of two equivalent formulations, and the sponsor of the application for equivalence, since the right decision has been made. In similar manner, if the formulations are not bioequivalent, the consumer loses if a decision of bioequivalence is made, since the consumer may be exposed to a formulation that

		TRUTH	
D E C I S I O N		Bioequivalent	Not Bioequivalent
	Bioequivalent	Right Decision Everyone Gains	Wrong Decision Consumer Loses
	Not Bioequivalent	Wrong Decision Sponsor Loses	Right Decision Consumer Gains

Figure 4 A truth table for bioequivalence decisions.

is not as efficacious as it should be, or is perhaps more toxic than thought. If a wrong decision is made, and an equivalent formulation is declared **not bioequivalent**, the table indicates that the sponsor loses, since an equivalent formulation is rejected, but the consumer may also lose if deprived of an equivalent formulation that may be cheaper.

When evaluating decision rules for deciding bioequivalence, it is important to keep this table in mind, so that it can be determined who is at risk and how large that risk is.

Characterizing and Evaluating Rules

Decision rules based on statistical procedures can be evaluated by computing the probability of rejecting equivalence for true values of Θ, the relative bioavailability. A desirable characteristic of a decision rule would be that the probability of rejection at the limits of acceptable relative bioavailability would not depend on the data. That is, the probability of rejection at A and B would depend on the rule, not on the sample size or variability. If PR is used for the probability of rejecting equivalence, then for the usual rule of thumb of $\pm 20\%$, and $\bar{\Theta} = \bar{X}_{test}/\bar{X}_{ref}$, we would like to know that PR given $\Theta = A = 0.8$ or $\Theta = B = 1.2$ are set by the decision rule. It is not clear what level of protection a regulatory agency should require to protect consumers. In this chapter we will use 95%; that is, the probability of rejecting equivalence at the endpoints is $0.95 = PR$ (given $\Theta = 0.80$ or $\Theta = 1.20$). All of the decision rules discussed here have an even higher probability of rejection if Θ is outside the acceptable interval.

It is possible to characterize a decision rule for all values of Θ by a PR curve (*p*robability of *r*ejection curve), analogous to the power curves used in statistics for characterizing hypothesis tests. An nearly ideal PR curve is shown in Figure 5. For this curve, it is assumed that the desired level of protection at the ends of the acceptable equivalence interval is 0.95. This curve is called "nearly ideal" because an ideal curve would have PR equal to zero for $0.8 < \Theta < 1.2$, and PR equal to 1 everywhere else. But when making decisions based on incomplete information (a sample) we know we cannot have an ideal curve with finite sample sizes.

Four Decision Rules

For many years decisions were made about bioequivalence without a strong statistical foundation for those decisions. Examples were the 75/75 rule and decisions based on testing the "no difference" null hypothesis and power. Since these are no longer used, they are not discussed here (see Metzler [6,10] for such a discussion). Four decision rules with a sound statistical basis will be discussed. These rules are described, illustrated, and evaluated in the context of crossover

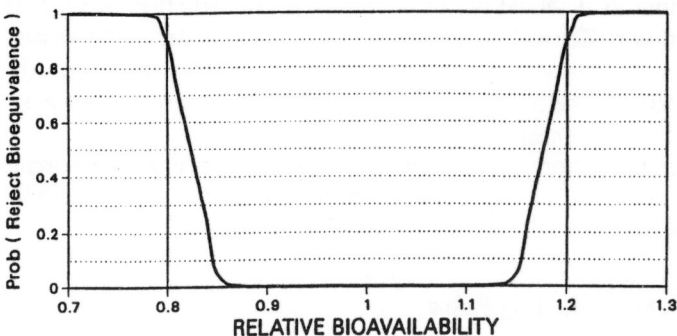

Figure 5 Nearly ideal PR curve.

studies, but they can all be adapted to parallel studies. In general, however, non-crossover studies will require much larger sample sizes.

For all these rules, if **bioequivalence** is not decided, then **not bioequivalence** is decided. Unlike conventional hypothesis testing, there is no withholding of a decision. Of course, if not bioequivalence is decided because the sample size is too small, then the drug sponsor might want to do another, larger bioavailability trial in the hope of being able to show equivalence.

Classic Confidence Intervals

The use of confidence intervals to evaluate relative bioavailability was proposed by Westlake [4] soon after bioequivalence became a widely recognized problem in the pharmaceutical sciences. Metzler [1] stated the problem, in somewhat different notation than used here, as follows:

> If B_s is the bioavailability of the standard formulation, and B_n the bioavailability of the new formulation, we don't want to show that $B_s = B_n$; we want to assess the difference $B_s - B_n$ and determine if it is acceptably small. . . . For example, it might be specified that, with 95% confidence, the new formulation should be between 80% and 120% as available as the standard.

In the notation of this book, it was suggested that a $(1 - a)\%$ confidence interval (C_1, C_u) for the relative bioavailability be computed and compared with (A,B), the acceptable interval for bioequivalence. If the confidence interval is completely contained in the acceptable interval, then bioequivalence is declared. That is, the test formulation is declared bioequivalent if and only if $A < C_1 < C_u < B$.

To have a 95% protection level at the endpoints, a 90% confidence interval is used. Applied to data sets A and B, the test formulation of A is not bioequivalent to the reference formulation, since the lower end of the interval, -24.1%, is less than -20%. The test formulation of B is bioequivalent, because the 90% confidence interval is within -20% to 20%.

This test is exactly equivalent to the two one-sided tests rule proposed by Schuirman [11].

Symmetric Confidence Intervals

If one follows Westlake [4], a decision rule can be based on symmetric confidence intervals. The rule is the same as that for the classic intervals, except a symmetric interval is computed. To have a 95% protection level, a 95% symmetric confidence interval is computed.

This rule agrees with the previous rule when applied to sets A and B; the 95% symmetric interval for A extends beyond both ends of the acceptable interval, whereas that for B is contained within the acceptable interval.

Anderson–Hauck Hypothesis Test

In 1983, Anderson and Hauck [12] provided the correct test for the bioequivalence decision problem. Their statement of the hypothesis test is

H_0: $\Theta < A$ or $\Theta > B$

H_A: $A < \Theta < B$

This is exactly the right statement of the hypotheses and in the right order for making bioequivalence decisions. In general, one hopes to show H_A. If H_0 is rejected at the chosen level of protection ($\alpha = 0.05$ in this section), then the alternate hypothesis of bioequivalence is accepted. The authors obtained the distribution of this test and also derived easily computed approximations to the distribution. The decision rule based on the Anderson–Hauck test is: Compute the probability of H_0; if this probability is less than 1 minus the protection level (taken to be 0.05 in this chapter), then reject H_0 and declare **bioequivalent**. If the probability is greater than 1 minus the protection level declare **not bioequivalent**.

As applied to set A, the probability of the null hypothesis is 0.273, so it cannot be rejected and bioequivalence cannot be declared. As applied to set B, the probability of H_0 is 0.001, so it is rejected, and the test formulation is declared bioequivalent.

Although the Anderson–Hauck statement of the bioequivalence problem is the exactly correct hypothesis test, it has some problems. It requires a major shift in the way one thinks about hypothesis tests. When compared with the classic test of a null hypothesis of equality, or no difference, the acceptance and rejection regions have been interchanged. With the classic hypothesis test the power may be made as large as is desired (up to the limit of 1.00) by choosing a difference far out in the tails of the distribution. But with the Anderson–Hauck test, power is maximum at zero, and can be increased only by increasing sample size. However, classic power considerations are not as important with this test and should not keep the test from being useful for providing a basis for a decision rule.

A theoretical problem has been pointed out by Rocke [13] and Schuirmann [11]: If the variance is larger (much larger) than the acceptable interval (A,B), then bioequivalence will always be concluded, regardless of the sample result. These authors seem to overlook that all bioavailability parameters, such as AUC and C_{max}, are positive and, thus, the variance cannot be large enough for the anomaly to occur.

Bayesian Procedures

Rodda and Davis [14] suggested the use of Bayesian analysis to compute the probability that Θ is in (A,B), given the sample results. Rodda and Davis gave the details of the analysis and indicated that this analysis is more useful than a test of the classic null hypothesis, but they did not explicitly state a decision rule. Their development is as follows: Assume that the error terms are normally distributed and that the prior distributions of $\tilde{\Theta} = \bar{X}_{test} - \bar{X}_{ref}$ and s, the standard deviation of the errors, are locally uniform (vague or uninformative). Then the posterior distribution of the sample mean difference, $\tilde{\Theta} = \bar{X}_{test} - \bar{X}_{ref}$, is the t-distribution. Thus, for any a and b, Pr (a < Θ < b) is the integral of the t-distribution from t_a to t_b, where

$$t_a = (a - \tilde{\Theta})(N/2)^{1/2}/s$$
$$\text{and } t_b = (b - \tilde{\Theta})(N/2)^{1/2}/s$$

In particular, if a = A < B = b are the ends of the acceptable bioequivalence interval, then Pr(a < Θ < b) is the probability that the test formulation is bioequivalent to the reference formulation.

We have seen that usually we would like to write A and B as percentages; this introduces the same problem here as in constructing confidence intervals: The sample mean rather than the population mean must be used. The Mandallaz and Mau [7] correction is also used here. The correct limits of integration are

$$t_a = (\bar{X}_{test} - p\bar{X}_{ref}) \{N/(1 + aa)\}^{1/2}/s$$
$$\text{and } t_b = (\bar{X}_{test} - q\bar{X}_{ref}) \{N/(1 + bb)\}^{1/2}/s.$$

The a and b values correspond to the ends of the acceptable interval and, in this chapter, are a = 0.8 and b = 1.2. These limits, which are used for all Bayesian analyses in this chapter, have been given by a number of authors, who also showed the equivalence of the Bayesian analysis, for a = A and b = B, to the symmetric confidence interval analysis. The posterior Bayesian analysis will depend on (1) the sample estimate of the relative bioavailability and of the error variance, (2) the number of observations, and (3) the limits of integration.

A decision rule based on Bayesian estimation is: Compute the posterior probability that Θ is between A and B; if this probability is at least the level of protection (0.95), declare **bioequivalent**. If it is less than the protection level declare **not bioequivalent**.

A useful property of the Bayesian analysis is that it not only provides a rule for deciding bioequivalence, but it also provides information about the location of the true relative bioavailability. Table 5 shows for the two data sets the posterior probabilities that Θ lies in the indicated intervals.

For Set A the probability that Θ, the true relative bioavailability is between 80 and 120% is only 0.747. The probability that the true relative bioavailability is less than 80% is 0.252. Thus, one would not want to declare the two formulations equivalent. The table also indicates that a larger study might not enable one to show bioequivalence, since the probability is 0.252 that the true relative bioavailability is less than 80%.

For set B the posterior probability that Θ is between 80 and 120% is 0.977; thus, the test formulation should be declared bioequivalent.

Comparison of Decision Rules

In addition to the exact equivalences already mentioned, inequalities can, under certain assumptions, be established for the probabilities associated with these rules. These have been discussed by several authors [13,15-17].

There are a number of factors that make it difficult or impossible to obtain closed form expressions for the PR curves of these rules: (1) For some, the mathematics is intractable, (2) all have assumptions of normality, (3) changing

Table 5 Bayesian Analysis of Relative Bioavailability

	Interval	Probability
Set A	60–70%	0.002
	70–80%	0.250
	80–90%	0.710
	90–100%	0.036
	100–110%	0.001
	80–120%	0.747
Set B	80–90%	0.001
	90–100%	0.122
	100–110%	0.744
	110–120%	0.130
	120–130%	0.003
	80–120%	0.997

from units of AUC or C_{max} to percentages introduces the problems already discussed. Consequently, a useful method of computing PR curves is by computer simulation.

Metzler [6,10] has reported numerous simulations comparing these rules. To compute PR curves by simulation of bioequivalence trials, the statistical model of Eq. (4) was assumed for the bioavailability parameters, but for simulation purposes all of the effects, except formulation were assumed to be normally distributed with zero means.

The simulated data were analyzed by AOV; because of the two-way design, only the error could be assumed random in the analysis. As discussed in the section on identifying sources of variation, for statistical purposes it is the distribution of the error term that is important, not the distribution of AUC. Many comparisons were reported in [6] and [10], only two are shown here.

Figure 6 shows the PR curves for the four decision rules for the case of error CV = 10% and N = 8, and with a stated protection level of 95% at the endpoints. The decision rules all have very similar performance, it is difficult to say that one is best. Note that all of them are a little skewed, the protection level at $\Theta = 1.2$ is only about 90%. The results of many simulations [6,10] all confirm that in those situations of sample size and variability where any of the decision rules is reasonable, all of them perform about the same.

Figure 7 shows, for the rule based on classic confidence intervals, the performance at two situations of CV and N for protection levels of 90 and 95%. For both cases of (CV,N) the upper PR curve gives the greater protection at the endpoints of acceptable relative bioavailability. These curves also show the price

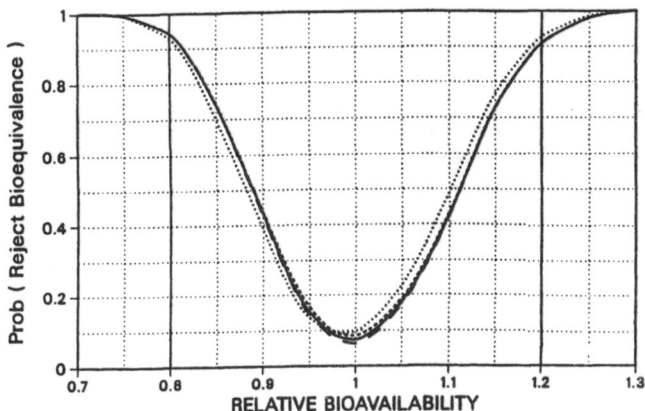

Figure 6 Probability of rejection (PR) curves for bioequivalence decision rules. $\alpha = 0.05$, N = 8, CV = 10%.

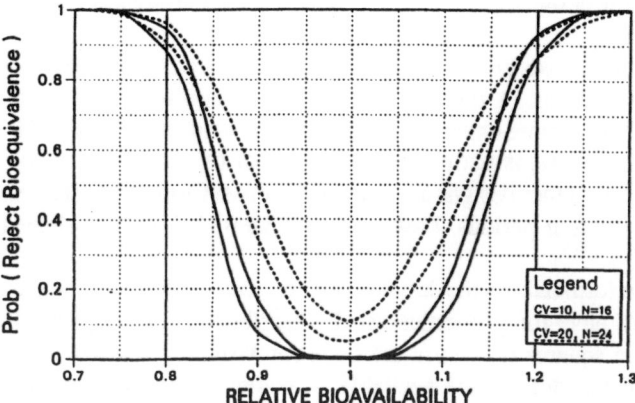

Figure 7 Probability of rejection (PR) curves for bioequivalence decision rules. $\alpha = 0.05$ or 0.10.

paid, in terms of wrongly rejecting bioequivalence when in the acceptable range, for greater protection at the endpoints or outside.

These figures also give an indication of the sample sizes needed to give the sponsor assurance that an equivalent formulation will not be wrongly declared not bioequivalent. The structure of these decision rules is such that the usual sample size calculations based on power are not useful. But it is easy to simulate conditions and, thereby, get a good idea of what N will give protection against wrongly declaring not equivalent. (Remember, the structure of the rules determines the protection level at the endpoints and outside the acceptable interval, so regulatory agencies do not need to be concerned with sample size.) Metzler [10] presents PR curves for error CVs of 10, 20%, and 30% and protection levels of 90 and 95%. Very few bioavailability studies conducted as crossovers have error CV greater than 30%.

OTHER STATISTICAL ISSUES

Experimental Designs for Bioequivalence

As has been illustrated in previous sections, the two-formulation, two-period design is very poor. It does not permit estimation of interactions, and analyses cannot be adjusted for carryover. Carryover can be much more than just residual drug still in the body from the previous formulation. Carryover is all those things, including metabolism and state of the system, that may have been altered by exposure to drug. These designs do not permit evaluation of within-subject variance of the two formulations.

There are a number of experimental designs that use more than two periods to evaluate two formulations. A possible three-period design uses the two sequences ABB and BAA. A more extensive design uses the sequences ABA, ABB, BAB, and BAA. These designs permit the estimation of carryover and within subject variability. Many other designs are available for two-formulation studies, including some that use four periods. Laska and associates [17], have evaluated a number of these.

For more than two formulations the designs used are often called Latin squares, although they do not have the properties usually ascribed to Latin squares in statistical texts. Latin squares may form the basis for assigning subjects to sequences, but often better designs are available. A common three-formulation, three-period design uses the sequences ABC, BCA, and CAB, and assigns one-third of the subjects to each of these sequences. This design always has A following C, B always follows A, and C always follows B. If N is a multiple of 6 (12,18,24,...), as is often the case, a much better design uses all six possible sequences: ABC, ACB, BAC, BCA, CAB, and CBA; and replicates these as needed. There are also designs that use four or more periods to evaluate three formulations [18].

If numerous formulations are to be studied, it may be necessary to use fewer periods than formulations. Westlake [5] discusses balanced incomplete block designs that are appropriate for these situations.

Dose-Response Studies

A class of bioavailability studies that are not strictly bioequivalence studies are those in which more than one dose level is used to evaluate linearity of the system. Although not usually called "dose-response," since a pharmacologic response is not observed, these are an attempt to evaluate the response—drug concentrations—to different doses of the formulation. They are often designed as though the doses were different formulations; the analysis is done by "normalizing" the responses, most often AUC and C_{max}, to some common dose. For evaluation of linearity multiple comparisons of the data must be made; always a troublesome statistical practice.

Analysis by linear regression has many advantages, since it uses the fact that the doses are indeed ordered. With three or more dose levels deviations from linearity can be tested. It should be understood that even though the data, AUCs for example, show no deviation from a linear regression, the system may not be "linear." For the system to be linear, the intercept of the straight line must be no different from zero; this can also be tested.

Transformations of Data

As mentioned earlier, often bioavailability data, such as AUCs, are transformed by taking the logarithms of the data. The reason usually given is the asymmetric appearance of the data. Very seldom are bioavailability data sets large enough to use statistical tests to determine the distribution of the data. We have shown that the use of nonparametric estimates can give estimates of average variability, even with outliers in the data. Most of these nonparametric tools are based on the ranks of the data. The use of ranks is also a way of transforming the data; it makes no assumptions about distributions. The use of AOV often removes those effects that skew the data.

There is one good reason for transforming to logarithms. It makes it easier to work with individual ratios, since the logarithm of a ratio is the difference of the two logarithms. This in itself does not justify the use of logarithms, however. The argument is sometimes made for AUCs that since one pharmacokinetic expression for AUC is

$$AUC = f \cdot dose/clearance,$$

where f is the fraction of dose absorbed, taking the logarithm of this expression gives an additive model. But it is not clear that there is any relation between the pharmacokinetic model and the statistical model used to evaluate the data.

Whenever analysis is done on transformed data, it is usually necessary to transform the results back to the original variable space. This transformation may cause problems in interpretation of the results.

REFERENCES

1. C. M. Metzler. Bioavailability—A problem in equivalence. *Biometrics* 30:309 (1974).
2. D. Freedman, R. Pisani, and R. Purves. *Statistics*. W. W. Norton, New York (1980).
3. G. W. Snedecor and W. G. Cochran. *Statistical Methods*, 6th ed. Iowa State University Press, Ames (1967).
4. W. J. Westlake. Symmetrical confidence intervals for bioequivalence. *Biometrics* 32:741 (1976).
5. W. J. Westlake. Bioavailability and bioequivalence of pharmaceutical formulations. In *Pharmaceutical Statistics for Drug Development* (K. E. Peace, ed.) Marcel Dekker, New York (1988).
6. C. M. Metzler. Statistical methods for deciding bioequivalence of formulations. In *Oral Sustained Release Formulations: Design and Evaluation* (A. Yacobi and E. Halperin-Walega, eds.) Pergamon Press, New York (1988).

7. D. Mandallaz and J. Mau. Comparison of different models for decisionmaking in bioequivalence assessment. *Biometrics 37*:213 (1981).
8. V. W. Steinijans and E. Diletti. Generalization of distribution-free confidence intervals for bioavailability ratios. *Eur. J. Clin. Pharmacol. 28*:85 (1985).
9. M. Hollander and D. A. Wolfe. *Nonparametric Statistical Methods*. John Wiley & Sons, New York (1973).
10. C. M. Metzler. Sample sizes for bioequivalence studies. *Stat. Med.* (in press) (1990).
11. D. J. Schuirmann. A comparison of the two one-sided tests procedure and the power approach for assessing the equivalence of average bioavailability. *J. Pharmacokinet. Biopharm. 15*:657 (1987).
12. S. Anderson and W. W. Hauck. A new procedure for testing equivalence in comparative bioavailability and other clinical trials. *Commun. Stat. Theory Methods 12*:2663 (1983).
13. D. M. Rocke. On testing for bioequivalence. *Biometrics 40*:225 (1984).
14. B. E. Rodda and R. L. David. Determining the probability of an important difference in bioavailability. *Clin. Pharmacol. Ther. 28*:247 (1980).
15. J. O'Quigley and C. Baudion. General approaches to the problem of bioequivalence. *Statistician 37*:51 (1988).
16. H. Peil and V. Haselbarth. Statistical testing of bioequivalence. *Arzneim. Forsch. 35*:1489 (1985).
17. E. Laska, M. Meisner, and H. B. Kushner. Optimal crossover designs in the presence of carryover effects. *Biometrics 39*:1087 (1983).
18. V. M. Chinchilli. Clinical efficacy trials with quantitative data. In *Pharmaceutical Statistics for Drug Development* (K. E. Peace, ed.) Marcel Dekker, New York (1988).

4
Influence of Disease on Bioavailability

Wolfgang A. Ritschel and Donald D. Denson
University of Cincinnati Medical Center
Cincinnati, Ohio

INTRODUCTION

Bioavailability in general serves two purposes: (1) the *absolute* bioavailability reveals how much of an extravascularly given drug product is actually absorbed, and (2) the *relative* bioavailability gives information on the rate and extent of absorption of a given drug product when compared with an approved standard formulation when both are administered by the same route. In both cases, the "performance" of a drug product (i.e., its formulation) is tested, keeping all the other parameters that may influence the pharmacokinetics of the drug constant. Therefore, bioavailability is tested in healthy volunteers, who do not receive any other drug; who are carefully screened for age, height, body weight, blood chemistry, and medical history; and who receive the products to be tested at the same time of day, with identical conditions of fasting, food, activity, and so forth. However, drugs are usually not intended for healthy people, but for those suffering from one or more ailments, arising from disease processes. And diseases are processes that *alter* the normal functions of the body. Therefore, the normal functions involved in or leading to absorption of an extravascularly administered drug may be altered by disease, thereby affecting the bioavailability of the drug. Most drugs are given perorally. Changes in absorption of a drug from the gastrointestinal tract may be a result of gastrointestinal disease, or it could be secondary to cardiovascular, hepatic, or renal diseases. Consequently, a decrease in absorption can lead to a decrease in the bioavailability of a drug and may reduce efficiency of a given regimen.

The bioavailability of perorally administered drugs can be affected by the extent of their metabolism during the first pass through the gastrointestinal tract and the liver. In hepatic and renal diseases, where first-pass metabolism is often reduced or absent, bioavailability may be substantially increased.

In all cases, not only the effect of disease states on the bioavailability of peroral drugs, but also by other extravascular routes, must be taken into consideration when administering a dose to the patient, as the bioavailability may be increased or decreased.

Because the body handles many drugs and endogenous substances similarly, diseases that alter the pharmacodynamics of endogenous substances may also alter the pharmacodynamics of the drugs. Disease states can also modify a number of kinetic parameters and, thereby, alter steady-state concentrations. The ability to predict or understand how pathological conditions can modify drug kinetics requires an understanding of the interrelationship among the various parameters. Bioavailability, distribution, and clearance (loss) represent three major pharmacokinetic variables. The pattern of the area under the concentration–time curve (AUC) is a function of the bioavailability, distribution, and loss factors.

Bioavailability studies are usually designed and analyzed as is done for an Abbreviated New Drug Application (ANDA). Even studies that specifically evaluate the effects of various types of intervention on the bioavailability of dosage forms are usually designed as though they were ANDA studies [Metzler, 1989]. Yet, they are very different. Primarily, interventions (physiological–pathological conditions), rather than the dosage form are changed. A crossover design to study the intervention "disease" is not possible; hence, a parallel design may be appropriate. Disease itself is not a constant, rather it is changing, dependent on the state of the disease, which makes it difficult to find a population of patients who are homogenous for the disease, disease state, therapy, and other factors. Accordingly, the question of bioavailability and bioequivalence in disease is much more complex than is that of a single ANDA evaluation for marketing a drug product.

PHARMACOKINETIC PHASES AND DISEASE

The pharmacokinetic phases, i.e., drug liberation from the dosage form, absorption, distribution, metabolism, and excretion, may be influenced by changes in physiological functions and in pathological conditions. The effect of various disease states on the pharmacokinetic behavior of numerous drugs has been studied clinically. Several excellent reviews are available [Benet, 1976; Bodenham et al., 1988; Evans et al., 1986; Koup, 1989; Sjoquist et al., 1980]. In addition to altering the pharmacokinetics of drugs, certain diseases and disease states may also alter corresponding pharmacodynamics by influencing bioavailability and intrinsic sensitivity of receptors. For instance, hypokalemia increases the toxicity of digoxin and potentiates the action of nondepolarizing muscle relaxants.

At this point, it is important to summarize the various pharmacokinetic phases before discussing the specific diseases and disease states, as well as to emphasize the appropriate selection criteria, methodology, and design of studies to evaluate the true effect of a pathological condition on a drug's uptake and fate in the body. There are numerous clinical reports in the literature germain to this topic; however, their conclusions are not always uniform, and often their results may lead to misinterpretation. For instance, the terminal half-life or elimination half-life ($t_{1/2}$) used as the only value in dosage regimen calculations, may be totally inappropriate. Often the $t_{1/2}$ is dependent on body or plasma clearance and volume of distribution. Hence, a prolonged $t_{1/2}$ in disease may be the result of a normal clearance if the volume of distribution is increased, and thus no change in dosage should be made. However, the time to reach steady state for clinical assessment and drug monitoring will be prolonged.

Liberation

Liberation or release of a drug from a dosage form is the first and sometimes rate-limiting step in the absorption of drugs. Liberation applies to all dosages forms except those in aqueous solution. In peroral administration, achlorhydria, hyperacidosis, and impaired gastric secretion may change the time for dissolution of the drug and the amount dissolved because of change in the pH or volume of gastric fluid, which may delay or reduce absorption. In intramuscular and subcutaneous administration, hypo- or hyperthermia, and resultant changes in the blood flow rate in the area of injection will influence the rate of dissolution of an injected suspension and the rate of absorption of the dissolved drug. It seems that the methodology for evaluating the process of liberation is to use the same subject to study both the rate and extent of absorption of the drug in solution and the dosage form.

Absorption

The absorption of any drug given extravascularly is characterized by two terms: rate and extent. For rate, one may simply compare the time to reach the peak, t_{max}, and the peak concentration C_{max}, or more elaborate, the rate of absorption can be determined by curve-fitting. For this, two or more populations, such as healthy versus a given disease can be compared. The extent of absorption is the only way to compare the area under the curve (AUC) after administration by the extravascular (EV) route with that after IV administration (corrected for dose size given) and obtain the absolute bioavailability F:

$$F = \frac{AUC_{Extravascular} \cdot D_{Intravascular}}{AUC_{Intravascular} \cdot D_{Extravascular}} \tag{1}$$

The results from a population with a certain disease can be compared with those obtained in healthy subjects. However, a comparison between healthy and diseased subjects of the AUCs obtained after EV administration is not permissible, because one has to assume that the total or plasma clearances, Cl_{tot}, are different in the two population groups. Differences in Cl_{tot} have an inversely proportional effect on AUCs [Koup, 1989]. Even if the $t_{1/2}$ is the same for both population groups, one cannot assume similar Cl_{tot} because, as described previously, $t_{1/2}$ depends on both clearance and volume of distribution. These parameters can be determined only from IV studies.

A comparison of the total amount of drug excreted in urine at infinite time (i.e., $> 7 \times t_{1/2}$) between healthy and diseased subjects is not permissible for the same reason, namely disease may alter the clearance and the percentage of dose eliminated in unchanged form *through* the kidney.

Distribution

Three different volumes of distribution can be used, depending on the scientific question being asked. All volumes of distribution can accurately be calculated from IV data with either compartment model-independent or model-dependent procedures. The volume of the central compartment, V_c, is the proportionality constant between an IV dose and the initial plasma concentration. V_c is used to calculate loading doses. The volume of distribution during the terminal phase or β-phase, V_β, is the proportionality constant between the amount of drug in the body postdistribution and the plasma concentration during the elimination phase. The volume of distribution at steady state, V_{ss}, is the proportionality constant between the amount of drug in the body and the plasma concentration at steady state during constant-rate IV infusion.

V_β depends on the rate of elimination from the central compartment, whereas V_{ss} is independent of the elimination process. Hence, V_β will be influenced in disease-altered elimination, whereas distributional changes independent of elimination are reflected in V_{ss}.

Because the onset and duration of action of a drug is dependent on the rate and extent of distribution, a change in the apparent volume of distribution, V_d, (or V_β) may change the drug concentration in blood or plasma and at the receptor site. With increasing V_d, the concentration in blood or plasma decreases, and vice versa. Several diseases affect the V_d, which may occur by quite different mechanisms, such as alterations in blood flow, pH changes, protein binding, and others. Tissue perfusion is dependent on the cardiac output. In myocardial infarction, shock, and heart failure, V_d for many drugs is reduced, primarily owing to reduced blood supply to peripheral tissues. This results in an increased drug concentration in blood, which may lead to toxicity. At the same time, clearance is often reduced, aggravating the situation by causing unwanted drug accumulation.

Many drugs are weak electrolytes. Relatively small changes in the acid-base balance may have a disproportionate effect on the degree of ionization of weak organic acids and bases the pK_a of which is close to the physiological pH of 7.4. For example, the myocardial uptake and efficacy of lidocaine (pK_a 7.9) is reduced by severe acidosis [Hayes, 1971].

The binding of drugs to proteins may be altered in diseases. Among the consequences are changes in V_d, displacement from binding, saturation of binding sites, and changes in the free/total durg concentration ratio.

Acidic drugs preferentially bind to albumin, the paramount importance of which is the maintenance of colloid osmotic pressure and the transport of endogenous and exogenous substances. In decreased hepatic protein synthesis and increased capillary permeability, the concentration of free or unbound drug increases. This may lead to increased hepatic extraction or renal excretion [Koch-Weser, 1973; Piafsky et al., 1978]. Changes in binding characteristics may be brought about in hepatic and renal failure and in changes of blood pH.

α_1-Acid glycoprotein, to which predominantly basic substances bind, may be drastically increased in plasma after acute stress, trauma, severe illness, and surgery.

Drugs are not bound only to plasma proteins (about 180 g in a 70-kg person), but also to tissue proteins (about 10 kg in a 70-kg person). Plasma albumin and α_1-acid glycoprotein are important tissue proteins. Alterations in plasma and tissue protein binding may have a significant effect on V_d. Koup [1989] performed a series of simulations in which it was assumed that both clearance and distribution act only on free-drug concentration. Koup demonstrated that total plasma drug concentration was higher with higher plasma binding. The time course of free-drug concentrations is affected by the extent of plasma and tissue binding, but the areas under the free plasma concentration curve and the time curve were identical. Total AUC and clearance, based on total drug concentration, are only affected by plasma binding, with an increase in plasma clearance as the free fraction in plasma increases. V_{ss} is affected by both plasma and tissue binding, increasing as the free fraction in plasma and in tissue decreases. The AUC and plasma clearance when based on unbound concentrations are always identical. A clinical example is phenytoin, the clearance of which depends on the free concentration. In reduced binding, such as in renal disease, the total concentration is decreased, whereas the free concentration is unchanged. In renal failure, an adjustment of a dosage regimen that is based on total phenytoin plasma concentration may result in toxicity.

Drugs with a high hepatic clearance that primarily bind to α_1-acid glycoprotein, such as propranolol or lidocaine, may behave differently [Piafksy, 1980]. Increased α_1-acid glycoprotein levels may increase plasma binding. However, the clearance of these drugs is limited by hepatic blood flow and not by the free-drug concentration. Here, the total drug concentration in plasma will not change, whereas the free-drug concentration decreases, reducing the clinical response.

Metabolism

The influence of diseases and disease states on drug metabolism has been extensively reviewed [Houston, 1985; Jenner and Testa, 1980; Kato, 1977]. It is very difficult to establish general patterns because of the variety of enzymatic processes and pathways available, as well as the wide range of hepatic diseases. Also, there are no universally applicable endogenous or exogenous markers or indicators available that will permit prediction of the metabolic capacity. This refers to compounds that have either low or high hepatic clearance. For compounds with low hepatic clearance, the clearance is proportional to, and limited by, enzyme activity, whereas for those with high clearance, the clearance is limited by hepatic blood flow. It was hoped that the indocyanine green clearance might evolve as a valuable tool in predicting metabolic capacity for low-clearance compounds. At present, this method is still controversial and needs more study [Bauer et al., 1989; Bax et al., 1980]. Cirrhosis has often been found to significantly increase the bioavailability of high-clearance compounds.

Excretion

In diseases involving the kidney, the extent of reduction in glomerular filtration rate (GFR) can be quantified by the creatinine clearance; hence, prediction of the renal elimination of drugs by glomerular filtration can be made. Usually, the GFR is also a good predictor for drugs actively secreted, since the nephron acts as a unit [Bricker et al., 1960], except in the case of mild interstitial nephritis, in which the active tubular secretion declines without change in GFR. Determination of creatinine clearance seems to have a 25–35% error range [Wilson, 1984], whereas the error range of inulin clearance is below 10% [Koup, 1989]. The use of serum creatinine concentrations instead of creatinine clearance to predict renal impairment needs careful consideration and is useful only in stabilized renal function. It should not be used for elderly patients, for those who are bedridden, or for those with cachexia or uremia [Ritschel, 1986]. The correlation between serum creatinine concentration and creatinine clearance has been reexamined recently [Robertshaw et al., 1989].

In renal diseases, the extent of protein binding is often reduced. For kinetic

DISEASE IN RELATION TO BIOAVAILABILITY

The previous section dealt with the general influence of disease and disease states on the basic pharmacokinetic phases. These influences are not necessarily limited to one phase alone, but may involve two or more. A basic understanding of this complex situation is necessary to appreciate the possible consequences diseases may have on bioavailability.

Bioavailability Aspects

Bioavailability testing for the governmental drug approval process is usually done with each subject as his or her own control. Thus, one assumes identical handling of the drug by the body, allowing the difference in formulation to be tested. This concept is based on the assumption that total or plasma clearance (Cl) is unchanged. However, in evaluating the influence of disease on bioavailability, we usually have only one drug product, and the disease or the disease state becomes the variable. *Absolute* bioavailability describes the absolute extent of absorption, whereas *relative* bioavailability describes the rate and extent of absorption in relation to a standard. The extent of absorption is estimated from the AUC. The total AUC, however, is influenced by the terminal rate constant, λ_z, the apparent volume of distribution, V_d, and the plasma clearance, Cl, as given in Eqs. (2) and (3).

$$\text{AUC } (0 \rightarrow \infty) = (D \cdot F)/(\lambda_z \cdot V_d) \tag{2}$$

$$\text{AUC } (0 \rightarrow \infty) = (D \cdot F)/\text{Cl} \tag{3}$$

The terminal rate constant λ_z is related to the plasma half-life, $t_{1/2}$, as given in Eq. (4)

$$\lambda_z = 0.693/t_{1/2} \tag{4}$$

As discussed in the previous section, all three kinetic parameters (i.e., $t_{1/2}$, V_d, Cl) may change because of disease.

The Cl can not be determined from EV administration because the bioavailability, F, is not known; the disease factor is studied by comparing the AUC after IV and EV in the same subject under the assumption of unchanged Cl [see Eq. (1)].

If F is then compared between healthy and diseased subjects, it is either the Cl that is responsible for differences, or a change in the first-pass effect (FPE), according to Eq. (5).

$$\text{Cl} = \frac{F \cdot F_{\text{FPE}} \cdot D}{\text{AUC}(0 \rightarrow \infty)} \tag{5}$$

where F_{FPE} is the fraction of drug reaching systemic circulation in the presence of FPE.

The rate of bioavailability can be expressed by the time, t_{max}, when peak concentration is observed after EV administration. The t_{max} depends on both the input and the output rates, as shown in Eq. (6).

$$t_{max} = \frac{\ln(k_a/\lambda_z)}{k_a - \lambda_z} \tag{6}$$

where k_a is the absorption rate constant.

Hence, even if the rate of absorption is unchanged, if the terminal disposition rate constant decreases, such as the hepatic or renal impairment, t_{max} will be shifted to the right (i.e., it will increase).

Disease Aspects

In context with bioavailability, both the severeness of the disease and the route of administration of drugs need to be considered. The major routes are listed as follows:

IV = intravascular
IM = intramuscular
SC = subcutaneous
IB = intrabronchial
O = oral (sublingual, buccal)
PO = peroral
R = rectal

In **acute severe illness** or in critically ill patients, most conditions, if untreated, will eventually lead to a state of shock, which is characterized by hemodynamic centralization and impairment of capillary microcirculation, which, in turn, impairs absorption owing to circulatory failure. Hence, in those patients, drug administration is usually by IV, which gives 100% bioavailability, by definition. Also IB formulations are available for catecholamines in cardiac arrest, bronchodilators in asthma, and inhalation of toxins, anesthetic gases, and O for nitroglyerin sublingually in angina pectoris or myocardial infarction. The IM route is seldom used because of vasoconstriction, resulting in unpredictable absorption or hematoma formation if a bleeding tendency is present. The R route may be used for nonsteroidal and antipyretic preparations. The PO route is never used because of erratic absorption caused by collapse of microcirculation.

The discussions presented in this chapter are primarily applicable to **chronic illness** in which impaired organic function is at least somewhat stabilized, and the PO route of administration is applicable. General guidelines are difficult to establish because it is not only a given disease, but also, the state of disease and other coexisting pathologic conditions that may create addition or counteracting effects.

In one survey, it was found that, for 124 drugs studied, bioavailability was reduced by disease in 27.4%, increased in 37.9%, and unchanged in 34.7% [Ritschel, 1987].

DISEASES AND DISEASE STATES AFFECTING RATE AND EXTENT OF ABSORPTION

Numerous papers have been published on the subject of disease and bioavailability of drugs. Only a few of many examples of disease states that either increase or decrease bioavailability of drugs will be given here.

In many cases, an alteration in bioavailability may be the result of an interaction between more than one pathological state (i.e., cardiovascular and gastrointestinal diseases, or gastrointestinal and neurological diseases).

The effect of disease states on the bioavailability of drugs must always be taken into consideration when administering a dose to the patient. Table 1 gives a summary of drugs that have been studied for their rate and extent of bioavailability in certain diseases. Excellent reviews have been published [Parsons, 1977; Welling and Craig, 1976; Welling, 1984; Welling and Tse, 1984; Gubbins and Bertch, 1989].

Gastrointestinal Diseases

In acute, severe conditions, such as bowel obstruction and paralytic ileus after acute pancreatitis or ulcer perforation, PO administration is contraindicated. In acute transient conditions, such as food poisoning (toxins) and acute infective enteritis, symptomatic treatment is given. Bioavailability may be influenced by drugs prescribed for symptoms as well as for other drugs used concomitantly. The largest group are the chronic gastrointestinal diseases, which may alter the bioavailability of a drug administered perorally by producing variation in both the amount of drug absorbed and rate of drug absorption. Many conditions involving the gastrointestinal tract are likely to cause changes in the absorption of drugs [Welling, 1984].

Gastrointestinal motility
Diseases of the stomach
Gastric and intestinal surgery
Diseases of the small intestine
Diseases of the large intestine
Gastrointestinal infections
Interactions with other substances

Table 1 Influence of Disease on Bioavailability

Disease	Drug	C_{max}	t_{max}	Rate	Extent	Ref.
Gastrointestinal						
Stomach						
Achlorhydria	Aspirin	↓	↓	↓	↓	Siurala et al., 1969
Hypochlorhydria	Salicylamide	-	-	U	U	Hartiala et al., 1963
	Tetracycline	↓	↑	↓	↓	Kramer et al., 1978
Postgastrectomy	Acetaminophen	-	-	↓	↓	Wojcik et al., 1984
	Cephalexin	-	-	↑	↑	Lode et al., 1974
	Digoxin	U	U	U	U	Beerman et al., 1973
	Ethambutol	↓	U	↓	↓	Venho et al., 1975
	Ethanol	↑	↓	↑	↑	Cotton et al., 1973
	Isoniazid	-	-	U	U	Mattila et al., 1969
	Quinidine	↓	↓	↓	↓	Venho et al., 1975
	Sulfafurazole	↓	U	↓	↓	Venho et al., 1975
	Tetracycline	U	U	U	U	Ochs et al., 1978
Pancreas	Phenoxymethyl penicillin	-	-	U	U	Lupinsky et al., 1973
Cystic fibrosis	Cephalexin	-	-	↓	↓	Parsons et al., 1975
	Cloxacillin	↓	↑	↓	↓	Spino et al., 1984
	Dicloxacillin	↓	U	-	↓	Jusko et al., 1975
Atrophy of villi	Chloramphenicol	-	-	U	U	Matilla et al., 1973
	Cycloserine	-	-	U	U	Matilla et al., 1973
	Isoniazid	-	-	U	U	Matilla et al., 1973
	Salicylate	-	-	U	U	Matilla et al., 1973
	Pindolol	↓	↑	↓	↓ U	Evard et al., 1984
Celiac disease	Acetaminophen	↓	-	↓	↓	Holt et al., 1981
	Amoxicillin	U	U	-	U	Parsons et al., 1975a
	Ampicillin	-	-	U	U	Parsons et al., 1975a
	Cephalexin	↑	↓	↑	↑	Parsons et al., 1975
	Clindamycin	-	-	↑	↑	Parsons et al., 1973
	Erythromycin ethyl succinate	U	U	U	U↓	Parsons et al., 1975a; Parsons et al., 1976
	Erythromycin stearate	U	U	U	U↓	Parsons et al., 1975a; Parsons et al., 1976
	Folic acid	↓	↑	↓	↓	Kitis et al., 1982
	Indomethacin	-	-	U	U	Parsons et al., 1977
	Lincomycin	-	-	U	U	Parsons et al., 1975a; Parsons et al., 1976
	Methyldopa	↑	-	↑	↑	Renwick et al. 1983
	Propranolol	↑	↓	↑	↑	Schneider et al., 1976
	Salicylate	U	-	↑	U	Parsons et al., 1977
	Sodium fusidate	↑	↓	↑	↑	Parsons et al., 1975a; Parsons, 1977

Continued

Table 1 *Continued*

Disease	Drug	C_{max}	t_{max}	Rate	Extent	Ref.
Celiac disease *continued*	Sulfamethazole	↑	-	↑	↑	Parsons et al., 1975a; Parsons et al., 1976
	Trimethoprim	↑	-	U	U	Parsons et al., 1975a; Parsons et al., 1976
Diverticulitis	Amoxicillin	-	-	U	U	Parsons et al., 1973
	Amipicillin	-	-	U	U	Parsons et al., 1973
	Cephalexin	↑	-	↑	↑	Parsons et al., 1975
	Clindamycin	-	-	↑	↑	Parsons et al., 1973
	Lincomycin	-	-	U	U	Parsons et al., 1973; Parsons et al., 1975
	Rifampin	-	-	U	U	Parsons et al., 1973; Parsons et al., 1975
Crohn's disease	Acetaminophen	↓	-	↓	↓	Holts et al., 1981
	Cephalexin	↓	↑	↓	↓	Parsons et al., 1975
	Clindamycin	-	-	↑	↑	Parsons et al., 1976a
	Co-trimoxazole	↑	↓	↑	↑	Parsons et al., 1975
	Erythromycin ethyl succinate	-	-	U	U	Parsons et al., 1976a
	Erythromycin stearate	↓	↑	↓	↓	Parsons et al., 1976a
	Hydrocortisone	-	-	U	U	Mlynark et al., 1963
	Methyldopa	↓	↓	-	↓	Renwick et al., 1983
	Metranidazole	↑	U	-	↑	Bergan et al., 1981
	Prednisolone	↑	U	-	↑	Tanner et al., 1981
	Propranolol	↑	↓	↑	↑	Schneider et al., 1976
	Rifampin	-	-	U	U	Parsons et al., 1976a
	Sodium fusidate	-	-	↑	↑	Parsons et al., 1976a
	Sulfamethazole	-	-	↑	↑	Renwick et al. 1983
	Trimethoprim	↓	↑	↓	↓	Parsons et al., 1975
Pernicious anemia	Cephalexin	↓	↑	↓	↓	Davies et al., 1970
	Penicillin V	-	-	↓	↓	Lupinsky et al., 1973
Resection	Ampicillin	-	↑	↓	↓	Kampman et al., 1984
	Aminopencilline	↓	↑	↓	↓	Menardi et al., 1984
	Digoxin	-	-	U	U	Beerman et al., 1973
	Hydrochloro-thiazide	↓	-	↓	↓	Beckman et al., 1979
	Phenytoin	↓	↑	↓	↓	Kennedy et al., 1949
Large Intestine Colitis	Hydrocortisone	-	-	U	U	Mlynark et al., 1973
	Metronidazole	↑	U	-	↑	Bergan et al., 1981
Ileostomy	Prednisolone	-	-	↓	-	Al-Habet et al., 1984
Cardiovascular Congestive heart failure	Aminopyrin	-	-	-	↑	Hepner et al., 1970

Continued

Table 1 *Continued*

Disease	Drug	C_{max}	t_{max}	Rate	Extent	Ref.
Myocardial infarction	Cephalexin	-	-	U	U	Parsons et al., 1975
	Digoxin	↓	↑	↓	↓	Korhonen et al., 1979
	Dihydroquinidine	↑	↓	↑	↑	Veda et al., 1979
	Disopyrmide	-	-	-	↑	Bryson et al., 1982
	Enalapril	↑	↑	↓ U	U↑	Dickstein et al., 1986; Dickstein et al., 1987
	Furosemide	-	-	U -	↑	Bryson et al., 1982
	Mexiletine	-	-	U	U	Vozeh et al., 1982
	Prazosin	↑	U -	-	↑	Baughman et al. 1980; Jaillon et al., 1979
	Procainamide	-	- -	U	↑	Lalka et al., 1978; Wyman et al., 1981
	Quinidine	-	-	-	↑	Veda et al., 1978
	Theophylline	-	-	-	↑	Powell et al., 1978
Hypertension	Hydrochlorothiazide	↑	U	-	↑	Williams et al., 1986
	Triamterine	↑	↑	-	↑	Williams et al., 1986
Liver Cirrhosis	Amobarbital	-	-	-	↑	Mawer et al., 1972
	Ampicillin	-	-	↑	↑	Lewis et al., 1975
	Antipyrine	-	-	-	↑	Brauch et al., 1973
	Buspirone	↑	U ↑	↑	↑	Gammans et al., 1986
	Cefoperazone	-	-	-	↑	Saudek et al., 1989
	Chloramphenicol	-	-	-	↑	Kunin et al., 1959
	Clormethiazole	-	-	-	↑	Pentikainen et al., 1978
	Diazepam	-	-	-	↑	Kiotz et al., 1975
	Encainidine	-	-	-	↑	Berstrand et al., 1986
	Labetalol	-	-	-	↑	Homeida et al., 1978
	Meperidine	-	-	-	↑	Klotz et al., 1974; Neal et al., 1979; Pond et al., 1979
	Nitrendipine	↑	U	↑	↑	Dylewicz et al., 1987
	Pentazocine	-	-	-	↑	Neal et al., 1979
	Propranolol	-	-	-	↑	Wood et al., 1978; Branch et al., 1976
Hepatitis	Antipyrine (A)	-	-	-	↑	Branch et al., 1973
	Antipyrine (C)	-	-	-	↑	Branch et al., 1973
	Diazepam (C)	-	-	-	↑	Klotz et al., 1975
	Hexobarbital (A)	-	-	-	↑	Breimen et al., 1975
	Nitrendipine (C)	↑	↓	↑	↑	Dylewioz et al., 1987
Obstructive Jaundice	Antipyrine	-	-	-	↑	Branch et al., 1973
Kidney Renal Failure	Ampicillin	-	-	-	↑	Jusko et al., 1973

Continued

Table 1 *Continued*

Disease	Drug	C_{max}	t_{max}	Rate	Extent	Ref.
	Carbenicillin	-	-	-	↑	Hoffman et al., 1970
	Cefazolin	↑	U	-	↑	Welling et al., 1974
	Cephalexin	↑	↑	-	↑	Bailey et al., 1970
	Digoxin	-	-	-	↑	Rasmussen et al., 1971
	Gentamicin	-	-	-	↑	Chan et al., 1972
	Netacillin	-	-	-	↑	Jusko et al., 1973
	Propranolol	↑	↓ U ↑		↑	Lowenthal et al., 1974
	Vancomycin	-	-	-	↑	Lindhohn et al., 1966
Lung						
Chronic obstructive lung disease	Sulfamethazine	↓	U	U U	↓	DuSouich et al., 1983
Chronic respiratory failure	Furosemide	-	-	-	↓	Ogato et al., 1985
Fever	Pranoprofen	U	U	U	U	Fijimura et al., 1989
Rheumatoid arthritis	Naproxen (total)	↓	↑	↓	↓	Duweland et al., 1987
	Naproxen (unbound)	↑	U	↑	↑	Duweland et al., 1987

↑, increased; ↓, decreased; U, unchanged; -, not reported; A, Acute; C, chronic

Physiological factors within the gastrointestinal tract that affect peroral drug absorption include gastric-emptying rate, intestinal motility, pH of gastrointestinal fluids, activity of gastrointestinal drug-metabolizing enzymes or drug-metabolizing bacteria, and surface area of the gut. All of these factors can be affected by pathological states.

Gastrointestinal Motility

The absorption of drugs from the gastrointestinal tract is predominantly dependent on passive diffusion, for which the drug should be nonionized as well as sufficiently lipophilic to diffuse across the lipoid epithelial lining of the gastrointestinal tract into the splanchnic circulation. Absorption of weak acids is considered optimal in the acidic environment of the stomach, whereas that of bases is in the weakly alkaline medium of the intestine. The presence of macro- and microvilli in the ileum facilitates absorption of most drugs from this site. Hence, any condition or state that would increase or decrease stomach emptying might, respectively, increase or decrease the rate at which a drug is absorbed.

Disease states, such as atrophic gastritis, gastric carcinoma, pyloric stenosis, pancreatitis, and gastric ulcer, delay the gastric emptying, whereas other conditions, such as celiac disease, cholecystitis, duodenal ulcer, stress, and gastroenterostomy, accelerate stomach emptying [Nimmo, 1976].

A case of inhibited drug absorption because of delayed stomach emptying occurred in a 68-year-old woman with adult hypertrophic pyloric stenosis, who had ingested 66 enteric-coated aspirin tablets over an 11-day period. Sixty-one of the tablets were recovered intact from the stomach by emergency gastrostomy [Harris, 1973].

A change in the rate of gastric emptying is not a disease in itself, but may be a consequence of several diseases. Factors that influence gastric emptying rate are listed in Table 2 [Nimmo, 1976].

Drugs, the absorption of which is influenced by altered gastric emptying, are listed in Table 3 [Nimmo, 1976]. Rapid intestinal transit owing to diarrhea may inhibit drug absorption. This would present a problem for slow-release and enteric-coated formulations, and has been implicated in reduced absorption of sulfisoxazole and delayed absorption of aspirin [Jussila et al., 1970]. Pregnancy has

Table 2 Factors That Influence the Rate of Gastric Emptying

	Gastric-emptying rate	
Pathological factors	Increased	Decreased
Acute abdomen		+
Chronic calculary cholecystitis	+	
Laparotomy		+
Trauma and pain		+
Labor		+
Myocardial infarction		+
Gastric ulcer		+
Duodenal ulcer	+	
Hepatic coma		+
Hypercalcemia		+
Diabetes mellitus		+
Myxedema		+
Malnutrition		+
Migraine		+
Raised intracranial pressure		+
Atrophic gastritis		
Solids		+
Liquids	+	
Pyloric stenosis		+
Gastric volvulus		+
Intestinal obstruction		+
Gastroenterostomy	+	

Source: Nimmo, 1976.

Table 3 Drugs the Absorption of Which is Influenced by Altered Gastric Emptying

Drug	Gastric-emptying rate	Effect
L-Dopa	Decreased	L-Dopa metabolized in stomach
L-Dopa	Increased by metoclopramide or gastrectomy	Increased rate and total absorption
Methyl digoxin	Decreased	Methyl digoxin inactivated in stomach
Penicillin	Decreased	Pencillin inactivated in stomach
Acetaminophen (paracetamol)	Increased by metoclopramide	Increased rate of absorption
	Decreased by propantheline, pyloric stenosis, food, or narcotic analgesics	Decreased rate of absorption
Tetracycline; pivampicillin; alcohol	Increased by metoclopramide	Increased rate of absorption
	Decreased by propantheline or food	Decreased rate of absorption
Lidocaine	Decreased by atropine	Decreased rate of absorption
Phenylbutazone	Decreased by desmethylimipramine	Decreased rate of absorption
p-Aminosalicylic acid	Decreased by diphenhydramine	Decreased rate of absorption
Digoxin tablets	Increased by metoclopramide	Decreased rate of absorption
Digoxin tablets	Decreased by propantheline	Increased rate of absorption
Riboflavin	Decreased by propantheline or food	Delayed absorption but total amount absorbed is increased
Ethionamide	Increased by gastrectomy	Failure of absorption
Phenobarbital	Decreased by food	Failure of hypnotic action in rats
Griseofulvin	Decreased by fatty meal	Absorption enhanced
Amoxicillin; pivampicillin; ampicillin	Decreased in women in labor	Decreased absorption
Mexiletine	Decreased by myocardial infarction and narcotic analgesics	Decreased absorption; failure to attain therapeutic plasma concentrations
Aspirin	Decreased by migraine	Decreased absorption; therapeutic failure

Continued

Table 3 *Continued*

Drug	Gastric-emptying rate	Effect
Furosemide	Decreased by phenytoin	Patient insensitivity
Isoniazid	Decreased by aluminum salts	Delayed absorption
Pentobarbital	Decreased by aluminum-containing antacids	Delayed absorption and failure of hypnotic action in rats
Quinine	Delayed by aluminum hydroxide	Delayed absorption

Source: Nimmo, 1976.

occurred following the use of peroral contraceptives during a bout of diarrhea, as absorption of the drug was reduced [John and Jones, 1975].

In studies on the influence of gastric-emptying time (GET) and small-bowel transit time (SBTT) on bioavailability, GET was modified by use of propantheline and metoclopramide, and SBTT was modified by use of loperamide and metoclopramide. Both shortening and increasing the GET resulted in significant changes in t_{max}, but had no influence on the extent of bioavailability of droxicam [Sanchez et al., 1989]. A prolonging of SBTT by loperamide decreased the rate of absorption of sustained-release theophylline, but not its extent; shortening of the SBTT by metoclopramide had no effect on either the rate or extent of absorption [Bryson et al., 1989].

Diseases of the Stomach

Achlorhydria has been studied for its effect on drug absorption. Its effect on the gastric-emptying rate is uncertain [Pottage et al., 1974], but it influences drug absorption by a direct pH effect. Absorption of aspirin in patients with achlorhydria increased significantly [Pottage et al., 1974]. It is generally expected that increased gastric pH, as in achlorhydria, would inhibit aspirin absorption because more of drug is in the ionized form. It is possible that dissolution, which is rate-limiting for absorption, may be increased in achlorhydric patients.

Diseases of the Small Intestine

Celiac disease, or gluten enteropathy, is an inflammatory condition of the proximal intestine that is characterized by the presence of total or subtotal villous atrophy. This is due to the destruction of numerous villi or microvilli by ingestion of gluten, a viscous protein contained in cereals [Rubin et al., 1962]. Thus, the overall surface area available for absorption is reduced considerably as a result of the destruction of villi and microvilli. Also associated with celiac disease, is a deficiency of enzymes, such as nonspecific esterases. The rate of gastric emptying is increased. Crohn's disease is an inflammatory condition of unknown etiology that is associated primarily with the distal small intestine and proximal large bowel. Both of these diseases are associated with malabsorption syndromes. Factors that affect drug absorption are shown in Table 4 [Parsons, 1977].

There are four different patterns of antibiotic absorption in celiac disease: increased, delayed, reduced, and normal [Parsons and Paddock, 1975; Parsons et al., 1975a; 1976]. The absorption of pivampicillin is reduced. This may be due to enzyme deficiencies of small-gut esterases necessary for the hydrolysis of the inactive to the active drug [Parsons et al., 1975a]. The timing of the peak plasma concentration after peroral administration of lincomycin and amoxicillin is delayed in celiac disease (Fig. 1) [Parsons et al., 1975a]. This may present a problem

Table 4 Abnormalities in Celiac Disease and Crohn's Disease That Can Affect Drug Absorption

Celiac disease		Crohn's disease	
Abnormality	Possible effect	Abnormality	Possible effect
Increased rate stomach emptying	Drugs delivered more rapidly to small intestine	Reduced surface area available for absorption	Malabsorption of drugs the major absorption site of which is at the site of disease
Increased permeability of gut wall	Increased transport of passively absorbed drugs	Thickening of bowel wall	Impaired drug diffusion
Enzyme deficiencies at brush border	Impaired hydrolysis of esterified drugs to their constituents	Bowel flora changed to predominantly anaerobic population	Absorption patterns of drugs active against anaerobes would be important
Altered intestinal drug metabolism	Increased absorption of unchanged drug	Slower intestinal transit rate	Unpredictable patterns of absorption
Steatorrhea	Malabsorption of fatsoluble drugs and vitamins		
Reduced enterohepatic cycling of bile acids	Impaired absorption of drugs that require micelle formation for optimal absorption	Diarrhea	Impaired absorption

Source: Parson, 1977.

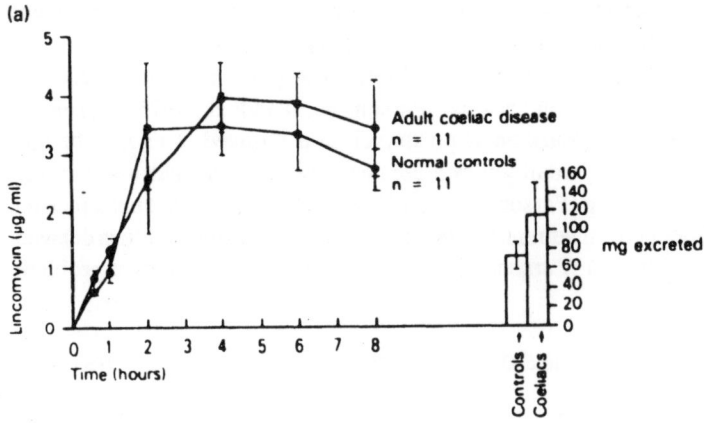

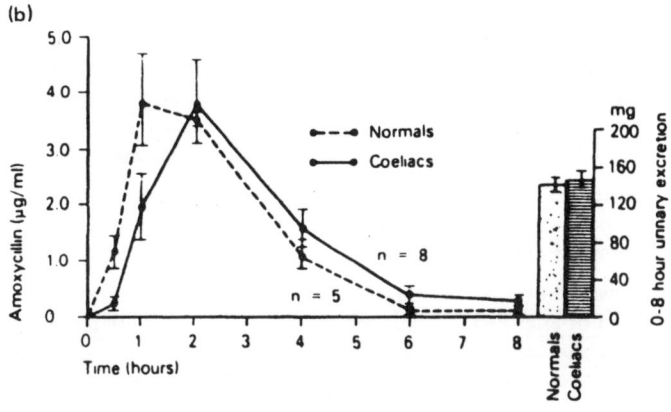

Figure 1 Drugs for which the timing of the peak plasma concentration is delayed in celiac disease. (a) Plasma lincomycin (± SEM) in normal subjects and adult celiac disease after 1 g lincomycin; (b) plasma amoxicillin (± SEM) in normal subjects and adult celiac disease after 250 mg amoxicillin. [From Parsons, 1977.)

because the time at which the organism is most susceptible to the drug and the time of the peak plasma concentration may not coincide.

In Crohn's disease, marked alterations in plasma AUCs have been observed after peroral administration of lincomycin, trimethoprim, and sulfamethoxazole [Parsons and Paddock, 1975]. The plasma C_{max} after administration of these drugs normally occurs at 2 hr, but, in Crohn's disease, it occurs at 4 hr. There is a disproportionate increase in the absorption of sulfamethoxazole from cotrimexazole, compared with trimethoprim, which alters the optimum synergistic trimethoprim/sulfamethoxazole ratio such that there is a relative excess of sulfamethoxazole (Fig. 2).

Plasma levels of propranolol are increased in celiac disease and markedly increased in Crohn's disease (Fig. 3) [Schneider et al., 1976] and may be due to either improved absorption of propranolol or to altered hydrogen ion concentration at the surface of the intestinal epithelium. Propranolol levels after peroral administration are also increased significantly in diseases such as ulcerative colitis, rheumatoid arthritis, and staphylococcal pneumonia. This casts doubt on the foregoing reasoning that the absorption efficiency is increased. Schneider et al. [1979] and Kendall et al. [1979] have identified elevated levels of α_1-acid glycoprotein in plasma in all disease conditions. Propranolol is a basic drug and, similar to most other basic drugs, binds to α_1-acid glycoprotein. Piafsky et al. [1978] have demonstrated a high correlation between levels of α_1-acid glycoprotein and binding of propranolol. Thus, it is likely that in Crohn's disease, in which α_1-acid glycoprotein levels are elevated, the increased binding of propranolol causes a distribution shift that favors drug concentrations in plasma, giving rise to increased circulating drug concentrations.

Drug absorption in patients with intestinal villous atrophy has been studied by Mattila et al. [1973]. For isoniazid, chloramphenicol, salicylates, and cycloserine, no differences were found from normal controls.

Diseases of the Large Intestine

For drugs absorbed throughout the gastrointestinal tract, diseases of the large bowel may be important. Colitis, diarrhea, bowel obstruction, amebic dysentery, and constipation may influence drug absorption, although there have been no reports of substantially altered drug absorption under these conditions [Welling, 1984].

Gastrointestinal Infections

Shigellosis, salmonella gastroenteritis, cholera, staphylococcal food poisoning, and infestation by worms or protozoa can cause diarrhea, which can give rise to drug malabsorption, resulting in decreased bioavailability [Welling, 1984]. The absorption of both ampicillin and nalidixic acid is reduced by diarrhea [Nelson et al., 1972].

Absorption of these two drugs is reduced, but the extent of reduction depends on the severity of the condition. There are either "good" absorbers or "poor" absorbers of these compounds, and the drug concentrations are markedly reduced in poor absorbers, but not in good absorbers. The poor absorbers are usually younger, low-body-weight infants, with severe diarrhea.

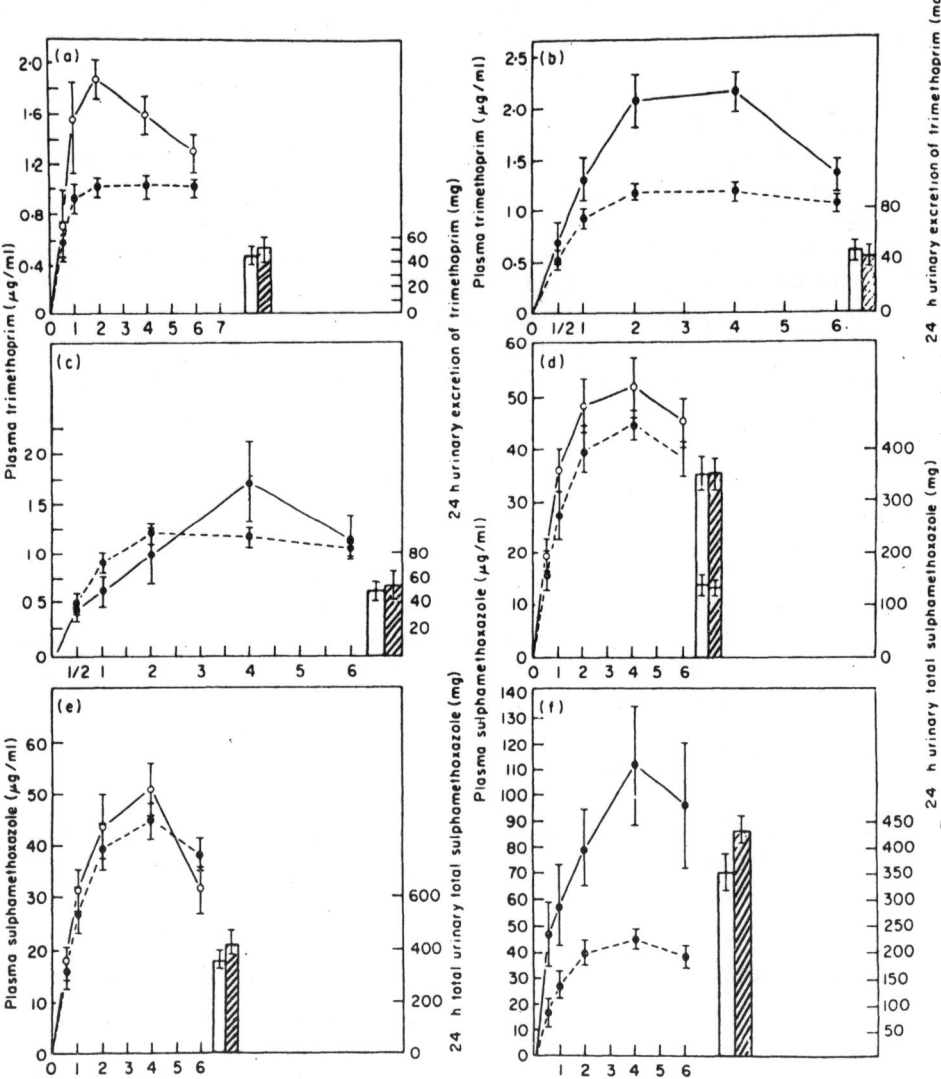

Figure 2 Absorption of trimethoprim and sulfamethoxazole in malabsorption syndromes. *Trimethoprim*: (a) Adult celiac disease [●--●, normals (n=13); ○—○, celiacs (n=11); □ normals; ▨ celiacs]. (b) Small-bowel diverticulosis [●--●, normals (n=14); ○—○, diverticulosis (n=8); □ normals; ▨, diverticulosis]. (c) Crohn's disease [●--●, normals (n=14); ○—○, Crohn's (n=10); □ normals; ▨ Crohn's]. *Sulfamethoxazole*: (d) Adult celiac disease [●--●, normals (n=14); ○—○, celiacs (n=15); □ normals; ▨ celiacs]. (e) Small-bowel diverticulosis [●--●, normals (n=14); ○—○, diverticulosis (n=8); □ normals; ▨ diverticulosis]. (f) Crohn's disease [●—● normals (n=14); ●—● Crohn's (n=10); □ normals; ▨ Crohn's]. (From Parsons and Paddock, 1975.)

The activity of sulfasalazine in treatment of Crohn's disease is dependent on bacterial microflora in the colon [Das and Dubin, 1976]. Some of the drug is absorbed intact, whereas most is cleaved by the bacteria to release the active moiety 5-aminosalicylate.

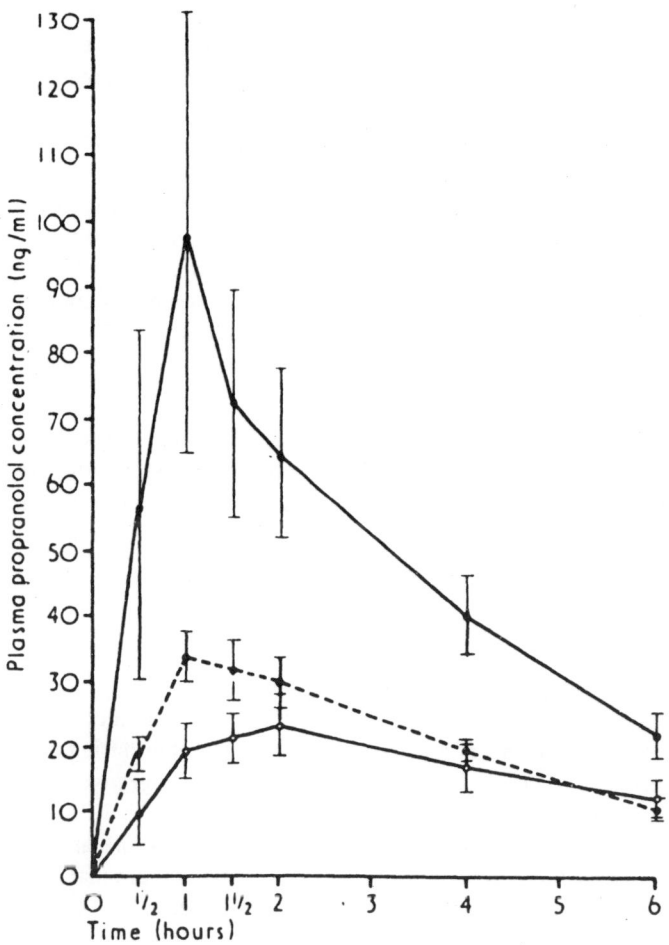

Figure 3 Mean plasma propranolol concentrations (± SEM) in controls (o—o), treated patients with celiac disease (•---•), and patients with Crohn's disease (•—•) after a 40-mg peroral dose. (From Schneider et al., 1976.)

Gastrointestinal Surgery

Partial removal of the stomach and connection of the remaining gaster to the duodenum [Bilroth I] or the jejunum [Bilroth II] may result in dumping syndrome (loss of reservoir function) and, particularly after Bilroth II which creates a blind loop, results in bacterial overgrowth and reduced activity of pancreatic enzymes. Gastrectomy may result in osmotic diarrhea and decreased intestinal transit time.

Massive intestinal resection following vascular insult, regional enteritis, jejunoileal bypass for morbid obesity, or ileostomy for distal malignancy are well tolerated up to a 50% resection, if the proximal duodenum and the distal ileum are spared, including the ileocecal valve. In general, absorption by passive diffusion can be reduced by massive resection owing to concomitant decrease in mucosal surface area.

Massive resection of the small intestine may deprive the bowel of both activity of mucosal enzymes and of bacterially produced enzymes, which may result in reduction of biotransformation of ester prodrugs to the active moiety, such as erythromycin, chloramphenicol, pivampicillin, steroid, and other esters.

Sulfasalazine is ineffective in patients with Crohn's diseases who have a relapse after colonic resection, but it is effective in patients with intact colon [Anthonisen et al., 1974]. This may be due to bacterial loss with resection.

Interactions with Other Drugs

Drugs given for treatment of a certain disease may interact with other drugs, often given for different, unrelated diseases. Such interactions are numerous, but are related only indirectly to the topic discussed here. The reader is referred to the literature, such as a compilation of drug interactions with antacids in humans, or drug interactions with cimetidine [Ritschel, 1984].

Cardiovascular Diseases

Cardiac failure is that pathophysiological state in which an abnormality of cardiac function is responsible for the failure of the heart to pump blood at a rate in accordance with the requirements of metabolizing tissues at rest or during normal activity. The spectrum of cardiac failure ranges from mild congestive heart failure to cardiogenic shock [Benowitz and Meister, 1976].

Most drugs taken on a long-term basis by patients with heart failure are administered perorally. There are several consequences of cardiac failure that may impair the rate and extent of absorption of peroral drugs [Benet et al., 1976].

Pathological changes of intestinal wall (i.e., edema of the bowel)
Decreased splanchnic blood flow
Delayed gastric emptying
Changes in gastrointestinal pH

Changes in gastrointestinal secretions
Change in bacterial flora of the gut

Cardiac failure could be either a forward failure, characterized by insufficient arterial blood supply to vital organs, or a backward failure owing to insufficient venous drainage from dependent organs. Congestive heart failure is due to stasis and edema in dependent areas.

A reduced blood flow from decrease in cardiac output or sympathetically mentioned vasoconstrictors reduces the rate of drug absorption [Benowitz, 1984].

As a consequence of sympathetic nervous stimulation, blood flow is redistributed so that higher fractions of cardiac output go to the brain and heart, and smaller fractions go to the kidney, skin, and splanchnic tissues [Benowitz and Meister, 1976]. Alterations of the autonomic nervous system (increased sympathetic and decreased parasympathetic activity) or tissue hypoperfusion could reduce gastrointestinal motility and increase transit time, thereby resulting in delayed peroral absorption and a decrease or increase in bioavailability, depending on the drug [Benowitz, 1984].

Edema of the intestinal wall leads to malabsorption of fat in patients with congestive heart failure [Berkowitz et al., 1963]. Mucosal edema might reduce epithelial permeability, thereby affecting drug absorption.

Reduced mesenteric and intestinal villus blood flow is associated with cardiac failure [Higgins et al., 1974]. For drugs that are highly permeable to the intestinal mucosa, reduced villus blood flow could delay diffusion and the rate of absorption. Thus, gastrointestinal blood flow may be the rate-limiting step in the absorption of drugs.

Fick's law, as specifically applied to gastrointestinal absorption, describes the transfer of substances by simple diffusion across a thin membrane [Ther and Winne, 1971].

$$\frac{dX_b}{dt} = P_m A_m (C_g - C_b) \tag{7}$$

where

X_b = the amount of drug in the blood or serosal solution at any time, t
P_m = the permeability coefficient for diffusion between the intestinal lumen and the blood
A_m = the area of membrane available for free diffusion
C_g = concentration of drug in the gut or mucosal solution at any time, t
C_b = concentration of drug in the blood or serosal solution at any time, t

Drugs cross the intestinal epithelium primarily as a function of blood flow. If there were no blood flow, then the concentration in the blood, C_b, would rapidly approach C_g, and net transfer of drug across the intestine would cease, as illustrated in Eq. (7). Therefore, a decreased flow may diminish the rate of removal of passively absorbed drugs [Ther and Winne, 1971].

Decreased blood flow could possibly interfere with active transport of drugs owing to reduction of the oxygen supply to tissues [Winne, 1975].

Winne and Remischovsky [1970] demonstrated the influence of blood flow on the rate of intestinal absorption of substances from the jejunum of the rat. Absorption of highly permeable substances, such as tritiated water, is very sensitive to blood flow, whereas the absorption rate of substances with low epithelial permeability, such as ribitol, are unaffected by changes in intestinal blood flow.

In patients with acute myocardial infarction, intestinal absorption of procainamide is markedly delayed [Koch-Weser and Klein, 1971]. Procainamide may not appear in the serum for 2 hr after administration, and peak concentrations may not be reached until 5 hr later. Sometimes patients absorb less than 50% of the peroral dose and reach therapeutic plasma concentrations only when the peroral dose is greatly increased.

A difference in plasma AUCs after peroral administration of aprindine to normal subjects and to patients with acute myocardial infarction was found by Hagemeijer [1975]. Despite high initial peroral doses, absorption of aprindine was so slow that more than half the patients failed to achieve effective plasma levels during the first 12 hr of treatment. The threshold for therapeutic efficacy is a blood concentration exceeding 0.70 μg/mL. In normal healthy volunteers, therapeutic levels were observed within 2 hr of peroral administration of aprindine. Possible reasons for this finding are that (1) upper gastrointestinal upsets are extremely common in acute myocardial infarction; (2) absorption may be markedly delayed in the presence of congestive heart failure; and (3) redistribution of blood flow from the gastrointestinal tract may interfere with uptake.

Hepatic drug-metabolizing activity may be reduced in patients with cardiac failure, which not only alters systemic clearance, but also, by reducing first-pass metabolism, could increase bioavailability of drugs with high hepatic extraction ratios [Benowitz, 1984]. Baughman et al. [1980] found that the blood AUC, the peak plasma prazosin concentration, and the terminal $t_{1/2}$ for peroral prazosin are substantially greater in patients with congestive heart failure than in normal subjects (Fig. 4). Possible explanations max include: (1) a reduction in hepatic blood flow, (2) altered gastrointestinal absorption of the drug, and (3) diminished intrinsic hepatic metabolic activity. Such an increase in bioavailability of prazosin may result in orthostatic hypotension and other adverse effects.

Examples of drugs the absorption of which is altered in cardiac failure are procainamide, quinidine, digoxin, and diuretics.

Procainamide is 85% absorbed in healthy subjects, but it is erratically and slowly absorbed in patients with acute myocardial infarction [Koch-Weser, 1971]. In fasting normal subjects, procainamide is rapidly absorbed from the gastrointestinal tract. Peak serum concentrations are achieved within 1 hr and absorption

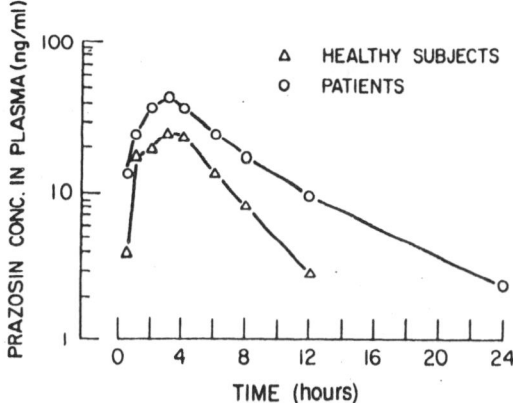

Figure 4 Prazosin concentration in plasma following peroral administration of 5 mg to nine individuals during congestive heart failure (open circles) and to five healthy control subjects (open triangles). Average values of each sampling time are shown. (From Baugham et al., 1980.)

is complete. However, in patients with myocardial infarction, intestinal absorption is markedly delayed and erratic. No detectable amount of procainamide may appear in blood for 2 hr after ingestion, and peak concentrations may not be reached until the third hour.

The time to peak drug concentration following peroral administration of quinidine to patients with congestive heart failure shifts to the right of that seen in normal subjects. Blood levels in these patients are higher than those seen for normal subjects at 4, 6, and 24 hr. The time to peak would shift to the right as a result of a decreased drug elimination rate or a decreased absorption rate. Crouthamel [1975] has reported elimination $t_{1/2}$ of 6.5 and 6.7 hr in normal persons and in patients with heart failure, respectively. Thus, the change in peak time may be attributed to a decreased rate of absorption in patients with heart failure, and it can be concluded that congestive heart failure reduces the rate and amount of quinidine absorption after peroral dosage.

Benet et al. [1976] reviewed the absorption of digoxin after peroral dosing. Postabsorptive digoxin levels in patients with congestive heart failure and, later, after congestive failure had disappeared, have been measured. Figure 5 shows the results obtained in one subject during congestive heart failure. There is a very slow increase in serum digoxin levels until a peak value is reached at 3 hr. However, in the same patients, given an identical dose of digoxin after congestive heart failure had cleared, an immediate marked increase in digoxin levels is

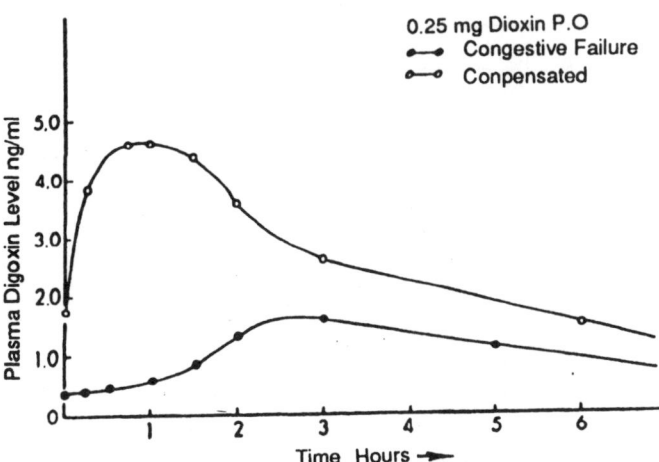

Figure 5 Serum digoxin levels achieved during and after clearing of congestive failure in an 85-lb female patient. (From Oliver et al., 1973, through Benet, 1976.)

found. This study suggests delayed absorption, but no information about the absorption was available. In contrast, another study reviewed by Benet et al. [1976] reported no difference in digoxin absorption, elimination rate constants, or cumulative 5-day urinary excretion after peroral administration of tritiated digoxin solution in seven patients during heart failure and after recompensation. Because the drug was not injected intravenously, absolute bioavailability and total clearance could not be determined. A study by Korhonen et al. [1979] demonstrated reduced absorption rate with lower C_{max} of diogxin after ingestion of tablets in patients with myocardial infarction, when compared with controls. The bioavailability, estimated from the AUC at 24 hr, was unaffected by myocardial infarction and cardiac failure. It appears, given the aforementioned studies, that digoxin absorption is not reduced by cardiac failure to the extent that higher-than-usual doses should be administered to achieve (or maintain) therapeutic concentrations.

Studies on furosemide in patients with congestive heart failure by Benet et al. [1976], Greither et al. [1976] and Kelly et al. [1974] suggest unchanged volume of distribution, clearance, and bioavailability. Studies on the converting enzyme inhibitor, enalapril, in patients with congestive heart failure did not show any significant differences in mean absorption, hydrolysis, bioavailability, urinary recovery, or FPE, although t_{max} was prolonged and FPE was reduced [Dickstein, 1986].

Hepatic Disease

The influence of hepatic disease on bioavailability of drugs may be highly variable and generally unpredictable. Depending on the stage and progress of the specific disease, the drug, and the individual patient, bioavailability may be increased, decreased, or unchanged.

In terms of drug absorption and disposition, the liver occupies a unique position, both functionally and anatomically. It is positioned between the systemic circulation and the vasculature that drains the absorptive areas of the gastrointestinal tract. Therefore, virtually all the blood perfusing the areas of the gastrointestinal tract, from which perorally administered drugs are absorbed, passes into the portal vein and through the liver before entering the general systemic circulation. For drugs that are slowly cleared by the liver, the position of the liver between the portal and general systemic circulations is of minimal importance; the availability of a drug is not altered appreciably if it is poorly extracted by the liver [Williams and Benet, 1980]. For drugs that are highly extracted by the liver, the position of the liver relative to drug absorption is crucial, and entry into the systemic circulation may be negligible for such drugs; therefore, they are subject to extensive first-pass metabolism following peroral administration.

In liver disease, there is a portosystemic shunting of blood; blood is shunted past functioning hepatocytes, resulting in a decrease or absence of first-pass metabolism [Williams and Benet, 1980]. The degree of shunting varies widely in individuals with acute and chronic hepatic disease. It has been estimated that as much as 60% of portal venous blood flow may be directed to the systeic circulation in severe liver disease [Groszmann et al., 1972]. In addition, in chronic liver disease, the drug-metabolizing capacity of the liver is reduced because of decreased microsomal enzyme content or activity [Homeida et al., 1978]. Thus, impairment of drug-metabolizing enzyme systems might account for decreased first-pass metabolism.

Minor alterations in the ability of the liver to extract a drug can have a major influence on the bioavailability of that drug because of the relationship between the extraction ratio (ER) and the fraction of a drug (F) that traverses the liver (F = 1−ER) [Wilkinson and Branch, 1984]. A small reduction in the extraction ratio for a highly extracted drug may double the fraction of drug available from the gastrointestinal tract. Clinical investigations of highly extracted drugs have shown increased bioavailability in patients with liver disease.

Neal et al. [1979] examined the effect of moderate cirrhosis on the bioavailability of three model analgesic compounds (meperidine, pentazocine, and salicylamide) with substantial first-pass metabolism, in eight cirrhotic patients and four aged-matched healthy controls. There was a 46% decrease in clearance of pentazocine and a 278% increase in bioavailability. The corresponding figures for meperidine were 36% and 81%. This study demonstrated that drugs with the highest hepatic clearances will have the largest relative increase in bioavailability in cirrhotic patients because of portosystemic shunting. These changes have a synergistic effect on the total AUC because both the amount of unchanged drug reaching the systemic circulation and duration of time over which drug remains in the body are increased.

When given peroral verapamil, peak plasma concentrations were higher and occurred earlier in cirrhotic patients, compared with normal subjects (Fig. 6) [Smogyi et al., 1981]. Bioavailability was greatly increased to a mean of 53%, more than double that of 22% in normal subjects. This was due to development of intra- and extrahepatic shunts in cirrhotic patients, as well as to a reduced ability of the liver to clear the drug. An unusual finding in this study was a shortening of the plasma t_{max}. Whereas in normal subjects, t_{max} occurred at approximately 1 hr after dosing, in cirrhotic patients, t_{max} was reduced to 30 min. This is attributed to the development of intra- and extrahepatic shunts in these patients,

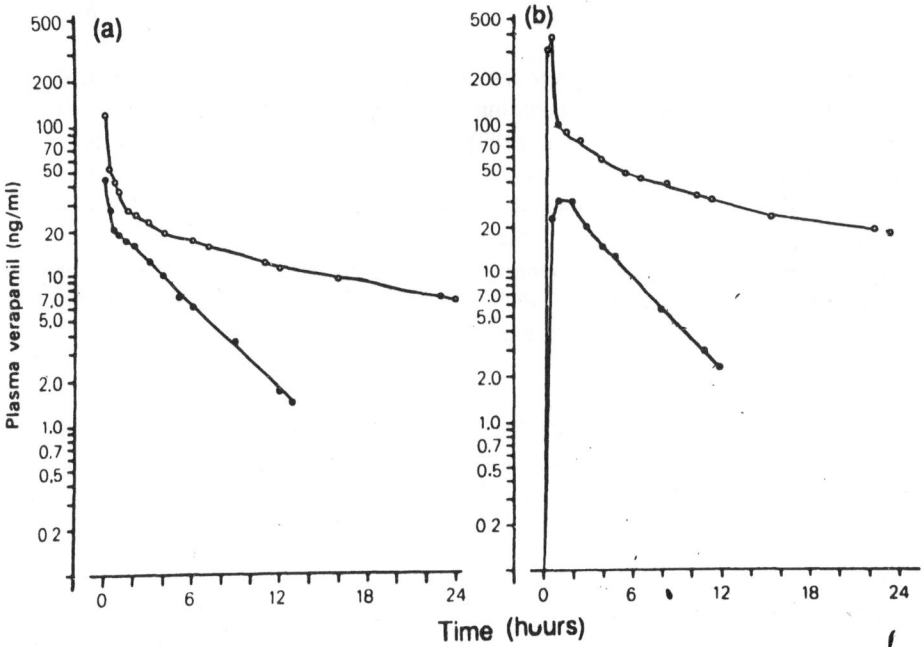

Figure 6 Plasma concentrations of verapamil as a function of time following intravenous administration of 10 mg verapamil (a) and peroral administration (b) of 40 mg d_3-verapamil in a patient with liver cirrhosis (○) and 80 mg d_3-verapamil in a normal subject (●). (From Somogyi et al., 1981.)

whereas in normal subjects, all the drug must first be taken up by the liver and then released into the venous circulation. In cirrhosis, therefore, a larger-than-expected fraction of the absorbed dose is immediately presented to the general systemic circulation.

The bioavailability of clormethiazole (chlormethiazole) has been increased tenfold in patients with advanced cirrhosis of the liver [Pentikainen et al., 1978]. Bioàvailability was calculated as the ratio of AUCs after peroral and intravenous administration of clormethiazole. Increased bioavailability was due to decreased first-pass metabolism of clormethiazole by the cirrhotic liver.

The effect of chronic liver disease on the extent of first-pass metabolism of labetalol was studied by Homeida et al. [1978]. The plasma AUC profile was approximately three times greater in patients than in controls after peroral administration (Fig. 7). Bioavailability of labetalol in patients was about twice that of the controls.

The $t_{1/2}$, AUC, and V_d of nitrendipine were significantly increased after IV administration in patients with cirrhosis or with chronic or acute hepatitis, when compared with controls. There were no significant differences in protein binding between patients and normal subjects. Following PO administration, the absolute bioavailability of nitrendipine was increased from 0.4 in normal persons to 0.54 in cirrhotic patients and to 0.48 in chronic hepatitis patients. No change in F was observed in patients with acute hepatitis [Dylewicz et al., 1987].

The clinical relevance of changes in bioavailability owing to hepatic disease is clear. If drugs normally undergo extensive first-pass metabolism, large increases in bioavailability and decreases in clearance are expected. When such drugs are administered perorally, the increase in bioavailability and decrease in clearance will have a multiplicative effect on the total blood AUC profile. This means that a 50% decrease in clearance and fourfold increase in bioavailability results in an eightfold increase in the AUC $(0 \rightarrow \infty)$ in cirrhotic subjects.

Renal Diseases

Renal failure, manifested as impaired capacity to clear material from the circulation, can result from a variety of pathological conditions. If impairment of renal function is of rapid onset and of relatively short duration, then the renal failure is described as acute [Guisti, 1975]. The primary cause of this condition may be prerenal (i.e., acute congestive heart failure, or shock), intrarenal (i.e., acute tubular necrosis), or postrenal (i.e., hypercalcemia). Acute renal failure is completely reversible, although it may take from 6 to 12 months. Chronic renal disease is caused by intrinsic renal disease and is characterized by slow, progressive development. This is generally irreversible.

Renal disease is of particular concern in older patients who may require a variety

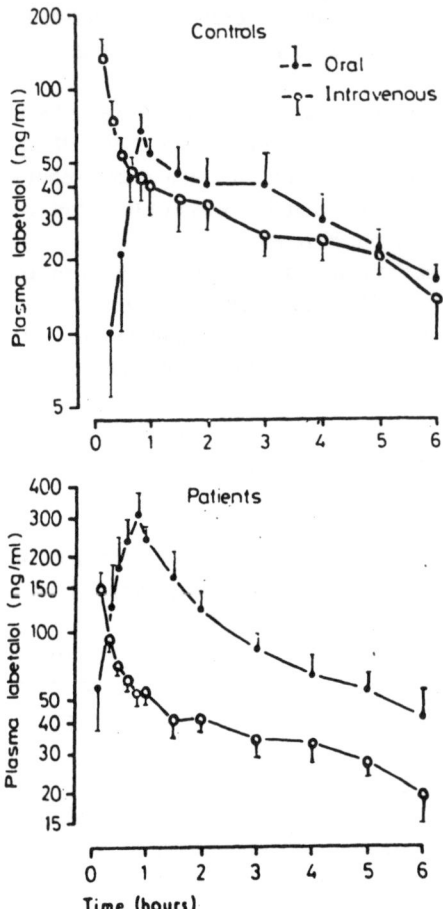

Figure 7 Mean (± SEM) labetalol concentrations after peroral and intravenous administration in seven normal healthy subjects and ten patients with chronic liver disease. (From Homeida et al., 1981.)

of medications, both for their basic renal condition and for variety of associated conditions [Welling and Craig, 1976].

Because of the physiological and biochemical changes associated with uremia, patients with renal failure may respond to a given dose of a drug differently from patients with normal renal function. It has been observed that there is an increased frequency of adverse drug reactions in patients with renal failure. The causes for drug toxicity in these patients may arise from either increased sensitivity to the drug because of uremia-induced alterations in target organs or from increased plasma drug concentrations owing to altered pharmacokinetics of the drug.

Renal failure, manifested as impaired capacity to clear material from the circulation, can result from several different pathological conditions. In terms of drug absorption and bioavailability, adequate information is lacking for patients with renal failure. Factors, such as gastrointestinal disturbance, altered gastric pH, and antacid administration, could affect drug bioavailability in the uremic patient [Gambertoglio, 1984]. Gastrointestinal disturbances of renal failure, such as nausea, vomiting, diarrhea, and edematous changes of the gastrointestinal tract, may alter drug bioavailability [Welling, 1984]. Patients with renal failure may also have uremic gastritis, colitis, and pancreatitis, which also may affect bioavailability.

As a result of elevated blood urea concentrations, uremic patients have elevated salivary urea levels that, when acted on by gastric ureases, cause an increase in gastric ammonia. This buffers the hydrochloric acid in the stomach, thereby increasing gastric pH. Consequently, drugs the absorption of which is favored in an acidic medium may have impaired absorption [Gambertoglio, 1984].

Drug metabolism may be impaired in the uremic patient, and this may result in changes in the bioavailability in the uremic patient, and this may result in changes in the bioavailability of drugs that are extensively metabolized during their first pass through the liver following peroral administration [Gibaldi et al., 1971].

The bioavailability of peroral propranolol in patients with chronic renal failure was significantly increased in comparison with patients undergoing regular dialysis treatment, and the dialysis patients showed an increase in bioavailability compared with healthy volunteers, as shown by the blood level curves in Figure 8 [Bianchetti et al., 1976]. The observed difference between the control group and the patients with renal failure was explained in terms of a reduced hepatic extraction in the terminal stages of uremia.

Propoxyphene, an analgesic, is subject to extensive first-pass metabolism upon PO administration. Maximum propoxyphene concentrations were much higher (177 ± 16 versus 81 ± 35 ng/mL), and the AUCs over 12 hr were much larger (4310 ± 1520 versus 2250 ± 1050 ng · hr^{-1} · mL^{-1}) in renal failure patients than in normal subjects [Gibson et al., 1980]. These differences were believed to be a result of decreased first-pass metabolism of propoxyphene and decreased elimination of norpropoxyphene (pharmacologically active metabolite) in patients with renal failure.

The biolavailability of digoxin in patients with renal failure was studied by Ohnhaus et al. [1979]. Following PO administration of 0.5 mg digoxin to patients with severe chronic renal failure, maximal plasma concentrations were significantly higher (4.1 ± 1.0 ng/mL) and were reached at 2 hrs, compared

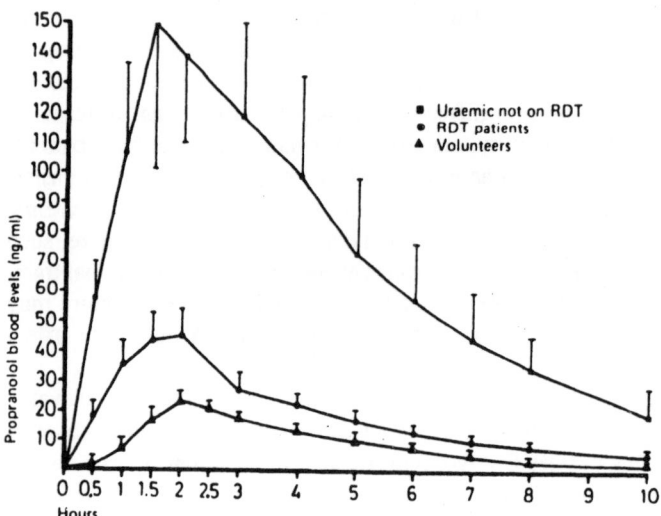

Figure 8 Average (± SEM) blood levels after a single peroral dose of 40 mg propranolol to healthy volunteers (lower curve), uremic patients not receiving dialysis treatment (upper curve), and uremic patients receiving regular dialysis treatment (middle curve). (From Bianchetti et al., 1976.)

with healthy volunteers, in whom the peak level was only 2.3 ± 0.1 ng/mL at 1 hr. Also, patients with renal failure had significantly lower absorption rate constants. The mean was 2.8 ± 0.6 hr^{-1} in volunteers and 0.76 ± 0.3 hr^{-1} in patients. However, determination of absolute bioavailability showed no significant differences between the two groups. The higher maximal plasma levels observed in patients with renal failure was due to a smaller volume of distribution.

Protein Binding

Bioavailability of a drug is minimally affected by alteration in binding to plasma proteins, except when extensive metabolism occurs in the liver or gut wall [Tozer, 1984]. Drugs undergoing first-pass clearance have low systemic availabilities because of the loss on first-pass through these organs. However, binding to plasma proteins impedes removal of drug from the blood on first-pass. Increased binding results in decreased extraction, thereby producing a large increase in the amount of drug available. Increased bioavailability may be accompanied by a decrease in volume of distribution and elimination half-life. The therapeutic consequences are minor because the increased availability after PO administration may be accompanied by decreased distribution and increased elimination rate constant for the drug.

Not only the absolute amount of protein in blood, but also possible structural changes that accompany disease must be considered.

Schneider et al. [1976] compared plasma concentrations of propranolol in patients with Crohn's disease with those in normal subjects after a single 40-mg peroral dose (see Fig. 3). The increased peak concentration in the diseased patients suggests increased bioavailability. The increased AUC, is due to either decreased volume of distribution or clearance. Elevated plasma levels are probably due to elevated levels of α_1-acid glycoprotein to which propranolol binds.

Pulmonary Diseases

The major pulmonary diseases that may influence drug bioavailability are

Chronic obstructive pulmonary disease (COPD)
Asthma
Bronchiectasis and cystic fibrosis
Acute respiratory failure
Cor pulmonale

In COPD, mucous gland hyperplasia, mucosal edema, and inflammation cause an airway narrowing. Thus, only with difficulty, may inhaled drugs reach alveoli. The situation is similar in asthma, in which additionally thickening of the basement membrane may hinder absorption. Patients with cystic fibrosis have many pathophysiological and biochemical abnormalities that may lead to altered drug absorption and disposition, including exocrine pancreatic insufficiency, hypoalbuminemia, cirrhosis, cor pulmonale, and altered turnover of bile salts; PO drug absorption may be decreased. Acute respiratory failure is characterized by an insult to the capillary epithelium, capillary congestion, intestitinal edema, and severe hypoxia. In cor pulmonale a structural and functional alteration of the right ventricle results, leading to hypoxia and acidosis.

For PO sulfamethazine, an acidic drug, decreased bioavailability was found in addition to an increased V_d secondary to decrease in binding [DuSouich et al., 1983]. In patients with COPD, a lower bioavailability was noted for furosemide, compared with healthy subjects. This was ascribed to enhanced glucuronidation and incomplete absorption. The F was 41.3% in patients versus 50–60% in healthy subjects [Ogata et al., 1985].

The absolute bioavailability of cloxacillin in cystic fibrosis was not significantly different from that in controls, albeit more variable. Renal clearance, and particularly the nonrenal clearance ($p < 0.07$), were increased [Spino et al., 1984].

In a study by Cohen et al. [1975], in newborns with respiratory distress, delayed and lower peaks of penicillin in plasma were obtained. Since renal and hepatic clearances are unlikely to be increased, this phenomenon would signify a decrease in absorption.

This fact is further confirmed by a study by DuSouich and Erill [1978]. They studied urinary elimination patterns of procainamide and metabolites in 20 subjects with chronic respiratory disease. A significant decrease in the total amount of drug and metabolite excreted was found in patients with respiratory failure, compared with the control group of healthy volunteers. These results suggest the possibility of delayed or incomplete absorption, since renal function in the two groups was comparable.

Neurological Diseases

Various neurological disorders influence the bioavailability of drugs, in terms of gastric emptying and absorption.

Migraine produces a significant delay in gastric emptying [Volans, 1974]. After 900 mg of effervescent aspirin, mean plasma salicylate levels at 30 min in 35 patients during an attack of migraine was only 4.97 ± 0.52 mg/100 mL, compared with a value of 7.11 ± 0.58 mg/100 mL ($\pm$ SE) in 14 patient controls. Impairment of absorption seemed to correlate with the severity of the headache and the gastrointestinal symptoms at the time of treatment. Delayed gastric emptying has been associated with brain tumor causing raised intracranial pressure [Rimmer, 1966].

Malabsorption of levodopa occurs in some patients with parkinsonism [Rivera-Calimli et al., 1970]. This is due to delayed gastric emptying, which increases the exposure of levodopa to destruction by gastric decarboxylase, thereby reducing its plasma concentration. This can lead to therapeutic failure.

Rheumatoid Arthritis

In patients with active rheumatoid arthritis, a chronic inflammatory disorder, hypoalbuminemia is present. Highly protein-bound drugs may therefore demonstrate differences in disposition. The AUC of total naproxen during a dosing interval at steady state was significantly smaller in patients than in volunteers. The unbound naproxen AUC was larger in these patients. The higher unbound naproxen concentrations in patients were accompanied by a 40% increase in Cl/F and a 60% increase in V_d/F [Van den Duwehand et al., 1987].

Hypothermia and Hyperthermia

Significant changes in both metabolism and renal function are observed in hypothermia. In rats, about a 40% reduction in the disappearance rate of uracil and L-dopa from the small intestine was observed with a 10°C reduction in rectal temperature. This was, at least partially, explained by a decrease of water efflux [Stavchansky and Tung, 1987]. In a study on the influence of temperature on morphine disposition in dogs, hypothermia (30°C) resulted in significantly higher plasma and cerebrospinal levels, increased $t_{1/2}$ and mean residence time, and decreased V_d and Cl. Hyperthermia did not result in significant changes [Bansihath et al., 1988].

In a human study with PO pranoprofen in febrile (38.3°C) and afebrile (36.3°C) subjects, the $t_{1/2}$ was significantly prolonged, and the AUC increased during fever. The authors concluded that the clearance was reduced during fever [Fujimura et al., 1989].

Radiopharmaceuticals in Diagnosis

Radiopharmaceuticals are used primarily in diagnostic procedures during which they are followed and located by detection of the gamma radiation emitted by the attached radionuclide. Most radiopharmaceuticals are freshly prepared just before administration from [^{99m}Tc]pertechnetate. Other radiopharmaceuticals are sodium [^{131}I]iodide, sodium [^{123}I]iodide, [^{201}Tl]thallium chloride, [^{67}Ga]gallium citrate, [^{133}Xe]xenon, [^{85}Kr]krypton, and several ^{99m}Tc-labeled compounds. A review has been published on radiopharmaceuticals and the alterations of their distribution in the body by other drugs and diseases [Shaw, 1985].

Chronic liver disease and nephrosis may cause increased ^{123}I or ^{131}I uptake in thyroid function studies. Uptake of ^{201}Tl in cardiac imaging is affected by chronic thyroiditis, cold thyroid nodule, excess endogenous thyroid-stimulating hormone, Graves disease, Hashimoto's disease, and hyperthyroidism. Uptake of ^{99m}Tc in myocardial studies is disturbed by amyloidosis, hyperphosphatemia, myocardial sarcoidosis, angina pectoris, gynecomastia, lactation, breast cancer, cardiomyopathy, and massive liver necrosis. Unexpected organ uptake of ^{99m}Tc in bone imaging is found in amyloidosis, carcinomas, hypercalcemia, leukemia and sickle cell disease, and repeated blood transfusions decrease skeletal uptake. Diseases affecting ^{99m}Tc liver-spleen studies are biliary cirrhosis, Crohn's disease, liver cirrhosis, infectious mononucleosis, and congestive heart failure. Conditions that may cause false-positive images with ^{99m}Tc in the detection of Meckel's diverticulum are abscess secondary to perforation of small bowel, appendicitis, Barrett's esophagus, Crohn's disease, ectopic gastric mucosa, hemangioma, intestinal lymphosarcoma, intestinal obstruction, lymphoma, peptic ulcer, regional enteritis, ulcerative colitis, and volvulus. Renal imaging with ^{99m}Tc may be affected by soft tissue sarcoma, bleeding gastric ulcer, cholecystitis, diabetic nephropathy, acid-base imbalance, and metastatic adenocarcinoma of the prostate.

PAIN, ANESTHESIA, AND SURGERY

Pain per se is a symptom, rather than a distinct disease entity. Consequently, pain will not exert any changes in bioavailability in addition to those exerted by the specific disease process. All of the peroral analgesic medications for both acute and chronic pain management will be affected by gastrointestinal, hepatic, and renal disease, as previously described.

Almost all drugs administered for surgical anesthesia are given intravenously. On accasion, however, transcutaneous or intramuscular routes are employed. The effect of anesthesia on the bioavailability of these drugs is limited to effects on the rate, rather than on the extent, of absorption. For example, intraoperative reductions or enhancements in blood flow will result in decreases or increases in the rate of absorption. The effects of the inhalation anesthetic agents themselves are limited to reversible decreases in the rates of oxidative drug metabolism by the hepatic mixed function oxidase system. For example, halothane reversibly inhibits the oxidative metabolism of bupivacaine, an aminoamide local anesthetic [Denson et al., 1982]. Such inhibition will result in increases in the serum AUC profile during the course of the anesthetic. This would be of greatest importance for drugs that have low hepatic extraction ratios, such as benzodiazepines. Inhalation anesthetics would be expected to produce elevated serum concentrations of benzodiazepines given perorally as a preoperative medication. These drugs could produce signs of toxicity secondary to accumulation from this reduction in metabolic rate.

Local anesthetics that are used for major surgery are usually administered by the epidural or subarachnoid routes. Tucker and Mather [1975; 1979] demonstrated that local anesthetic absorption was a biphasic and complete process, by comparing intravenous and epidural serum AUCs for lidocaine, etidocaine, and bupivacaine. Studies, using a stable isotope technique in humans, confirmed these results [Burm et al., 1987]. Studies have now demonstrated complete absorption for epidural bupivacaine and lidocaine in humans [Burm et al., 1988] and bupivacaine lidocaine, and ropivacaine in monkeys [Thompson et al., 1986; Denson et al., 1988; Katz et al., 1988]. Similar results have now been reported following subarachnoid administration for lidocaine and bupivacaine in humans [Burm et al., 1988] and lidocaine in monkeys [Denson et al., 1981; 1988]. The use of epidural infusions of local anesthetics, for the management of postoperative pain, reduce gastric-emptying time and, therefore, would be expected to influence bioavailability, as previously described.

ENANTIOSELECTIVE BIOAVAILABILITY

Recent advances in analytical methods have permitted separation and quantitation of several racemic mixtures of commonly prescribed drugs into their respective enantiomeric isomers [Nation, 1988]. Enantiospecific differences in pharmacokinetics have been the subject of two excellent reviews [Tucker and Lennard, 1990; Jamali et al., 1989]. *Enantiomer* is a synonym for *stereoisomer*, which is defined as an isomer that is not superimposable on its mirror image. This characteristic imparts the property of optical activity. Briefly, one enantiomer will rotate polarized light in one direction, whereas the other enantiomer will rotate polarized light in the opposite direction. This rotation can be dextrorotatory (*D* or *R*) or levorotatogry (*L* or *S*). In addition, each enantiomer will absorb polarized light in either a positive (+) or negative (−) direction. Although several common drugs are optically active, they are often administered as the *racemate* (combination of the two enantiomers). It should not be surprising that enantioselectivity of drug action is important, since the body exhibits a predominant entioselectivity for endogenous compounds. The preferred enantiomer is usually the levorotatory or L enantiomer.

Since absorption of many drugs is dependent on passive diffusion, enantioselective differences would not be expected. Few drugs exhibit enantioselective differences in membrane permeability. An exception is terbutaline. It has been proposed that the (−) enantiomer has a greater membrane permeability, resulting in a twofold increase in peroral availability over the (+) enantiomer [Borgstrom et al., 1989]. When a active transport process is important to the absorption profile, enantioselective differences can be anticipated. For example, absorption of dopa from the rat intestine favors the L enantiomer [Williams and Lee, 1985]. Enantioselective differences in bioavailability may depend on whether the drug is administered briefly or long-term. For example, the bioavailability of (−)-propranolol markedly increases with long-term administration [Bai et al., 1983].

In addition to the absorption profile, enantioselective differences in serum protein binding and first-pass metabolism are important determinants of bioavailability. The importance of enantioselective differences in protein binding has been the subject of a recent review [Muller, 1988]. For example, the binding of (−)-propranolol to human α_1-acid glycoprotein was similar to that noted for the racemate. In contrast, the (+) form exhibited two distinct binding sites, with binding affinites substantially different from those of the (−) enantiomer [Oravcova et al., 1989]. Such enantioselective differences in plasma protein binding will have overall effects on the bioavailability of each enantiomer, similar to those discussed previously. Enantioselective differences in protein binding could also lead to enantioselective differences in clearance. Without thorough investigation, such changes could lead to an erroneous conclusion that a particular drug exhibits enantioselective differences in bioavailability. The enantioselective differences in binding to plasma proteins may extend to binding with hepatic enzymes responsible for the metabolism of many drugs. Enantioselective metabolism for both phase I and phase II reactions is well documented [Jamali et al., 1989]. In addition, metabolic drug interactions can be enantioselective. For example, cimetidine causes an enantioselective inhibition of the metabolism of *R*-metoprolol, resulting in a reduction in first-pass extraction and a concomitant increase in bioavailability [Toon et al., 1988].

In addition to enantioselective effects within the liver, some drugs can undergo a unidirectional change in conformation. R-Ibuprofen undergoes transformation to the pharmacologically active S enantiomer in the gastrointestinal tract. Delays in gastric emptying should lead to increases in the concentration of the active enantiomer that reaches the systemic circulation. Such processes must be understood before concluding that there are enantioselective differences in bioavailability.

ACKNOWLEDGEMENT

The authors thank R. Panchagnula, J. Kappes, and P. Agrawala for their help in literature search and compilation.

REFERENCES

S. N. Agnihotri, R. A. Clark, S. Cooper, A. O. Iyun, and G. T. Tucker. Chronic pulmonary disease and antipyrine disposition. *Br. J. Clin. Pharmacol.* 5:275–277 (1978).

S. Al-Habet, H. C. Kinsella, H. J. Rogers, and J. R. Trounce. Malabsorption of prednisolone from enteric coated tablets after ileostomy. *Br. Med. J.* 281:843–844 (1980).

P. Anthonisen, F. Barnay, O. Folkenborg, A. Holtz, S. Jarnum, M. Kristensen, P. Riis, A. Walan, and H. Worning. The clinical effect of salaazosulfapyridine in Crohn's disease. A controlled double-blind study. *Scand. J. Gastroenterol.* 9:549–554 (1974).

S. A. Bai, M. J. Wilson, U. K. Walle, and T. Walle. Stereoselective increase in propranolol bioavailability during chronic dosing in the dog. *J. Pharmacol. Exp. Ther.* 227:360–364 (1983).

R. R. Bailey, P. E. Gower, and C. H. Dash. The effect of impairment of renal function and haemodialysis on serum and urine levels of cephalexin. *Postgrad. Med. J.* 46(Suppl.):60–64 (1970).

M. Bansinath, H. Turndorf, and M. M. Puig. Influence of hypo and hyperthermia on disposition of morphine. *J. Clin. Pharmacol.* 28:860–864 (1988).

L. A. Bauer, J. R. Horn, and K. E. Opheim. Variability of indocyanine green pharmacokinetics in healthy adults. *Clin. Pharm.* 8:54–55 (1989).

R. A. Baughman, Jr., S. Arnold, L. Z. Benet, E. T. Lin, K. Chatterjee, and R. L. Williams. Altered prazosin pharmacokinetics in congestive heart failure. *Eur. J. Clin. Pharmacol.* 17:425–428 (1980).

N. D. S. Bax, G. T. Tucker, and H. F. Woods. Lignocaine and indocyanine green kinetics in patients following myocardial infarction. *Br. J. Clin. Pharmacol.* 10:353–361 (1980).

L. Beckman, B. Beerman, M. Groschinsky-Grind, D. Hallberg. Malabsorption of hydrochlorothiazide following intestinal shunt surgery. *Clin. Pharmacokinet.* 4:63–68 (1979).

B. Beerman, K. Hellstrom, and A. Rosen. The gastrointestinal absorption of digoxin in 7 patients with gastric or small intestinal reconstructions. *Acta Med. Scand.* 193:293-297 (1973).

L. Z. Benet. *The Effect of Disease States on Drug Pharmacokinetics.* American Pharmaceutical Association, Washington, D.C. (1976).

L. Z. Benet, A. Greither, and W. Meister. Gastrointestinal absorption of drugs in patients with cardiac failure. In *The Effect of Disease States on Drug Pharmacokinetics* (L. Z. Benet, ed.) American Pharmaceutical Association, Washington, D.C., pp. 33-50 (1976).

L. Z. Benet and N. Massoud. Pharmacokinetics. In *Pharmacokinetic Basis for Drug Treatment* (L. Z. Benet, N. Massoud, and J. G. Gambertoglio, eds.) Raven Press, New York, pp. 1-28 (1984).

N. L. Benowitz. Effects of cardiac disease on pharmacokinetics: Pathophysiologic consideration. In *Pharmacokinetic Basis for Drug Treatment* (L. Z. Benet, N. Massoud, and J. G. Gambertoglio, eds.) Raven Press, New York, pp. 89-103 (1984).

N. L. Benowitz and W. Meister. Pharmacokinetics in patients with cardiac failure. *Clin. Pharmacokinet.* 1:389-405 (1976).

T. Bergan, P. E. M. Bjerke, and O. Fausa. Pharmacokinetics of metranidazole in patients with enteric disease compared to normal volunteers. *Chemotherapy* 27:233-238 (1981).

R. H. Bergstrand, T. Wang, D. M. Roden, G. Arant, W. W. Sulton, L. A. Siddoway, H. Wolfendsen, R. L. Woosley, G. R. Wilkinson, and A.J.J. Wood. Encainide disposition in patients with chronic cirrhosis. *Clin. Pharmacol. Ther.* 40:148-154 (1986).

D. Berkowitz, M. N. Droll, and W. Likoff. Malabsorption as a complication of congestive heart failure. *Am. J. Cardiol.* 11:43-47 (1963).

G. Bianchetti, G. Graziani, D. Brancaccio, and A. Morganti. Pharmacokinetics and effects of propranolol in terminal uraemic patients and in patients undergoing regular dialysis treatment. *Clin. Pharmacokinet.* 1:373-384 (1976).

T. F. Blaschke. Protein binding and kinetics of drug in liver disease. *Clin. Pharmacokinet.* 2:32-44 (1977).

T. F. Blaschke and P. C. Rubin. Hepatic first-pass metabolism in liver disease. *Clin. Pharmacokinet.* 4:423-432 (1979).

A. Bodenham, M. P. Shelly, and G. R. Park. The altered pharmacokinetics and pharmacodynamics of drugs commonly used in critically ill patients. *Clin. Pharmacokinet.* 14:347-373 (1988).

S. W. Boobiş. Alteration of plasma albumin in relation to decreased binding in uremia. *Clin. Pharmacol. Ther.* 22:147-153 (1977).

L. Borgstrom, L. Nyberg, S. Jonsson, C. Lindberg, and J. Paulson. Pharmacokinetic evaluation in man of terbutaline given as separate enantiomers and as the racemate. *Br. J. Clin. Pharmacol.* 27:49-56 (1989).

R. A. Branch, C. M. Herbert, and A. E. Read. Determinants of serum antipyrine half-lives in patients with liver disease. *Gut* 14:569-573 (1973).

R. A. Branch, J. James, and A. E. Read. A study of factors influencing drug disposition in chronic liver disease, using the model drug (+)-propranolol. *Br. J. Clin. Pharmacol.* 3:243-249 (1976).

B. B. Breimer, W. Zilly, and F. Richter. Pharmacokinetics of hexobarbital in acute hepatitis and after apparent recovery. *Clin. Pharmacol. Ther.* 18:433–440 (1975).

N. S. Bricker, P. A. F. Morrin, and S. W. Kine. The pathologic physiology of chronic Bright's disease. *Am. J. Med.* 28:77–98 (1960).

S. M. Bryson, G. J. Cairms, and B. Whiting. Disopyramide pharmacokinetics during recovery from myocardial infarction. *Br. J. Clin. Pharmacol.* 13:412–421 (1982).

J. C. Bryson, G. E. Dubes, M. G. Kirby, W. D. Heizer, and J. R. Powell. Effect of altering small bowel transit time on sustained release theophylline absorption. *J. Clin. Pharmacol.* 29:733–738 (1989).

A. G. L. Burm, J. W. Van Kleef, N. P. E. Vermeulen, G. Olthof, D. D. Breimer, and J. Spierdijk. Pharmacokinetics of lidocaine and bupivacaine following subarachnoid administration in surgical patients: Simultaneous investigation of absorption and disposition kinetics using stable isotopes. *Anesthesiology* 69:584–592 (1988).

A. G. L. Burm, N. P. E. Vermeulen, J. W. Van Kleef, A. G. DeBoer, and J. Spierdijk. Pharmacokinetics of lidocaine and bupivacaine following epidural administration in surgical patients: Simultaneous investigation of absorption and disposition kinetics using stable isotopes. *Clin. Pharmacokinet.* 13:191–203 (1987).

R. A. Chan, E. J. Benner, and P. D. Hoeprich. Gentamicin therapy in renal failure: A nomogram for dosage. *Ann. Intern. Med.* 76:773–778 (1972).

M. D. Cohen, J. A. Raeburn, J. Devine, J. Kirkwood, B. Elliot, F. Cockburn, and J. O. Forfar. Pharmacology of some oral penicillins in the newborn infant. *Arch. Dis. Child.* 50:230–234 (1975).

P. B. Cotton and G. Walker. Ethanol absorption after gastric operations and in the coeliac syndrome. *Postgrad. Med. J.* 49:27–28 (1973).

W. G. Crouthamel. The effect of congestive heart failure on quinidine pharmacokinetics. *Am. Heart J.* 90:335–339 (1975).

W. G. Crouthamel, L. Diamond, L. W. Dittert, and J. T. Doluisio. Drug absorption VII: Influence of mesentric blood flow on intestinal drug absorption in dogs. *J. Pharm. Sci.* 64:661–667 (1975).

J. F. Cumming. The effect of arterial oxygen tension on antipyrine half-time in plasma. *Clin. Pharmacol. Ther.* 19:468–471 (1976).

K. M. Das and R. Dubin. Clinical pharmacokinetics of sulphasalazine. *Clin. Pharmacokinet.* 1:406–425 (1976).

J. A. Davis, J. M. Holt, and B. Mullinger. Absorption of cephalexin in diseased and aged subjects. *J. Antimicrob. Chemother.* (Suppl.):69–70 (1975).

J. A. Davis, J. E. M. Strangeways, and J. M. Holt. Absorption of cephalexin from the gastrointestinal tract in diseased subjects. *Postgrad. Med. J.* 46(Suppl.):16–19 (1970).

D. D. Denson, J. A. Myers, C. Watters, and P. P. Raj. Selective inhibition of the aromatic hydroxylation of bupivacaine by halothane. *Anesthesiology* 57:A242 (1982).

D. D. Denson, W. A. Ritschel, P. A. Turner, D. F. Ohlweiler, and P. O. Bridenbaugh. A comparison of intravenous and subarachnoid lidocaine pharmacokinetics in the rhesus monkey. *Biopharm. Drug Dispos.* 2:367–380 (1981).

D. D. Denson, P. A. Turner, P. O. Bridenbaugh, and G. A. Thompson. CSF pharmacokinetics following intravenous and epidural lidocaine. In *New Aspects in Regional Anesthesia* (H. J. Wust and M. Stanton-Hicks, eds.) Verlag Medizin, Heidelberg, pp. 54–63 (1988).

K. Dickstein. Pharmacokinetics of enalapril in congestive heart failure. *Drugs* 32(Suppl.):40–44 (1986).

K. Dickstein, A. E. Till, T. Aarsland, K. Tjelta, A. M. Abrahamsen, K. Kristianson, H. J. Gomez, H. Gregg, and M. Hichens. The pharmacokinetics of enalapril in hospitalized patients with congestive heart failure. *Br. J. Clin. Pharmacol.* 23:403–410 (1987).

J. E. Doherty, J. J. Kane, J. R. Phillips, and J. S. Adamson. Digitalis in pulmonary heart disease (cor pulmonale). *Drugs* 13:142–151 (1977).

O. DuSouich, R. Amyot, M. Julien, S. Desjardin, J. Latouri, and P. Leblanc. Influence of chronic obstructive lung disease on the disposition of an acidic drug (sulfamethazine). *Arch. Intern. Med.* 143:233–236 (1983).

P. DuSouich and S. Erill. Metabolism of procainamide in patients with chronic heart failure, chronic respiratory failure and chronic renal failure. *Eur. J. Clin. Pharmacol.* 14:21–27 (1978).

P. Dylewicz, W. Kirch, S. R. Santos, H. J. Hult, H. Monig, and E. E. Ohnhus. Bioavailability and elimination of nitrendipine in liver disease. *Eur. J. Clin. Pharmacol.* 32:563–568 (1987).

G. H. Evans and D. G. Shand. Disposition of propranolol VI: Independent variation in steady-state circulating drug concentrations and half-life as a result of plasma drug binding in man. *Clin. Pharmacol. Ther.* 14:494–500 (1973).

W. E. Evans, J. J. Schentag, and W. J. Jusko. *Applied Pharmacokinetics, Principles of Therapeutic Drug Monitoring*. Applied Therapeutics, Spokane, (1986).

D. Evard, J. P. Aubry, Y. LeQuintrec, G. Cheymol, and A. Cheymol. Study of the bioavailability of pindolol in malabsorption syndromes. *Br. J. Clin. Pharmacol.* 18:632–637 (1984).

A. Fujimura, H. Kajiyama, and A. Ebihara. The influence of fever on the pharmacokinetics of pranoprofen in elderly subjects. *J. Clin. Pharmacol.* 29:500–503 (1989).

J. G. Gambertoglio. Effects of renal disease: Altered pharmacokinetics. In *Pharmacokinetic Basis for Drug Treatment* (L. Z. Benet, N. Massoud, and J. G. Gambertoglio. eds.) Raven Press, New York, pp. 149–171 (1984).

R. E. Gammans, R. F. Mayol, and J. A. Labudde. Metabolism and disposition of buspirone. *Am. J. Med.* 80(Suppl. 3B):41–51 (1986).

M. Gibaldi, R. M. Boyes, and S. Feldman. Influence of first-pass effect on availability of drugs on oral administration. *J. Pharm. Sci.* 60:1338–1340 (1971).

T. P. Gibson, K. M. Giacomini, W. A. Briggs, W. Whitman, and G. Levy. Propoxyphene and norpropoxyphene plasma concentrations in the anephric patient. *Clin. Pharmacol. Ther.* 27:665–670 (1980).

T. P. Gibson, E. J. Matusik, and W. A. Briggs. N-Acetylprocainamide levels in patients with end-stage renal failure. *Clin. Pharmacol. Ther.* 19:206–212 (1976).

A. Greither, S. Goldman, J. S. Edelen, K. Cohn, and L. Z. Benet. Erratic and incomplete absorption of furosemide in congestive heart failure. *Am. J. Cardiol.* 37:139 (1976).

R. Groszmann, B. Kotelanski, J. N. Cohn, and I. B. Khatri. Quantitation of portasystemic shunting from the splenic and mesenteric beds in alcoholic liver disease. *Am. J. Med.* 53:715–722 (1972).

P. O. Gubbins and K. E. Bertch. Drug absorption in gastrointestinal disease and surgery. *Pharmacotherapy* 9:285–295 (1989).

R. Gugler, P. Lain, and D. L. Azarnoff. Effects of portocaval shunt on the disposition of drugs with and without first-pass effect. *J. Pharmacol. Exp. Ther.* 195:416–423 (1975).

J. P. Guignard, A. Torrado, S. M. Mazouni, and E. Gautier. Renal function in respiratory distress syndrome. *J. Pediatr.* 88:845–850 (1976).

D. L. Guisti. Acute renal failure. In *Clinical Pharmacy and Therapeutics* (E. T. Herfindal and J. I. Hirschman, eds.) Williams & Wilkins, New York, p. 80 (1975).

F. Hagemeijer. Absorption, half-life, and toxicity of oral aprindine in patients with acute myocardial infarction. *Eur. J. Clin. Pharmacol.* 9:21–25 (1975).

F. C. Harris. Pyloric stenosis: Hold-up of enteric coated aspirin tablets. *Br. J. Surg.* 60:979–981 (1973).

K. Hartialia, A. Kasanen, and M. Raussi. The absorption of salicylamide in pernicious anaemia, gastric achylia and paplic ulcer. *Ann. Med. Exp. Biol. Fenn.* 41:549–533 (1963).

A. Hass, H. Lullman, and T. Peters. Absorption rates of some cardiac glycosides and portal blood flow. *Eur. J. Pharmacol.* 19:366–370 (1972).

A. H. Hayes. Intravenous infusion of lidocaine in the control of ventricular arrhythmias. In *Lidocaine in the Treatment of Ventricular Arrhythmias* (Scott and Julian, eds.) Livingstone, Edinburgh, p. 189 (1971).

G. W. Hepner, E. S. Vesell, and K. R. Tantum. Reduced drug elimination in congestive heart failure. Studies using aminopyrine as a model drug. *Am. J. Med.* 65:271–276 (1978).

C. B. Higgins, S. F. Vatner, D. Franklin, and E. Braunwald. Pattern of differential vasoconstriction in response to acute and chronic low-output states in the conscious dog. *Cardiovasc. Res.* 8:92–98 (1974).

T. A. Hoffman, R. Cestero, and W. E. Bullock. Pharmacodynamics of carbenicillin in hepatic and renal failure. *Ann. Intern. Med.* 73:173–178 (1970).

S. Holt, R. C. Heading, J. A. Clements, P. Tothill, and L. F. Prescott. Acetaminophen absorption and metabolism in celiac disease and Crohn's disease. *Clin. Pharmacol. Ther.* 30:232–238 (1981).

M. Homeida, L. Jackson, and C. J. C. Roberts. Decreased first-pass metabolism of labetalol in chronic liver disease. *Br. Med. J.* 2:1048–1050 (1978).

J. B. Houston. Kinetics of drug metabolism and diposition: Physiological determinants. In *Drug Metabolism and Disposition: Considerations in Clinical Pharmacology* (G. R. Wilkinson and M. D. Rawlins, eds.) MTP Press, Boston, pp. 63–90 (1985).

P. Jaillon, P. Rubin, Y. G. Yee, R. Ball, R. Kates, D. Harrion, and T. Blaschke. Influence of congestive heart failure on parazosin kinetics. *Clin. Pharmacol. Ther.* 25:790–794 (1979).

F. Jamali, R. Mehvar, and F. M. Pasutto. Enantioselective aspects of drug action and disposition: Therapeutic pitfalls. *J. Pharm. Sci.* 78:695–715 (1989).

P. Jenner and B. Testa. Altered drug disposition in disease states: The first pieces of a jigsaw. In *Concepts in Drug Metabolism*, Part A. (P. Jenner and B. Testa, eds.) Marcel Dekker, New York, pp. 423–513 (1980).

A. H. John and A. Jones. Gastroenteritis causing failure of oral contraception. *Br. Med. J.* 3:207–208 (1975).

W. J. Jusko, G. P. Lewis, and G. W. Schmilt. Ampicillin and netacillin pharmacokinetics in normal and anephric subjects. *Clin. Pharmacol. Ther.* 14:90–99 (1973).

W. J. Jusko, L. L. Mosovich, L. M. Gerbarcht, M. E. Mattar, and S. J. Yaffie. Enhanced renal excretion of dicloxacillin in patients with cystic fibrosis. *Pediatrics* 56:1038–1044 (1975).

J. Jussila, M. J. Matilla, and S. Takki. Drug absorption during lactose-induced intestinal symptoms in patients with selective lactose malabsorption. *Ann. Med. Exp. Biol. Fenn.* 48:33–37 (1970).

J. P. Kampman, H. Klein, B. Lumholtz, and J. E. Molhohm Hansen. Ampicillin and propylthiouracil pharmacokinetics in intestinal by pass patients followed up to a year after operation. *Clin. Pharmacokinet.* 9:168–176 (1984).

R. Kato. Drug metabolism under pathophysiological and abnormal physiological states in animals and man. *Xenobiotica* 7:25–92 (1977).

J. Katz, C. S. Sehlhorst, D. Denson, D. Coyle, and P. O. Bridenbaugh. Intravenous and epidural pharmacokinetics of ropivacaine in the rhesus monkey. *Reg. Anesth.* 13(2S):80 (1988).

M. R. Kelly, R. E. Cutler, A. W. Forrey, and B. M. Kimpel. Pharmacokinetics of orally administered furosemide. *Clin. Pharmacol. Ther.* 15:178–186 (1974).

M. J. Kendall, L. P. Quaterman, H. Bishop, and R. E. Schneider. Effects of inflammatory disease on plasma oxprenolol concentrations. *Br. Med. J.* 2:465–468 (1979).

M. C. Kennedy and D. N. Wade. Phenytoin absorption in patients with ileojejunal bypass. *Br. J. Clin. Pharmacol.* 7:515–518 (1979).

G. Kitis, M. L. Lucas, H. Bishop, A. Sargent, R. E. Schareider, J. A. Blair, and R. N. Allan. Altered jejunal surface pH in coeliac disease: Its effects on propranolol and folic acid absorption. *Clin. Sci.* 63:373–360 (1982).

U. Klotz, G. R. Avant, A. Hoyumpa, S. Schewker, and G. R. Wilkinson. The effects of age and liver disease on the disposition and elimination of diazepam in adult man. *J. Clin. Invest.* 55:347–35 (1975).

U. Klotz, T. S. McHorse, G. R. Wilkinson, and S. Schenker. The effect of cirrhosis on the disposition and elimination of meperidine (Pethidine) in man. *Clin. Pharmacol. Ther.* 16:667–675 (1974).

J. Koch-Weser. Pharmacokinetics of procainamide in man. *Ann. N.Y. Acad. Sci.* 179:370–382 (1971).

J. Koch-Weser. Correlation of serum concentrations and pharmacological effects of antiarrhythmic drugs. In *Proceedings of the 5th International Congress on Pharmacology*. San Francisco 1872, Vol. 3. Karger, Basel, p. 69 (1973).

J. Koch-Weser and J. W. Klein. Procainamide dosage schedules, plasma concentrations, and clinical effects. *JAMA* 215:1454–1460 (1970).

U. R. Korhomen, A. J. Jounela, A. J. Pakarinen, P. J. Pentikainen, J. T. Takkunen. Pharmacokinetics of digoxin in patients with acute myocardial infarction. *Am. J. Cardiol.* 44:1190–1194 (1979).

P. I. Korner. Effects of low oxygen and of carbon monoxide on the renal circulation in unanesthetized rabbits. *Circulation Res.* 12:361–373 (1963).

J. R. Koup. Disease states and drug pharmacokinetics. *J. Clin. Pharmacol.* 29:674–679 (1989).

P. A. Kramer, D. J. Chapron, J. Benson, and S. A. Mercik. Tetracycline absorption in elderly patients with achlorhydria. *Clin. Pharmcol. Ther.* 23:467–472 (1978).

G. M. Kunin, A. J. Glazko, and M. Finland. Persistence of antibiotics in blood of patients with acute renal failure. II. Chloramphenicol and its metabolic products in blood of patients with severe renal disease or hepatic cirrhosis. *J. Clin. Invest.* 38:1498–1508 (1959).

D. Lalka, M. G. Wyman, B. N. Goldreyer, T. M. Ludden, and D. S. Cannon. Procainamide accumulation kinetics in the immediate post myocardial infraction period. *J. Clin. Pharmacol.* 18:397–401 (1978).

J. M. Letteri, H. Mellk, S. Louis, H. Kutt, P Durante, and A. Glazko. Diphenylhydantoin metabolism in uremia. *N. Engl. J. Med.* 285:648–652 (1971).

G. Levy and A. Yacobi. Effect of plasma protein binding on elimination of warfarin. *J. Pharm. Sci.* 63:805–806 (1974).

G. P. Lewis and W. J. Jusko. Pharmacokinetics of ampicillin in cirrhosis. *Clin. Pharmacol. Ther.* 18:475–484 (1975).

D. D. Lindholm and J. S. Murray. Persistence of vancomycin in the blood during renal failure and its treatment by hemodialysis. *N. Engl. J. Med.* 274:1047–1047 (1966).

H. Lode, D. Frisch, and P. Maumann. Oral antibiotic therapy in patients with partial gastrectomy. In *Progress in Chemotherapy*, Vol. 1 (Daikas, ed.) Hellenic Society of Chemotherapy, Athens, pp. 543–546 (1974).

D. T. Lowenthal. Pharmacokinetics of propranolol, quinidine, procainamide, and lidocaine in chronic renal disease. *Am. J. Med.* 62:532–538 (1971).

D. T. Lowenthal, W. A. Briggs, T. P. Gibson, H. Nelson, and W. J. Cirksena. Pharmacokinetics of oral propanolol in chronic renal disease. *Clin. Pharmacol. Ther.* 16:761–769 (1974).

J. Lupinsky and S. Berthoud. Absorption of pencillin V in relation to digestive disorders. *Schweiz. Rundsch. Med. Prax.* 62:959–963 (1973).

M. J. Matilla, A. Friman, T. K. I. Larmi, and R. Koskinen. Absorption of ethionamide, isoniazid and aminosalicylic acid from post-resection gastrointestinal tract. *Ann. Med. Exp. Biol. Fenn.* 47:209–212 (1969).

M. J. Matilla, J. Jussila, and S. Takki. Drug absorption in patients with intestinal villous atrophy. *Arzneim. Forschung* 23:583–585 (1973).

G. E. Mawer, N. E. Miller, and L. A. Turnberg. Metabolism of amylobarbitone in patients with chronic liver disease. *Br. J. Pharmacol.* 44:549–560 (1972).

G. Menardi and J. P. Guggenbichler. Bioavailability of oral antibiotics in children with short bowel syndrome. *J. Pediatr. Surg.* 19:84–86 (1984).

C. M. Metzler. Bioavailability/bioequivalence: Study design and statistical issues. *J. Clin. Pharmacol.* 29:289–292 (1989).

P. Mlynark and J. B. Kissner. Absorption and excretion of $^{1\text{-}2}H^3$ hydrocortisone in regional enteritis and ulcerative colitis, with a note on hydrocortisone production rates. *Gastroenterology* 44:257–260 (1963).

W. E. Muller. Stereoselective plasma protein binding of drugs. In *Drug Stereochemistry, Analytical Methods and Pharmacology* (I.W. Wainer and D. E. Drayer, eds.) Marcel Dekker, New York, pp. 227–244 (1988).

R. L. Nation. Enantioselective drug analysis: Problems and resolutions. *Clin. Exp. Pharmacol. Physiol.* 16:471–477 (1989).

E. A. Neal, P. J. Meffin, P. B. Gregory, and T. F. Blaschke. Enhanced bioavailability and decreased clearance of analgesics in patients with cirrhosis. *Gastroenterology* 77:96–102 (1979).

J. D. Nelson, S. Shelton, J. T. Kusmiesz, and K. C. Haltalin. Absorption of ampicillin and nalidixic acid by infants and children with acute shigellosis. *Clin. Pharmacol. Ther.* 13:879–886 (1972).

A. S. Nies, D. G. Shand, and G. R. Wilkinson. Altered hepatic blood flow and drug disposition. *Clin. Pharmacokinet.* 1:135–156 (1976).

W. S. Nimmo. Drugs, diseases and altered gastric emptying. *Clin. Pharmacokinet.* 1:189–203 (1976).

H. R. Ochs, D. J. Greenblatt, and H. J. Dengler. Absorption of oral tetracycline in patients with Bilorth-II gastrectomy. *J. Pharmacokinet. Biopharm.* 6:295–303 (1978).

G. C. Oliver, R. Tazman, and R. Frederickson. Influence of congestive heart failure on digoxin levels. In *Symposium on Digitalis* (O. Strostein, ed.) Gyldenal Norsk Forlog, Oslo, Norway, pp. 336–347 (1973), through Benet et al. (1976).

H. Ogata, Y. Kawatsn, Y. Marnyama, K. Machida, and T. Haga. Bioavailability and diuretic effect of furosemide during long-term treatment of chronic respiratory failure. *Eur. J. Clin. Pharmacol.* 28:53–59 (1985).

E. E. Ohnhaus, S. Vozeh, and E. Neusch. Absolute bioavailability of digoxin in chronic renal failure. *Clin. Nephrol.* 11:302–306 (1979).

J. Oravcova, S. Bystricky, and T. Trnovec. Different binding of propranolol enantiomers to human alpha-1-acid glycoprotein. *Biochem. Phamacol.* 38:2575–2579 (1989).

R. L. Parsons. Drug absorption in gastrointestinal disease with particular reference to malabsorption syndroms. *Clin. Pharmacokinet.* 2:45–60 (1977).

R. Parsons, D. J. N. Hossack, M. J. Bywater, D. M. Humphreys, and D. M. Hailey. The absorption of trimethoprin, sulphamethoxazole, fucidin, lincomycin, clindamycin and rifamprin in adult coeliac disease. In *Progress in Chemotherapy: Proceedings of the 8th International Congress of Chemotherapy*, Vol 1. (Daikos, ed.) Hellenic Society for Chemotherapy, Athens, pp. 499–506 (1973).

R. L. Parsons, G. A. Hossack, and G. M. Paddock. The absorption of antibiotics in adult patients with coeliac disease. *J. Antimicrob. Chemother.* 1:39–50 (1975a).

R. L. Parsons, W. J. Jusko, and J. M. Young. Pharmacokinetics of antibiotic absorption in coeliac disease. *J. Antimicrob. Chemother.* 2:214–215 (1976).

R. L. Parsons, C. M. Kaya, and K. Raymond. Pharmacokinetics of salicylate and indomethacin in celiac disease. *Eur. J. Clin. Pharmacol.* 11:473–477 (1977).

R. L. Parsons and G. M. Paddock. Absorption of two antibacterial drugs, cephalexin and co-trimoxazole in malabsorption syndromes. *J. Antimicrob. Chemother.* 1(Suppl.):59–67 (1975).

R. L. Parsons, G. M. Paddock, G. M. Hossack, and D. M. Hailey. Antibiotic absorption in Crohn's disease. In *Chemotherapy*, vol. 4: *Pharmacology of Antibiotics* (J. D. Williams and A. M. Geddes, eds.) Plenum Press, New York, pp. 219–229 (1976a).

P. J. Pentikainen, P. J. Neuvonen, S. Tarpila, and E. Syvalanti. Effect of cirrhosis of the liver on the pharmacokinetics of chlormethiazole. *Br. Med. J.* 2:861–863 (1978).

D. Pessayre, D. Lebrec, V. Descatoire, M. Peignoux, and J. Benhamou. Mechanism for reduced drug clearance in patients with cirrhosis. *Gastroenterology* 74:566–571 (1978).

K. M. Piafsky. Disease induced changes in the plasma binding of basic drugs. *Clin. Pharmacokinet.* 5:246–262 (1980).

K. M. Piafsky, O. Borga, I. Odar-Cederlof, C. Johansson, and F. Sjoqvist. Increased plasma protein binding of propranolol and chlorpromazine mediated by disease-induced elevations of plasma α_1-acid glycoprotein. *N. Engl. J. Med.* 299:1435–1439 (1978).

A. Pottage, J. Nimmo, and L. F. Prescott. The absorption of aspirin and paracetamol in patients with achlorhydria. *J. Pharm. Pharmacol.* 26:144–145 (1974).

J. R. Powell, S. Vozeh, P. Hopewell, J. Costell, L. B. Sheiner, and S. Riegelman. Theophylline disposition in acutely ill hospitalized patients. *Am. Rev. Respir. Dis.* 118:229–238 (1978).

L. F. Prescott, K. K. Yamoah-Adjepon, and R. G. Talbot. Impaired lignocaine metabolism in patients with myocardial infarction and cardiac failure. *Br. Med. J.* 1:939–941 (1976).

K. Rasmussen, J. Jervell, L. Storstein, and K. Gjerdrun. Digitoxin kinetics in patients with impaired renal function. *Clin. Pharmacol. Ther.* 13:6–14 (1972).

A. G. Renwick, V. Higgins, K. Powers, C. L. Smith, and C. F. George. The absorption and conjugation of methyldopa in patients with coeliac and Crohn's diseases during treatment. *Br. J. Clin. Pharmacol.* 16:77–83 (1983).

D. G. Rimmer. Gastric retention without mechanical obstruction. *Arch. Intern. Med.* 117:287–299 (1966).

W. A. Ritschel. *Antacids and Other Drugs in GI Diseases*. Drug Intelligence Publications, Hamilton, Ill., pp. 64–70; 149–153 (1984).

W. A. Ritschel. *Handbook of Basic Pharmacokinetics*, 3rd ed. Drug Intelligence Publications, Hamilton, Ill., pp. 219–221 (1986).

W. A. Ritschel. Bioavailability: A critical evaluation. In *Biotechnology in Health Care*. Proceedings of the 37th Indian Pharmaceutical Congress, New Delhi. Printorium Press, Ahmedabad, India, pp. 111–142 (1987).

L. Rivera-Calimlim, C. A. Dujovne, J. P. Morgan, L. Lasagna, and J. R. Bianchine. L-Dopa treatment failure: Explanation and correction. *Br. Med. J.* 4:93–94 (1970).

M. Robertshaw, K. N. Lai, and R. S. Swaminathan. Prediction of creatinine clearance from plasma creatinine: Comparison of five formulae. *Br. J. Clin. Pharmacol.* 28:275–280 (1989).

M. Rowland, L. Z. Benet, and G. G. Graham. Clearance concepts in pharmacokinetics. *J. Pharmacokinet. Biopharm.* 1:123–136 (1973).

C. E. Rubin, L. L. Brandborg, A. L. Flick, P. Phelps, C. Parmentier, and S. Van Niel. Studies of celiac sprue. *Gastroenterology* 43:621–641 (1962).

J. Sanchez, L. Martinez, J. Garcia-Barbal, R. Roser, A. Bartlett, and R. Sagarra. The influence of gastric emptying on droxicam pharmacokinetics. *J. Clin. Pharmacol.* 29:739–745 (1989).

F. Saudek, J. Moravek, and Z. Modr. Cefoperazone pharmacokinetics in patients with liver cirrhosis: A predictive value of the ujoviridin test. *Int. J. Clin. Pharmacol. Ther. Toxicol.* 27:82–87 (1989).

R. E. Schneider, J. Babb, H. Bishop, M. Mitchard, A. M. Hoare, and C. F. Hawkins. Plasma levels of propranolol in treated patients with Crohn's disease. *Br. Med. J.* 2:794–795 (1976).

R. E. Schneider, H. Bishop, and C. F. Hawkins. Plasma propranolol concentrations and erythrocyte sedimentation rate. *Br. J. Clin. Pharmacol.* 8:43–47 (1979).

S. M. Shaw. Drugs and diseases that may alter the biodistribution or pharmacokinetics of radiopharmaceuticals. *Pharm. Int.* 6:293–298 (1985).

M. Siurala, O. Mustala, and J. Jussila. Absorption of acetylsalicyclic acid by normal and an atrophic gastric mucosa. *Scand. J. Gastroenterol.* 4:269–273 (1969).

F. Sjoquist, O. Borga, and M. L. E. Orme. Fundamentals of clinical pharmacology. In *Drug Treatment*, 2nd ed. (G. S. Avery, ed.) Adis Press, Sydney, New York, pp. 33–40 (1980).

A. Somogyi, M. Albrecht, G. Kliems, K. Schafer, and M. Eichelbaum. Pharmacokinetics, bioavailability and ECG response of verapamil in patients with liver cirrhosis. *Br. J. Clin. Pharmacol.* 12:51–60 (1981).

M. Spino, R. P. Chai, A. F. Isles, J. J. Thiessen, A. Tesoro, R. Gold, and S. M. MacLead. Cloxacillin absorption and disposition in cystic fibrosis. *J. Pediatr.* 105:829–835 (1984).

S. Stavchansky and T.-L. Tung. Effect of hypothermia on the intestinal absorption of uracil and L-dopa in the rat. *J. Pharm. Sci.* 9:688–691 (1987).

R. E. Stenson, R. E. Constantino, and D. C. Harrison. Interrelationships of hepatic blood flow, cardiac output and blood levels of lidocaine. *Circulation* 43:205–211 (1971).

S. M. Stewart, I. M. E. Anderson, G. R. Jones, and M. A. Calder. Amoxycillin levels in sputum, serum and saliva. *Thorax* 29:110–114 (1974).

A. R. Tanner, J. W. Halliday, and L. W. Powell. Serum prednisolone levels in Crohns disease and celiac disease following oral prednisolone administration. *Digestion* 21:310–315 (1981).

L. Ther, and D. Winne. Drug absorption. *Annu. Rev. Pharmacol.* 11:57–70 (1971).

G. A. Thompson, P. A. Turner, P. O. Bridenbaugh, R. C. Stuebing, and D. D. Denson. The influence of diazepam on the pharmacokinetics of intravenous and epidural bupivacaine in the rhesus monkey. *Anesth. Analg.* 65:151–155 (1986).

P. D. Thomson, K. L. Melmon, and J. A. Richardson. Lidocaine pharmacokinetics in advanced heart failure, liver disease and renal failure in humans. *Ann. Intern. Med.* 78:499–508 (1973).

W. J. Tilstone, H. Dargie, E. N. Dargie, H. G. Morgan, and A. C. Kennedy. Pharmacokinetics of metalazone in normal subjets and in patients with cardiac or renal failure. *Clin. Pharmacol. Ther.* 16:322–329 (1974).

S. Toon, E. M. Davidson, F. M. Garstang, H. Batra, R. J. Bowes, and M. Rowland. The racemic metoprolol H_2-antagonist interaction. *Clin. Pharmacol. Ther.* 43:283–289 (1988).

T. N. Tozer. Implications of altered plasma protein binding in disease states. In *Pharmacokinetic Basis for Drug Treatment* (L. Z. Benet, N. Massoud, and J. G. Gambertoglio, eds.) Raven Press, New York, pp. 173–193 (1984).

G. T. Tucker and M. S. Lennard. Enantiomer specific pharmacokinetics. *Pharmacol. Ther.* 45:309–329 (1990).

G. T. Tucker and L. E. Mather. Pharmacokinetics of local anesthetic agents. *Br. J. Anaesth.* 47:213-224 (1975).

G. T. Tucker and L. E. Mather. Clinical pharmacokinetics of local anaesthetic agents. *Clin. Pharmacokinet.* 4:241-278 (1979).

G. T. Ueda and B. S. Dzindzio. Quinidine kinetics in congestive heart failure. *Clin. Pharmacol. Ther.* 23:158-164 (1978).

G. T. Ueda and B. S. Dzindzio. Pharmacokinetics of dihydroquinidine in congestive heart failure patients after intravenous quinidine administration. *Eur. J. Clin. Pharmacol.* 19:187-197 (1979).

F. A. V. D. Van den Duweland, M. J. A. M. Franssen, L. B. A. V. D. Putte, Y. Tan, C. A. M. V. Ginneken, and F. W. J. Gribnau. Naproxen pharmacokinetics in patients with rheumatoid artheritis during active polyarticular inflammation. *Br. J. Clin. Pharmacol.* 23:189-193 (1987).

V. M. K. Venho, S. Aukee, J. Jussila, and M. J. Mattila. Effect of gastric surgery on gastrointestinal drug absorption in man. *Scand. J. Gastroenterol.* 10:43-47 (1975).

G. N. Volans. Absorption of effervescent aspirin during migraine. *Br. Med. J.* 4:265-269 (1974).

S. Vozeh, G. Katz, V. Steiner, and F. Follath. Population pharmacokinetic parameters in patients treated with oral mexiletine. *Eur. J. Clin. Pharmacol.* 23:445-451 (1982).

P. G. Welling. Effects of GI disease of drug absorption. In *Pharmacokinetic Basis for Drug Treatment* (L. Z. Benet, N. Massoud, and J. G. Gambertoglio, eds.) Raven Press, New York, pp. 29-47 (1984).

P. G. Welling and W. A. Craig. Pharmacokinetics in disease states modifying renal function. In *The Effect of Disease States on Drug Pharmacokinetics* (L. Z. Benet, ed.) American Pharmaceutical Association, Washington, D.C., pp. 155-187 (1976).

P. G. Welling, W. A. Craig, G. L. Amidon, and C. M. Kunin. Pharmacokinetics of cefazolin in normal and uremic subjects. *Clin. Pharmacol. Ther.* 15:344-353 (1974).

P. G. Welling and F. L. S. Tse. Factors contributing to variability in drug pharmacokinetics. I. Absorption. *J. Clin. Hosp. Pharm.* 9:163-179 (1984).

G. R. Wilkinson and R. A. Branch. Effects on hepatic disease on clinical pharmacokinetics. In *Pharmacokinetic Basis for Drug Treatment* (L. Z. Benet, N. Massoud, and J. G. Gambertoglio, eds.) Raven Press, New York, pp. 49-61 (1984).

K. Williams and E. Lee. Importance of drug enantiomers in clinical pharmacology. *Drugs* 30:333-354 (1985).

R. L. Williams. Drugs and the liver: Clinical applications. In *Pharmacokinetic Basis for Drug Treatment* (L. Z. Benet, N. Massoud, and J. G. Gambertoglio, eds.) Raven Press, New York, pp. 63-75 (1984).

R. L. Williams and L. Z. Benet. Drug pharmacokinetics in cardiac and hepatic disease. *Annu. Rev. Pharmacol. Toxicol.* 20:389-413 (1980).

R. L. Williams, M. D. Thornhill, R. A. Upton, C. Blume, T. S. Clark, R. Liw, and L. Z. Benet. Absorption and disposition of two combinations formulations of hydrochlorothiazide and triameterene: Influence of age and renal function. *Clin. Pharmacol. Ther.* 40:226-232 (1986).

D. M. Wilson, Tests of renal function. In *Clinical Medicine* (J. A. Spittell and P. P. Frohnert, eds.) Harper & Row, Philadelphia, pp. 1-36 (1984).

D. Winne. The influence of villous counter current exchange on intestinal absorption. *J. Theor. Biol.* 53:145–176 (1975).

D. Winne and J. Remischovsky. Intestinal blood flow and absorption of nondissociable substances. *J. Pharm. Pharmacol.* 22:640–641 (1970).

J. Wojciki, M. Ostrowski, and B. Gawronska-Szklarz. The effect of gastrosectomy on pharmacokinetics of orally administered paracetamol in man. *Pol. J. Pharmacol. Pharm.* 36:323–327 (1984).

A. J. J. Wood, R. E. Vestal, C. L. Spannuth, W. J. Stone, G. R. Wilkinson, and D. G. Shand. Propranolol disposition in renal failure. *Br. J. Clin. Pharmacol.* 10:561–565 (1980).

M. G. Wyman, B. N. Goldreyer, D. S. Cannom, T. M. Ludden, and D. Lalka. Factors influencing procainamide total body clearance in the immediate postmyocardial infarction period. *J. Clin. Pharmacol.* 21:20–25 (1981).

5
Factors Influencing Bioavailability and Bioequivalence

Arzu Selen
Parke-Davis Pharmaceutical Research Division
Warner-Lambert Company
Ann Arbor, Michigan

INTRODUCTION

Bioavailability is one of the key factors that may explain therapeutic success or failure. In Food and Drug Administration (FDA) regulations, the statute describes *bioavailability* as ". . . the rate and extent to which the active ingredient or therapeutic ingredient is absorbed from a drug and becomes available at the site of drug action" [1,2]. Thus, bioavailability of a compound can be determined by measuring the rate and extent of absorption of the active component, either by evaluating concentrations of the drug and/or its metabolites in biological fluids or by determining pharmacologic response.

Comparison of bioavailability from different formulations has resulted in a term, *bioequivalence*, which is defined as similar rate and extent of absorption of the active component [3]. An ambiguity in definitions of bioavailability and bioequivalence in the statute has been pointed out. It may be possible that, because of some physiological mechanism, two products with equal rates and extents of absorption of the active component may demonstrate differences in the rate and extent of active component reaching the site of drug action. Under the statutory definition, these formulations would not be equivalent in bioavailability, but they may be considered bioequivalent under the statute's bioequivalence criteria [4]. This has led to a petition asking for a change in FDA bioequivalence standards, applicable to a certain compound and its generic formulations, that equivalence in absorption might not equal equivalence at the site of drug action [4]. Currently, bioequivalence testing is based on assessment of rate and extent of drug absorption and, in some cases, there may be "guidances" provided by FDA for evaluation of bioequivalence for particular drugs or drug products.

The objective of this chapter is to review some of the factors that may influence drug bioavailability and, hence, bioequivalence assessment, when two formulations are being compared. Although a multitude of factors affect drug bioavailability, their origin can be traced mainly to physiological or physicochemical factors. Bioavailability of a compound will greatly depend on its route of administration. Routes of administration, such as oral, sublingual, and transdermal, and factors related to these routes, will be examined in detail. Other factors that affect drug bioavailability or contribute to its variability will be discussed because, to some extent, all contribute to the complexity of the process.

ROUTES OF DRUG ADMINISTRATION

The absorption characteristics of a drug will depend on the drug substance, its route of administration, and the dosage form. If intravenous, sublingual, or buccal dosage routes are used, onset of action will be rapid, whereas oral and topical administration would yield a slower onset of action. In general, drugs are most frequently taken by oral administration, swallowed or, in some instances, dissolved in the mouth. Systemic drug effect is usually desired, although some drugs are taken for their local effect in the gastrointestinal tract.

Table 1 shows the effect of different routes of drug administration on drug bioavailability. Depending on the route of administration, the onset and duration of effect of nitroglycerin varies, providing fastest onset after sublingual administration and slowest after transdermal application [5].

Oral

The oral route is still the preferred route of drug administration for systemic activity, as it is the most natural and convenient means of drug delivery. Possible disadvantages of drug delivery by this route include irregular drug absorption, slower onset of response than parenteral routes, loss of drug from gastric acidity or presence of gastrointestinal (GI) enzymes, and the presence of food, microorganisms, and other factors that may influence the physiology of the GI tract.

Factors Influencing Bioavailability

Table 1 Dosage Form and Route-Dependent Therapeutic Activity of Nitroglycerin

Dosage form	Dose (mg)	Onset (min)	Peak action (min)	Duration (min or hr)
Sublingual	0.3–0.8	2–5	4–8	10–30 min
Buccal	1–3	2–5	4–10	30–300 min
Oral	6.5–19.5	20–45	45–120	2–6 hr
Transdermal disks	5–10	30–60	60–180	Up to 24 hr

Source: From Ref. 5.

To provide an insight into physiological factors that may impact on drug absorption and bioavailability, a brief review of the physiology of the GI tract is warranted.

Physiological Basis of Absorption

For a drug to be absorbed, it has to cross several biological membranes or barriers. The structure of a biological membrane has been described as a "mayonnaise sandwich," in which a bimolecular layer of lipid substances is contained between two parallel monomolecular layers of protein [6]. Cell membranes appear to be perforated by vacuoles or pores, 4–10 Å in diameter, that are filled with water. Inorganic ions and small water-soluble organic ions can pass through these pores. Even small lipid-soluble molecules may pass through these vacuoles. However, it is more likely that all hydrophobic lipid-soluble molecules, penetrate the biological membrane through the fatlike portion of the lipoprotein membrane [7].

Structure and Innervation of Gastrointestinal Tract

The structure of the GI tract varies greatly from region to region. However, there are common features in the overall organization of the tissue. The general layered structure of the wall of the GI tract is illustrated in Figure 1. The *mucosa, submucosa, muscularis externa*, and the serosa make up the four main components of GI wall.

The *mucosa* consists of the muscularis mucosae, the lamina propria, and an epithelium. The thin innermost layer of intestinal smooth muscle is the muscularis mucosae that, in some parts of the GI tract, has an inner circular layer and an outer longitudinal layer. The lamina propria contains lymph nodules and capillaries, and is rich in several types of glands. The *submucosa* consists mainly of loose connective tissue with collagen and elastin fibrils. It also contains glands and the larger blood vessels of the intestinal wall. The muscularis externa consists of two substantial layers of smooth-muscle cells that form an inner circular

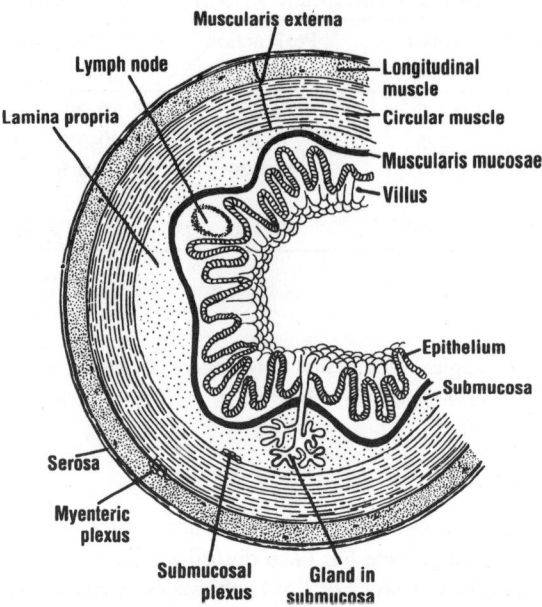

Figure 1 Structure of the wall of gastrointestinal tract. (From Ref. 8 redrawn with permission.)

layer and an outer longitudinal layer. Contractions of the muscularis externa provide mixing and propelling of the lumen contents. The outermost layer is the *serosa* or *advantitia*, which is covered with a layer of squamous mesothelial cells and consists mainly of connective tissue [8].

The wall of the GI tract contains many neurons that are highly interconnected. The submucosal and myenteric plexuses (intramural plexuses), together with other neurons of the GI tract, constitute the enteric nervous system, which facilitates the motor and secretory activities of the GI system. In the absence of input from the sympathetic and parasympathetic nerves, many of the motor and secretory activities would still continue because of the control exerted by the enteric nervous system. It was proposed by Langley, in 1921, that the plexuses of the wall of the GI tract function as a semiautonomous nervous system controlling motor and secretory activities of the digestive system [8].

The human enteric nervous system of the large and small intestines alone contains approximately 10^8 neurons, as many neurons as in the spinal cord [8]. Neurons sensitive to mechanical deformation, to particular chemical stimuli, and to temperature have been characterized. Since some of the neurons of the enteric ganglia are effector neurons that send axons to smooth-muscle cells of the circular and longitudinal layers, to secretory cells of the GI tract, or to GI blood vessels, a variety of stimuli or varying stimuli may have a substantial effect on bioavailability of a drug substance and may even confound bioequivalence assessment.

The number of neuromodulatory substances present in the wall of the GI tract is comparable with the number of similar compounds in the brain. Most of the known neuromodulators present in both gut and brain are listed in Table 2. Presence of met- and leu-enkaphalin, substance P, vasoactive intestinal peptide (VIP), and cholecystokinin in enteric neurons is well established. Angiotensin II-like peptide, dynorphin, γ-aminobutyric acid, motilin, neurotensin, and pancreatic polypeptide are anticipated to be present in enteric neurons [8,9].

Structure and Innervation of the Stomach

The basic structure of the gastric wall resembles the scheme illustrated in Figure 1, with a more prominent circular muscle layer than the longitudinal layer of muscularis externa.

The extrinsic nerves and neurons of the submucosal and myenteric plexuses innervate the stomach. Smooth muscle and secretory cells are innervated by the axons from the cells of the intramural plexuses. Extrinsic innervation is provided by the vagus nerves and from the celiac plexus. In general, cholinergic nerves stimulate gastric smooth-muscle motility and gastric secretions, and adrenergic fibers inhibit these functions. The presence of several other gastric transmitter and modulator substances has also been reported [8,9].

Structure of the Gastric Mucosa

The gastric mucosa can be divided into three regions, based on the structure of the glands. The region just below the lower esophageal sphincter is the cardiac glandular region; the remainder is called the oxyntic glandular region, above the notch, and the pyloric glandular region, below the notch.

The glands of cardiac glandular region contain primarily mucus-secreting cells. The structure of a gastric gland from the oxyntic glandular region is shown in Figure 2. The mucous neck cells secrete mucus, whereas parietal or oxyntic cells secrete HCl and intrinsic factor. Pepsinogen is secreted by chief or peptic cells. The glands of the pyloric glandular region contain mainly mucus-secreting cells and G cells, which secrete gastrin, and a few oxyntic and peptic cells [10-12].

Structure of the Intestine

The intestine at every level is made up of four layers: mucosa, submucosa, muscularis externa, and serosa, as illustrated in Figure 1.

The absorptive cells of the small intestine are highly polarized columnar cells the major function of which is absorption of water, electrolytes, and nutrients.

Table 2 Substances Present in Enteric Neurons

Acetylcholine
Adenosine triphosphate (ATP)
Bombesin-gastrin-releasing peptide
Cholecystokinin octapeptide (CCK8)
Leu-enkaphlin
Met-enkephalin
5-Hydroxytryptamine (5-HT)
Norepinepherine
Somatostatin
Substance P
Vasoactive intestinal polypeptide (VIP)

Source: Modified from Ref. 8.

The surface of the intestinal Kerckring folds is covered by fingerlike formations—intestinal villi, which consist of epithelium and stroma. The luminal, cytoplasmic, and basal parts of the epithelial cell can be easily distinguished. The basal part lies on the basal membrane, which is a close link between the cell and the lamina propria. The luminal part of the enterocytes consists of the microvilli. Microvilli increase the absorptive surface of the intestinal mucosa and also, together with the unstirred layer and glycocalyx, form the brush border, constituting the apical (microvillus) membrane of the enterocytes. Many enzymes (disaccharidases, peptidases, hydrolases), which play an important role in the final phase of carbohydrate, lipid, and protein digestion, are located in the brush border. Receptor proteins for vitamin B_{12} and Ca^{2+} transport proteins are associated with the brush border structures. The tight junctions are important pathways for the paracellular route of absorption of both water and solutes. The basolateral membrane constitutes the intercellular membrane of the enterocyte toward adjacent cells and has a specialized function in intestinal transport processes, quite distinct from the microvillus membrane. Sodium-potassium-ATPase is chiefly localized in this structure, whereas it is practically absent in the apical membrane [12,13]. The cells between the villi form the area known as the crypts or the gastric pits. Goblet cells are polarized mucus-producing cells present both in the lower part of the villus and in the crypts, with increasing numbers from proximal to the distal region of the small intestine. It is assumed that intragranular mucin is excreted by the goblet cells by exocytosis. Paneth cells, located at the base of crypts of Lieberkuhn in most mammalian species, secrete protein-rich secretory granules, and the secretory activity of these cells appears to be under cholinergic control [14]. These cells may play a role in regulation of the microbiological flora of the human small intestine [15].

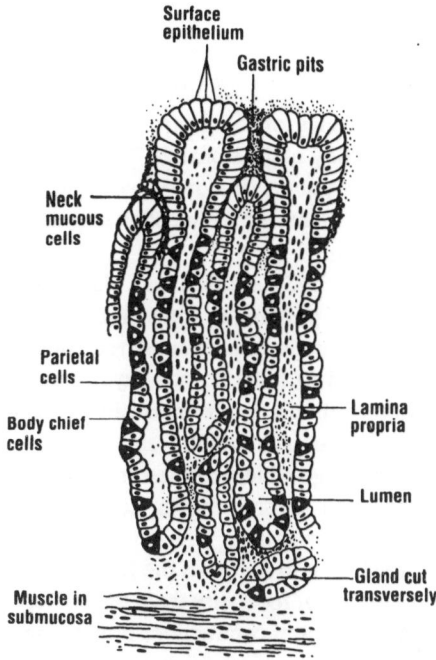

Figure 2 Structure of a gastric gland from the oxyntic glandular region. (From Ref. 11, redrawn with permission.)

Immunology of the Intestinal Tract

Another important function of the GI tract is that it is one of the largest organs in the body that protects against environmental agents entering by mouth. Luminal acidity, intestinal motility, structure of the epithelial surface, the protecting intestinal flora, and other factors are parts of nonimmunological defense. Gut-associated lymphoid tissue makes up the single largest organ of the immunological system. One-quarter of the intestinal mucosa is lymphoid tissue, which consists of T (thymus-dependent) and B (bursa-dependent) cells, carriers of cellular and humoral defense, respectively [13-15]. In humoral defense, the most important component is IgA, which has two subtypes: IgA1 and IgA2. Unlike serum, IgA2 is the major component in the immunoglobulin-producing cells of intestinal mucosa. Since IgA2 is also resistant to the action of proteolytic enzymes, it can effectively bind to antigens and prevent their absorption [16,17]. It can also inhibit binding of bacteria to epithelial cells and prevent bacterial colonization

[18,19]. If there is a deficiency in IgA secretion, there may be local inflammation, which may result in variable absorption of drugs.

Gastric Motility

The gastric peristaltic waves occur at the frequency of the gastric slow waves that are generated by the pacemaker zone in the body of the stomach. These waves travel toward the pylorus. In the human, the frequency of slow waves is about three per minute. The frequency of waves can be increased by injection of gastrin or may be reduced by administration of secretin.

The muscle layers in the fundus and stomach body are thin and, therefore, result in weak contractions. Thus, the contents of the fundus and stomach body tend to form layers, based on their density. The gastric contents may remain unmixed for as long as 1 hr after eating. Fats tend to form an oily layer on top and, consequently, are emptied later than other food components. Liquids can flow around the mass of food contained in the stomach and are emptied more rapidly into the duodenum, whereas large or indigestible particles are retained in the stomach for a longer period. After ingestion of food, regular contractions of the antrum occur at the frequency of gastric slow waves. The rate of gastric emptying is regulated by mechanisms that feed back to diminish the force of antral contractions. Antral contractions after ingestion of food vary from moderately forceful to weak. In a fasted animal, the pattern of antral contractions is different. The antrum is quiescent for 1-2 hr; then for a period of 10-20 min, an intense electrical and motor activity occurs that is characterized by strong contractions of the antrum, with a relaxed pylorus. During this period, even large remnant pieces of the previous meal are emptied from the stomach. A 1- to 2-hr period of quiescence follows the period of intense contractions. This pattern of cyclic contractile activity is called the *migrating myoelectric complex* (MMC). In humans, MMC occurs every 75-90 min. Although, it is inconclusive, motilin is expected to be the hormone responsible for initiation of MMC or the "housekeeper" activity [8]. Plasma motilin concentrations were shown to follow the occurrence of the MMC in dog [20,21].

Both neural and humoral mechanisms regulate emptying of gastric contents. The duodenal and jejunal mucosa have receptors that are sensitive to acidity, osmotic pressure, and fat content. The duodenum has a basic electrical rhythm of 10-12 contractions per minute. Transit time of food through the small intestine is generally measured in hours, whereas transit time through the large intestine is generally measured in days [22]. In healthy subjects, colonic contents move at a rate of 5 cm/hr under fasting conditions and increase to approximately 10 cm/hr after eating [8].

The effect of altered gastric-emptying rate on drug absorption has been studied for some time. Nimmo refers to a 1920 Agatha Christie novel *The Mysterious Affair at Styles* in which Hercule Poirot explains the delayed absorption of a fatal strychnine dose by delayed gastric emptying owing to presence of narcotic analgesics [23].

Gastric Acid Secretion

Fluid secreted into the stomach—the gastric juice—is a mixture of secretions of the surface epithelial cells and of gastric glands. Salts, water, HCl, pepsins, intrinsic factor, and mucus are the basic main components of gastric juice. Gastric secretions increase after a meal. The ionic composition of gastric juice is related to the rate of secretion. The higher the secretory rate, the higher the hydrogen ion concentration [H^+]. At lower secretory rates (< 1 mL/min), [Na^+] increases and [H^+] diminishes. The major anion in gastric juice, at all rates of secretion, is chlorine. The rate of gastric acid secretion varies considerably among individuals, possibly owing to variations in the number of parietal cells. In humans, the basal (unstimulated) rates of gastric acid production typically range from approximately 1 to 5 mEq/hr, and with histamine or pentagastrin stimulation, maximum acid output rises to 6–40 mEq/hr [12]. In general, patients with gastric ulcers secrete less HCl, and patients with duodenal ulcers secrete more HCl, than normal individuals. Gastric HCl secretion is reported to be less in patients with gastric cancer, compared with normal persons [24].

Control of Acid Secretion

There are distinct classes of receptors on the plasma membrane of parietal cells that bind acetylcholine, histamine, and gastrin and, thereby, directly stimulate the parietal cell to secrete HCl. Acetycholine is released near parietal cells by cholinergic nerve terminals, whereas gastrin, a hormone produced by G cells in the mucosa of the gastric antrum and duodenum, reaches parietal cells through the bloodstream. Histamine, released from cells in the gastric mucosa, diffuses into the parietal cells. Acetylcholine, histamine, and gastrin are important in the regulation of HCl secretion and act directly on parietal cells to enhance the rate of acid secretion. Acetylcholine binds to muscarinic receptors on the basal membrane of the parietal cell and stimulates acid secretion. The binding of acetylcholine to its receptors opens Ca^{2+} channels, allows Ca^{2+} to enter the cell, and increase the cytosolic level of free Ca^{2+}. Although, the mechanism is unclear, increased intracellular Ca^{2+} concentration results in increased secretion of HCl.

Histamine increases the cytosolic level of cyclic adenosine monophosphate (cAMP) when it binds to H_2-receptors on the parietal cell membrane and activates adenylate cyclase in the plasma membrane. The increased cAMP is proposed to stimulate a cAMP-dependent protein kinase that phosphorylates a protein that regulates acid secretion.

Gastrin, compared with acetylcholine and histamine, is not as potent a direct stimulant of parietal cells. Muscarinic antagonists such as atropine, and H_2-receptor blockers such as cimetidine, do not block the direct actions of gastrin, and the second messenger for gastrin action is unknown. However, cimetidine attenuates physiological response to elevated levels of gastrin in the blood, suggesting that physiological response to gastrin may be due to gastrin-stimulated histamine release [12]. When the stomach has been empty for several hours, HCl secretion is at approximately 10% of its maximal rate. The basal rate of HCl secretion varies diurnally and is highest in the evening and lowest in the morning [12]. The mechanisms responsible for diurnal variation are unknown.

Phases of Gastric Acid Secretion

After ingestion of a meal, the rate of acid secretion by the stomach increases promptly. The three phases of increased acid secretion in response to food are the cephalic phase (elicited before food reaches the stomach), the gastric phase (secretion elicited by the presence of food in the stomach), and the intestinal phase (elicited by input originating in the duodenum and upper jejunum) [12]. The major mechanisms that control gastric acid secretion are summarized in Table 3.

The cephalic phase. This phase of gastric secretion is elicited by sight, smell, and taste of food. The acid secretion rate during this phase can be as much as 40% of the maximum rate. Other stimuli sensed in the brain, in addition to those related to presence of food, may evoke acid secretion through vagal impulses. A decreased concentration of glucose in the cerebral anterial blood would elicit acid secretion. A low pH in the antrum will diminish the amount of HCl secreted during the cephalic phase, and the amount of acid secreted is limited by a direct effect on parietal cells.

The gastric phase. The presence of food in the stomach evokes this phase of gastric acid secretion. The principal stimuli include distension of the stomach and the presence of amino acids and peptides. Distension of the body or the antrum of the stomach results in stimulation of the mechanoreceptors that bring about secretion of acetylcholine, HCl, and gastrin.

The intestinal phase. The presence of chyme in the duodenum results in neural and endocrine responses that first stimulate and, later, inhibit secretion of acid by the stomach. The stimulatory influences dominate when the pH of gastric chyme is above 3; however, when the buffer capacity is exhausted and pH falls below 2, inhibitory influences prevail.

Regulation of Gastric Acid Secretion by the Central Nervous System

Gastric acid secretion may be regulated by several brain peptides, some of which may affect pathways that enhance secretion, whereas others may act centrally to inhibit acid secretion. Norepinephrine appears to be the neurotransmitter in some central pathways that inhibit gastric acid secretion, whereas γ-aminobutyric acid is the transmitter for certain pathways that stimulate acid secretion [12].

Factors Influencing Bioavailability

Table 3 Major Mechanisms Affecting Gastric Acid Secretion

Stimulus	Pathway/mediator	Stimulus to parietal cell for gastric acid secretion	Inhibit gastrin release	Inhibit acid secretion
Chewing, swallowing, etc. (cephalic phase)	Vagus nerve to: 1. Parietal cells 2. G cells	Acetylcholine Gastrin		
Gastric distension (gastric phase)	Local and vasovagal reflexes to: 1. Parietal cells 2. G cells	Acetylcholine Gastrin		
Protein digestion products in duodenum (intestinal phase)	1. Intestinal G cells 2. Intestinal endocrine cells	Gastrin Enterooxyntin		
Acid (pH < 3.0) in antrum	None, direct		+	
Acid pH in duodenum	Secretin, bulbogastrone, nervous reflex		+ +	+ + +
Hyperosmotic solutions, fatty acids, monoglycerides in duodenum and jejunum	Unidentified enterogastrone, gastric inhibitory peptide, cholecystokinin		+	+ + +

Source: Modified from Ref. 12.

Sublingual or Buccal

The major advantage of administering drugs by this route is that drugs directly and rapidly enter the systemic circulation, bypassing the liver. For drugs that are subject to first-pass metabolism, this route will provide higher systemic availability, compared with oral doses [25]. Nitroglycerin tablets are administered by this route to facilitate rapid therapeutic drug concentrations. Certain hormones, such as methyltestosterone and oxytocin, as well as other drugs that require small doses to elicit a biological response, can be administered by the buccal cavity.

Physicochemical properties of the drug and its dosage form must be compatible with the intended use by the sublingual or buccal route. In addition to nitroglycerin tablets, which are formulated to dissolve rapidly to provide prompt relief from angina attacks, buccal controlled-release nitroglycerin formulations have been developed and are popular in the clinic [26,27].

Some of the main disadvantages of administering drugs by buccal route would be unpleasant taste, inconvenience, and the need to retain drug formulation in the mouth for long periods. However, interest in this route of drug administration, particularly for controlled-release formulations, is apparent in the number of drugs that are being tested for this route. Nifedipine, isoproterenol (isoprenaline), oxytocin, and steroids are some compounds being evaluated as possible candidates for buccal administration [28].

Inhalation

Drugs administered by inhalation are generally given for their local effect, such as for treatment of airway obstruction. The objective of inhalation therapy is to deliver drugs to the site of maximum effect in the respiratory tract, and successful use of this route is dependent on efficiency in drug delivery.

The formulation selected for a drug aerosol depends on the intended use of the product. Aerosol contents may be expelled as a fine mist, a coarse, wet or a dry spray, a steady stream, or a stable or fast-breaking foam. In the treatment of asthma or emphysema, drug particles are presented as a fine liquid mist or finely divided solid particles. Particles smaller than 6 μm will reach the respiratory bronchioles, and those smaller than 2 μm will reach the alveolar ducts and alveoli. However, when deposition in the trachea and the primary and secondary bronchioles is desired, for localized effects, a particle range of 20–60 μm is necessary [29,30].

Lung endothelium provides a large surface area for absorption because of the dense network of capillaries and the many projections and indentations of the endothelial cells. Lipophilicity of the active drug would be another facilitating factor for drug absorption from the lungs.

Particles are removed from the respiratory tract by motion of the cilia, viscous mucous lining on the surface of the respiratory tract, coughing, and scavenging by alveolar macrophages [31]. In addition to physical removal of particles, systemic availability of drugs may be reduced by first-pass pulmonary metabolism. Capillary endothelial cells in the lungs, rich with enzymes, are anticipated to be possible sites for metabolic activity. Similar to the enzymes in the liver, a variety of drug-metabolizing enzymes, such as microsomal mixed function oxidases, amine oxidase, monoamine oxidase, reductases, esterases, and a variety of conjugases, are reported to be present in the lungs [32,33].

The major disadvantages in use of inhalation for most systemically acting compounds are inability to deliver drug substances to the optimal site, high intrinsic clearance, and metabolic defense mechanisms.

Terbutalin, metaproterenol, albuterol, fenoterol, bitolterol, and cromolyn sodium (disodium cromoglycate; DSG) are among compounds that are administered by this route [28].

Assessment of Lung Capacity

Respiratory disorders that obstruct the airways, decrease the expiratory airflow rates. The reduction is proportional to the severity of the airway obstruction. The resistive properties of the airways are commonly assessed from measurements of airflow rates out of the lungs during a rapid, forceful expiratory maneuver. The volume exhaled during the first second is called the forced expiratory volume in 1 sec (FEV_1), and FEV_3 represents the forced expiratory volume exhaled over 3 sec. These parameters are expressed as a percentage of the forced vital capacity (FVC), which is the total volume of air that can be rapidly and forcefully exhaled following a maximal inspiration. The mean airflow rate is measured over the middle half of the forced vital capacity, that is, between 25 and 75% of the vital capacity and is called the maximum midexpiratory flow rate, or the forced midexpiratory flow rate ($FEF_{25-75\%}$).

The $FEF_{25-75\%}$ is a sensitive index of airway obstruction, and this value may be decreased if the airway obstruction is mild or prolonged, with more severe obstruction depending on the time required to expel the vital capacity [34]. These pulmonary parameters, FEV_1, FVC, and $FEF_{25-75\%}$ are evaluated for bioavailability assessment of inhalants. In the FDA guidelines, evaluation of these pulmonary function parameters in asthmatic patients is recommended for comparison of inhalant products such as albuterol and metaproterenol.

Transdermal

Absorption of substances through the skin is known as *percutaneous absorption*. Percutaneous absorption of a drug is dependent not only on the physicochemical properties of the drug, but also on the condition of the skin.

Various layers of the skin are illustrated in Figure 3. Upon the surface of the skin is a film of emulsified material composed of sebum, sweat, and desquamating horny layer (epidermal cells, stratum corneum). Beneath the stratum corneum, in sequence, is a barrier layer (living epidermis or the stratum germinativum) and the dermis. Nerve fibers and capillaries travel from the subcutaneous adipose tissue into the dermis and up to the epidermis. Sebacious glands and, similarly, sweat glands and hair follicules originating in the subcutaneous tissue and dermis reach the skin surface as ducts or hairs.

Following topical application, drugs may penetrate intact skin through the walls of the hair follicles, through the sweat glands, sebaceous glands, or between the cells of the stratum corneum [35,36]. Stratum corneum is the principal barrier for most compounds. The skin from which stratum corneum was removed, was shown to be highly permeable, whereas stratum corneum was nearly as

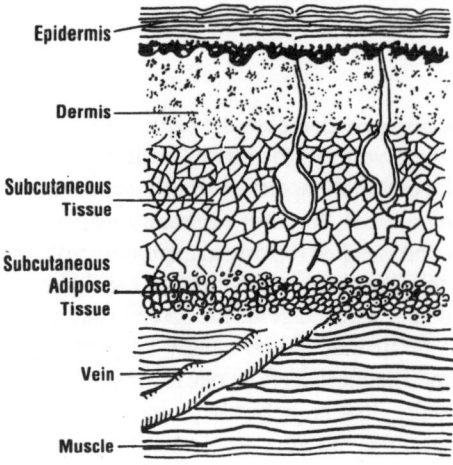

Figure 3 Stratified organization of skin. (From Ref. 35, redrawn with permission.)

impermeable as the entire skin [37]. The degree of hydration of the skin is also another important factor that facilitates transdermal drug absorption, possibly by hydration of lipid channels of the stratum corneum or simply by improving contact and wetting. Behl et al. have shown that hydration increases the penetration of polar molecules more than that of nonpolar ones [38].

Cutaneous metabolism for transdermal absorption of topically applied compounds is another factor that deserves attention. The significance of diffusional and metabolic processes contributing to percutaneous absorption of compounds has been investigated. The percutaneous fate of two model compounds, benzo[a]pyrene (BP) and testosterone, both lipophilic compounds, in skin samples maintained as short-term organ cultures was examined. For permeation of BP, viability of the skin preparation was important and played an essential role in transport of topical BP through the skin. Testosterone, on the other hand, readily permeated both viable and nonviable skin from six mammalian species. Transport of BP and testosterone through the skin was accompanied by varying degrees of cutaneous first-pass metabolism [39]. In another study, stereoselectivity of BP metabolism by human skin was investigated to determine its carcinogenic potential, and interindividual variations in stereoselective metabolism of BP was observed [40].

Both diffusional and metabolic processes are involved in percutaneous absorption. The relative importance of these processes is a function of the physicochemical properties of the compound and the ability of epidermal cells to

Factors Influencing Bioavailability

metabolize the compound. When considering percutaneous absorption, both diffusion of the compound through the skin and also cutaneous biotransformation of the compound should be examined.

Parenteral

Sir Christopher Wren, who was an amateur physiologist and also the architect of St. Paul's Cathedral, was the first person to inject drugs intravenously into dogs, in 1657. Intravenous medication was first given to humans in 1662, but was abandoned for a period because of occurrence of embolism and thrombosis [41].

Drugs administered by the intravenous route enter the systemic circulation directly and, consequently can provide quick clinical response. This route of administration also provides a reference for determining absolute drug availability by other routes. Drug distribution and disposition kinetics can be examined and the magnitude of dose, rate of drug administration, and plasma drug concentrations can be correlated with pharmacologic effect.

The use of jugular vein delivery when determining systemic availability of drugs in laboratory animals has been recommended. The effect of site of intravenous administration on assessment of cyclosporine bioavailability was demonstrated in the rat. The area under curve (AUC) value was highest following drug delivery by jugular vein and was approximately twofold greater than when administered by femoral or penile vein, and fivefold greater than after intraperitoneal administration [42].

Insoluble or suspended drug formulations cannot be administered intravenously, as they can cause embolism or thrombophlebitis. Nevertheless, they can be given by other extravascular routes (i.e., intramuscular, intradermal, and subcutaneous).

Drugs administered by the intramuscular route provide drug effects that are less rapid, but generally of longer duration, than those obtained from intravenous administration. Aqueous or oleaginous solutions or suspensions of drug substances may be administered. Usually, the volume of medication that may be administered by this route is limited; generally, a maximum of 5 mL if administered in the gluteal region and 2 mL in the deltoid muscle of the arm [35].

A number of substances may be injected intradermally. These include various agents for diagnostic determination, desensitization, or immunization. Approximately 0.1-mL volumes can be administered by this route.

The subcutaneous route is ideal for prolonged drug delivery from solutions or suspensions. However, because of less efficient regional circulation, absorption efficacy by this route is usually less than that by the intramuscular route. Commercial products administered subcutaneously include insulin, testosterone, progesterone, penicillin, and some sulfonamides. Volumes administered by this route should generally not exceed 2 mL [35].

Other Routes

Intranasal

The intranasal route of administration can be used for local or systemic effects. To facilitate absorption, a drug may be delivered to the nasal mucosa in the form of a solution as drops, as a nebulized spray, or as an aerosol. The optimal particle size for nasal deposition is 5–10 μm [43].

Nasal absorption of a variety of compounds, such as cardiovascular drugs, antimicrobials, pituitary hormones, gonadotropin-releasing hormones, adrenal and sex hormones, prostaglandins, antihistamines, CNS agents, and insulin, has been investigated [43–45]. Corticosteroids and antihistaminics result in local effects when used for conditions such as nasal allergy, rhinitis, and nasal decongestion.

Despite considerable interest in the use of intranasal route for systemic effects, the only products currently marketed are vasopressin analogues and oxytocin. The physiology of this administration route may be the reason for its limited use. Local toxicity, particularly with chronic use, and the need for surfactants to enhance drug bioavailability are the major disadvantages. However, direct access to pathways connecting the nasopharynx, sinus, and brain and avoidance of presystemic clearance by intranasal route, continue to keep interest alive for this route of administration.

Rectal

Suppositories, although not very popular in United States, are used extensively in European countries. Efficacy of suppositories depends on the drug, physiological factors, and the nature and composition of the vehicle used. Absorption rate of drugs given by rectal route is slower than for orally administered drugs because of reduced absorptive surface area. Rectal absorption is much faster if the drug is administered in solution, as in retention enemas, than as suppositories [7].

Absorption of insulin when administered by the rectal route, the physiological advantages of this route, and the use of absorption promoters were studied. Utilization of the first-pass effect inherent to the rectal anatomy is recommended as a viable means of physiological insulin input [46].

DRUG TRANSPORT

Drug transport across biological membranes occurs by passive diffusion, facilitated diffusion, active transport, pinocytosis, or ionic or electrochemical diffusion.

Passive or Nonionic Diffusion

Passive diffusion is the most common mechanism for drug transport whereby molecules move from a region of high concentration to a region of low concentration [7]. Movement of molecules is directly proportional to the concentration gradient, permeability of the membrane, and is inversely proportional to thickness of the membrane. Application of Ficks law of diffusion yields the following model to describe the rate of change of concentration of a drug diffusing from the mucosal side of the intestinal epithelium into the bloodstream:

$$-dC_g/dt = (DA/V_gh) \cdot (C_g - C_p)$$

where D is the diffusion coefficient, A is the absorptive surface area, C_g concentration of drug in gut, C_p concentration of drug in blood, V_g the effective volume of fluid in the gut, and h the effective thickness of the GI tract barrier.

By combining D and h into one permeability constant P, and for unit surface area (i.e., A = 1), the foregoing equation simplifies to

$$-dC_g/dt = (P/V_g) \cdot (C_g - C_p) = P'(C_g - C_p)$$

where P' is the first-order rate constant for absorption.

Since, during the absorption process, the concentration of drug in blood is much lower than that in the GI tract, a large concentration gradient is maintained throughout the absorption process. To the extent that $C_g >> C_p$, thus

$$-dC_g/dt = P' C_g$$

As diffusion continues and C_p approaches C_g, the net rate approaches zero and equilibrium is established between the two sites.

Facilitated Diffusion

Some compounds move through biological membranes at a rate and to an extent greater than that which can be accounted by simple diffusion. Carriers present within the membrane, which can be enzymes or some other components of GI epithelial cells, are assumed to form a complex with the drug, resulting in an improved membrane permeability for the complex over that of the drug alone. After the complex traverses the membrane, the complex is dissociated and drug is liberated. Facilitated diffusion occurs with the concentration gradient. Transport of vitamins B_1 and B_{12} are examples of compounds that cross membranes by facilitated diffusion processes [7].

Movement of glucose from plasma into erythrocytes is another example. Glucose moves down a concentration gradient from plasma into erythrocytes, without expenditure of energy. At equilibrium, glucose concentrations inside and outside the erythrocyte are equal. At high plasma glucose concentrations, however, the rate of glucose transport into erythrocytes reaches a limiting value, or transport maximum.

Active Transport

Active transport differs from facilitated diffusion in that it takes place when the drug is transported uphill, or against a concentration gradient [7,47], and this requires an energy source. Maintenance of this gradient requires metabolic energy. Active transport, accordingly, can be affected by metabolic inhibitors. Examples of active transport are renal and biliary secretion of many acids and bases; ions and organic substances, such as sodium, calcium, iron, glucose, some amino acids; and intestinal absorption of drugs such as fluorouracil and 5-bromouracil. Common characteristics with passive transport are specificity, competitive inhibition, and saturability.

In active transport processes, the amount of carrier may be limited. Therefore, absorption rate, if an active transport process is involved, will be affected not only by drug concentration, but also by the carrier availability.

Pinocytosis

A transport mechanism similar to phagocytosis, pinocytosis is anticipated to be a capability common to all cells. The cell walls invaginate into a saccular structure engulfing extracellular materials. The saccule is then pinched off from the cell wall and forms a vacuole within the interior of the cell. Transport of macromolecules that are absorbed in the gut is thought to be due to pinocytosis [7].

Ionic or Electrochemical Diffusion

The penetrability of ionized drugs across biological membranes depends on the potential difference or electrical gradient as well as the concentration gradient across the membrane. Because of the positive charge on the outside of membranes, there is a tendency to repel positively charged drug molecules. Thus, only cations with high kinetic energy will be able to penetrate the membrane. Once the cation is inside the epithelial cell, cations will be attracted to the negative charge on the intracellular surface of the membrane, thereby creating an electrical gradient. Movement of the drug will be downhill with the electrical gradient until equilibrium is reached between the intracellular and extracellular drug concentration. The Nernst equation describes the distribution of ionized drug molecules and is a function of intra- and extracellular molar concentration of drug, number of charges on the molecule, and the membrane potential [7].

FACTORS AFFECTING DRUG ABSORPTION

Effect of Blood Flow and Drug Permeability

The slowest, or rate-limiting, steps in drug absorption are blood flow (perfusion rate-limited) or drug penetration through the membrane (diffusion rate-limited).

By removing drug that passes through a membrane, blood flow maintains a concentration gradient and thus assures continuous absorption.

With highly lipid-soluble drugs, or those that pass freely through aqueous-filled pores, penetration through a membrane may be so rapid that equilibrium is promptly established between the drug concentration at the absorption site and that of the drug in blood. Under these conditions the slowest or rate-limiting step controlling drug absorption is blood flow. This is illustrated in Figure 4. Tritiated water moves freely through aqueous pores, and its absorption rate increases with increasing blood flow. Absorption of ethanol and many lipophilic compounds is similarly perfusion rate-limited.

In contrast, with polar compounds such as ribitol (see Fig. 4), absorption is controlled by diffusion through the membrane and is relatively insensitive to changes in blood flow.

Urea is a compound with intermediate permeability characteristics. At low blood flow rates, absorption of urea is perfusion rate-limited because the compound has sufficient time to diffuse across the membrane. However, at higher blood flow rates, membrane permeability becomes rate-limiting and the rate of urea absorption is then insensitive to changes in blood flow [47,48].

In general, absorption of drugs in solution from muscle and subcutaneous tissue is perfusion rate-limited. Increased blood flow increases drug absorption. The main barrier to drug absorption here is the capillary wall, which at these sites is a much more loosely knit structure than the epithelial lining of the GI tract. The capillary wall permits rapid passage of all molecules below a molecular weight of 5000, whether ionized or un-ionized. Neomycin, a relatively water-soluble polar base, is absorbed rapidly from the intramuscular site, whereas it has difficulty penetrating the GI mucosa [47].

Effect of pH

Most drugs are weak acids or weak bases. According to the pH partition hypothesis, only un-ionized nonpolar drug penetrates the membrane. At equilibrium, the concentration of un-ionized species is equal on both sides of the membrane. The fraction of un-ionized drug at the absorption site is controlled by both the pH and the pKa of the drug, according to the Henderson–Hasselbalch equation [49]. Since the gastric pH may vary from 1 to 7, a pH in this range would be suitable for studying the effect of pH changes on absorption. Very weak acids, such as phenytoin and many barbiturates, the pKa values of which are higher than 7.5, are essentially un-ionized at all pH values and, therefore, their absorption should be independent of pH. For acids with pKa values in the range of 2.5–7.5, the un-ionized fraction changes with pH, and the absorption rate of these compounds is pH-dependent. For weak bases with pKa values lower than 5,

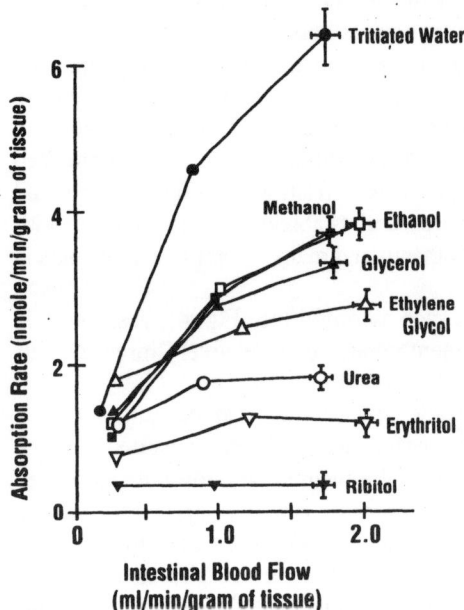

Figure 4 Effect of intestinal blood flow on absorption rate. (From Ref. 48, redrawn with permission.)

absorption would be independent of pH. With stronger bases, the pKa values of which range from 5 to 11, absorption would be pH-dependent.

It is important to recognize that the pH partition hypothesis does not explain all observations. Absorption of ionized species through the intestinal epithelium has been reported. A variety of quaternary ammonium compounds, which are always ionized, were shown to elicit systemic effects following oral dosing [47].

Dissolution Rate

The dissolution rate of solid dosage forms may be a major factor controlling the rate and extent of absorption, particularly for sparingly soluble drugs. There are numerous factors, such as particle size, blending time, differences in the amount of disintegrants, and binders, that would alter the dissolution rates and, possibly, in vivo bioavailability [50–52]. The effect of reducing the amount of disintegrant (Veegum) is illustrated in Figure 5. Oral administration of commercial tolbutamide tablets (Orinase) produced higher blood levels and lower blood glucose, whereas the experimental formulation, which contained half the amount of the disintegrant,

Factors Influencing Bioavailability

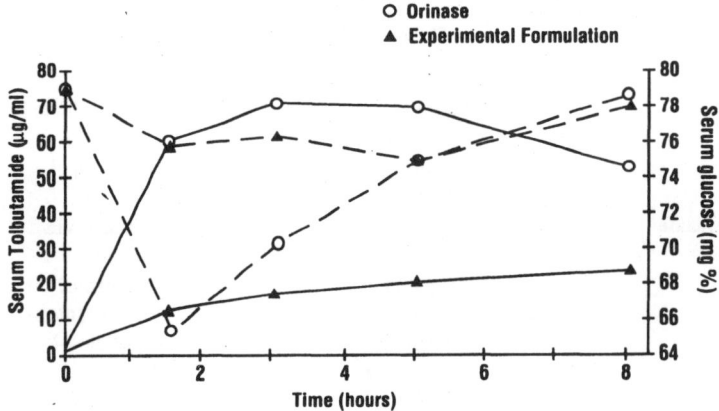

Figure 5 Serum tolbutamide (———) and serum glucose (- - -) concentrations following administration of Orinase and an experimental formulation. (From Ref. 52, redrawn with permission.)

yielded lower plasma tolbutamide concentrations and was not as effective in lowering blood glucose levels [52].

Food and Fluid Volume

The influence of food and diet on drug absorption has been recognized for some time and has been studied extensively during recent years. Food–drug interactions are difficult to predict and occur because of a variety of reasons such as effect of food on physiological function and/or because of physicochemical interactions. Changes in stomach-emptying rate, intestinal motility, splanchnic blood flow, acid or bile secretions, and changes in absorptive processes are examples of physiological food–drug interactions, whereas factors that alter dissolution or cause chelating and adsorption are examples of physicochemical interactions [28,53–55].

Drug absorption may be reduced, delayed, increased, or unaffected by the presence of food. A list of drugs, the absorption of which is altered in the presence of food, has been reviewed by Welling [28] and is summarized in Table 4.

The effect of food and type of diet on bioavailability of erythromycin is illustrated in Figure 6. The extent of erythromycin absorption is reduced when a single dose of 500-mg erythromycin stearate tablet is administered with food or with 20 mL of water, compared with when it is given with 250 mL of water under fasting conditions [56]. Figures 7 and 8 illustrate a significant food effect

Table 4 Example of Drugs the Absorption of Which Is Altered by Food

Reduced	Delayed	Increased
Ampicillin	Acetaminophen	Acitretin
Aspirin	Aspirin	Cholorothiazide
Atenolol	Cephalosporins	Diazepam
Captopril	(most)	Dicoumarol
Ethanol	Diclofenac	Diftalone
Hydrochlorothiazide	Digoxin	Griseofulvin
Iron	Furosemide	Labetalol
Levodopa	Indoprofen	Metoprolol
Penicillamine	Nitrofurantoin	Nitrofurantoin
Penicillins	Sulfadiazine	Propranolol
Sotalol	Sulfisoxazole	Riboflavin
Tetracylines	Valproate	
(most)		
Warfarin		

Source: Data compiled from Refs. 28, 53–55.

on cephradine and acitretin bioavailability. Food significantly reduces the rate and extent of cephradine absorption [57]. In contrast, the extent of acitretin absorption is doubled in the presence of food. This is thought to be due to increased drug solubility, increased lymphatic absorption, and prolonged residence time in the GI tract [58].

Drug administration with a larger fluid volume will improve its dissolution characteristics and may also result in rapid emptying of drug from the stomach. Rapid delivery of drug to an environment more suitable for absorption will provide better and more reproducible absorption. The effect of fluid volume on drug absorption has been reviewed [59] and an example is also provided in Figure 6.

Antacids

Drug-antacid interactions have been reported for many drugs. Absorption of chlorpromazine, digitoxin, digoxin, iron, isoniazid, naproxen, pentobarbital sodium, quinine sulfate, sulfadiazine sodium, and tetracyclines decreases in the presence of antacids. On the other hand, absorption of aspirin, bishydroxycoumarin, levodopa, naproxen, pseudoephedrine HCl, and sulfadiazine acid increases. Concomitant antacid administration does not affect absorption of chlordiazepoxide HCl, quinidine sulfate, and warfarin sodium [60].

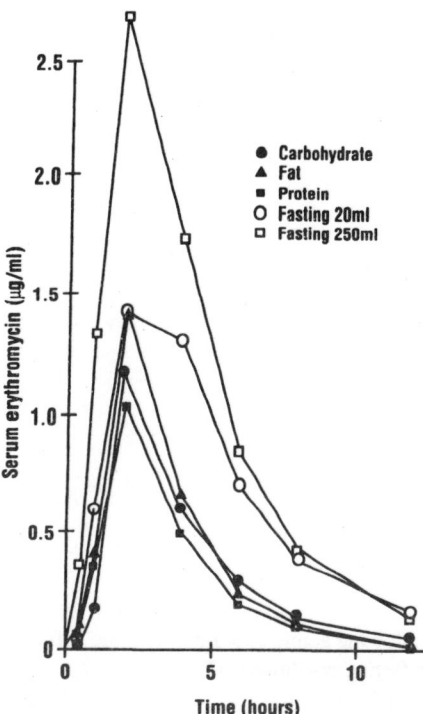

Figure 6 Serum erythromycin concentrations obtained following administration of a single dose of 500-mg erythromycin stearate tablet with food and under fasting conditions with different fluid volumes. (From Ref. 56.)

Drug Metabolism in Intestinal Mucosa

A variety of drugs are metabolized in the gut wall. Metabolism of drugs in the gut lumen and wall can decrease bioavailability and introduce significant variability in therapeutic efficacy of a wide range of drugs.

The role of gut wall metabolism on systemic bioavailability has been reviewed by Ilett et al. [61]. In vitro metabolism of ethinyl estradiol was studied using jejunal mucosa from healthy volunteers and patients with celiac disease who were on a gluten-free diet. The ability of the mucosa to form conjugates in celiac patients was significantly reduced, compared with healthy persons. In healthy females, the ratio of area under curve value of sulfate conjugate to unchanged drug, ethinyl estradiol, was almost three times higher after oral administration than after intravenous administration. Concentrations of ethinyl estradiol

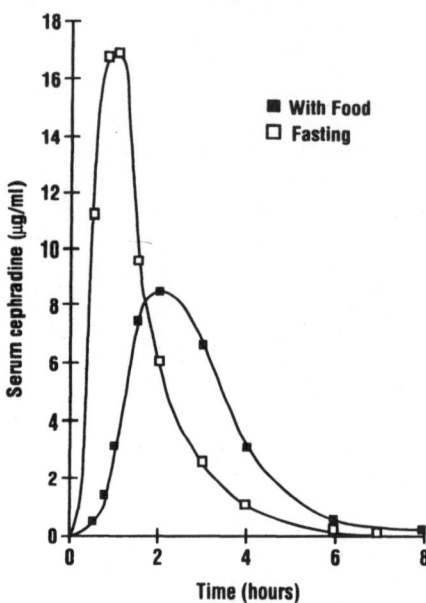

Figure 7 Serum cephradine concentrations following administration of a single 500-mg oral cephradine capsule with food and under fasting conditions. (From Ref. 57.)

metabolites in the portal vein, compared with the systemic circulation, suggested that a considerable proportion of absorbed ethinyl estradiol had been metabolized, presumably in the gut wall [62,63].

The extent of first-pass metabolism for orally administered drugs depends on the enzyme activity in the mucosal epithelial cells and the rate of drug transfer through the mucosal cells [64]. Drug pKa and oil/water partition coefficients are among the factors controlling transfer of drug from systemic circulation to the intestinal metabolic sites [65]. Villous tips had the highest enzyme activity, which decreased progressively toward the crypts [66]. Metabolic activity, in general, is higher at the epithelial cells of the duodenum and jejunum than in the ileum and colon [67–70]. However, metabolic activity is reported to be similar in the mouse duodenum and colon [61].

Metabolism in the gut wall may be inhibited or induced by dietary or environmental xenobiotics or by coadministered drugs. Phase 1 and phase 2 metabolic reactions occurring in the gut wall of the rat, dog, monkey, human, chimpanzee, cow, rabbit, guinea pig, hamster, pig, baboon, and mouse have been described by Ilett et al. [61]. Metabolic reactions occurring in gut wall of humans are listed in Table 5.

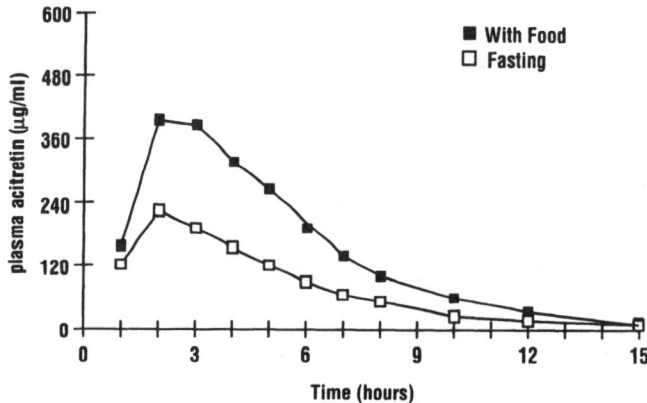

Figure 8 Plasma acitretin concentrations obtained following administration of 2 × 50-mg acitretin capsules with food and under fasting conditions. (From Ref. 58, redrawn with permission.)

Important drug interactions in the intestinal wall have been reported. Both acetaminophen (paracetamol) and ascorbic acid conjugate with intestinal mucosal sulfate and cause a 22 and 48%, respectively, increase an bioavailability of 30–50 µg of concomitantly administered oral ethinyl estradiol [71,72].

Metabolic Activity of the Intestinal Microflora

Metabolism by gut flora is quantitatively less important than that occurring presystemically in the gut wall. This is a consequence of the highest concentrations of metabolizing enzymes residing in the upper gut, where most drug absorption occurs.

Drug metabolism in gut lumen proceeds largely by organisms residing in the lower gut and, hence, has minimal effect on most orally administered drugs. However, slowly absorbed orally administered drugs and drugs administered by the rectal route may be subject to substantial bacterial metabolism. The large intestine contains billions of microorganisms.

Habitat and diet play major orles in determining the flora of each individual. The influence of diet on the number and type of bacteria found in the GI tract of humans is unclear. Two studies have shown that extreme variations in diet do not significantly alter the microflora [73,74], whereas other studies have shown the opposite effect [75,76].

Increased colonization of bacteria in the lower gut was observed when dietary refined carbohydrates and fat are increased and fiber is decreased, resulting in

Table 5 Phase 1 and Phase 2 Metabolic Reactions Occurring in Human Gut Wall

Reactions/enzyme	Substrate	Method[a]
Phase 1		
Oxidation	Ethanol	1, 2
C-Hydroxylation	Benzo[a]pyrene	1
	Ethinyl estradiol	3
N-Dealkylation	Flurazepam	2
Phase 2		
Glucuronidation		
Ester	Hyodeoxycholic acid	1
Ether	Ethinyl estradiol	3, 4
Sulfation		
	Ethinyl estradiol	1, 3
Glutathione conjugation	Isorbide dinitrate	1
O-Acetylation	N-Hydroxyamino fluorene	1
Nonspecific deesterification	N/A[b]	5
Deesterification	Pivampicillin	2
β-Glucuronidase	N/A	1, 5, 6
Sulfatases	p-Acetylphenyl or p-nitrophenyl sulfate	

[a]Methods used for determination of metabolic reaction: (1) Tissue homogenates, or subcellular fractions; (2) in vivo experiments; (3) Using chambers; (4) in situ perfused gut loops; (5) histochemical techniques; (6) intestinal mucosal cells.
[b]Not applicable.
Source: Data from Ref. 61.

a marked increase in intestinal transit time [77]. High levels of dietary cellulose increased fecal β-glucosidase, whereas there was a significant decrease in fecal β-glucuronidase activity for estrogen glucuronides in vegetarian than in omnivorous women [77,78].

Bacterial enzymes are important because of their participation in the conservation of nutrients, metabolism of endogenous and dietary substrates, and also metabolism of drugs. Systemic availability of sulfasalazine (salicylazosulfapyridine) is dependent on bacterial enzymes. Sulfasalazine, used for treatment of inflammation of the large bowel, is a sulfonamide linked to salicylate by an azo bond that is resistant to mammalian enzymes. However, in the colon, bacteria hydrolyze the azo bond to release sulfapyridine and salicylic acid. The components are thought to exert the therapeutic effect [79,80].

The diverse metabolic activities of the mammalian gut microflora are well documented. The role of microflora in altering toxicological properties of ingested compounds by catalyzing various reactions is well known. Certain nitro compounds, such as dinitrotoluene and nitrobenzene, which depend on microbial reduction for their toxic effects, might be expected to be more potent in rats, mice, and hamsters than in humans, since nitroreductase activity of the human microflora is much lower than that in rodents [81,82].

Another important role of the intestinal microflora is in the enterohepatic recycling of compounds, such as digoxin, ouabain, oral contraceptives, promazine, and endogenous compounds such as cholesterol, and bile acids. These compounds are well absorbed and are generally conjugated to more polar metabolites in the liver before their secretion into the bile. Hydrolysis of these conjugates are catalyzed in the small intestine by bacterial enzymes such as β-glucuronidase, sulfatase, and various glycosides.

Altered bioavailability because of the effect of antibiotics on bacterial enzymes that are responsible for hydrolysis of drug conjugates that undergo enterohepatic recycling has also been reported. Therapeutic failure of oral contraceptives containing norethindrone (norethisterone), ethinyl estradiol, and mestranol, when administered concurrently with antibiotics, has been suggested to be due to decreased enterohepatic recycling of steroid conjugates excreted in bile [83,84]. Other investigators have correlated therapeutic failure of the oral contraceptives with a decreased mass of intestinal microflora [85,86]. Therapeutic efficacy of digoxin in patients with cardiac failure was reported to increase after erythromycin therapy. Digoxin is inactivated by bacterial reduction of the lactone ring to its inactive metabolite dihydrodigoxin. Following erythromycin treatment of patients, a two- to threefold increase in digoxin steady-state concentrations, with decrease in urinary excretion of dihydrodigoxin, were observed [87]. Interethnic variations in occurrence of the bacteria that reduce digoxin and its effect on digoxin availability have also been reported [88].

CONCLUSIONS

Bioavailability and bioequivalence of drugs are influenced by the drug, the dosage form, and the interaction of these with the complex environment of the absorption site. For orally administered compounds, many factors including GI anatomy and physiology, bacterial, mucosal, and hepatic metabolism may affect absorption. The possible contribution of all of these factors must be considered when examining drug absorption, when interpreting the results of bioavailability and bioequivalence studies, and when designing drugs and dosage forms to optimize absorption characteristics to achieve desired therapeutic goals.

REFERENCES

1. FDCA Section 505(j)(7)(A), 21 U.S.C. 355(j)(7)(A).
2. 21 CFR 320.1(a)(1987).
3. Approved Drug Products with Therapeutic Equivalence Evaluations, 10th ed. U.S. Dept. of Health and Human Services, Public Health Service Food and Drug Administration Center for Drug Evaluation and Research Office of Management. Rockville, MD, pp. 1–9, 1990.
4. D. O. Beers. Abbreviated new drug applications and "Paper NDAs". In *Generic Drugs—A Guide to FDA Approval Requirements*. Prentice Hall Law & Business, p. 83–135 (1988).
5. H. C. Ansel and N. G. Popovich. Dosage form design: Biopharmaceutic considerations. In *Pharmaceutical Dosage Forms and Drug Delivery Systems*, 5th ed. Lea & Febiger, Malvern, Pa., pp. 51–91, (1990).
6. S. C. Harvey. Drug absorption, action, and disposition. In *Remington's Pharmaceutical Sciences* 15th ed. (A. Osol, D. Grafton, A. R. Gennaro, M. R. Gibson, C. B. Granberg, S. C. Harvey, R. E. King, A. N. Martin, E. A. Swinyard, and G. L. Zink, eds.) Mack Publishing, Easton, Pa., p. 680 (1975).
7. H. M. Abdou. Mechanism of drug absorption. In *Dissolution, Bioavailability and Bioequivalence*. Mack Publishing, Easton, Pa., pp. 303–314 (1989).
8. H. C. Kutchai. Gastrointestinal motility. In *Physiology*, 2nd ed. (R. M. Berne and M. N. Levy, eds.) C. V. Mosby, St. Louis, pp. 649–681 (1988).
9. M. Costa and J. B. Furness. Neuronal peptides in the intestine. *Br. Med. Bull.* 38:247–252 (1982).
10. J. H. Meyer. Motility of the stomach and gastroduodenal junction. In *Physiology of Gastrointestinal Tract*, 2nd ed. (L. R. Johnson, ed.) Raven Press, New York, pp. 613–629, (1987).
11. W. F. Ganong. Gastrointestinal secretion and motility. In *Review of Medical Physiology*, 10th ed. Lange Medical Publications, Los Altos, Calif., pp. 380–404, (1981).
12. H. C. Kutchai. Gastrointestinal secretions. In *Physiology*, 2nd ed. (R. M. Berne and M. N. Levy, eds.) C. V. Mosby, St. Louis, pp. 682–717 (1988).
13. V. Varro, T. Varkonyi, and P. V. Veghelyi. *Absorption and Malabsorption Clinical Aspects* (Akademiai Kiado, Budapest, 1988) Distr. H. Stilman Publishers, Boca Raton, Fl., pp. 13–55 (1988).
14. N. W. Weisbrodt. Motility of the small intestine. In *Physiology of the Gastrointestinal Tract*, 2nd ed. (L. R. Johnson, ed.) Raven Press, New York, pp. 631–663 (1987).
15. J. S. Trier. Structure of the mucosa of the small intestine as it relates to intestinal function. *Fed. Proc.* 26:1391–1404 (1967).
16. J. Bienenstock, M. McDermott, and D. Befus. A common mucosal immune system. In *Immunology of Breast Milk* (P. Ogra and D. Dayton, eds.) Raven Press, New York, p. 91–104 (1979).
17. M. F. Kagnoff. Immunology of the digestive system. In *Physiology of the Gastrointestinal Tract* (L. R. Johnson, ed.) Raven Press, New York, p. 1337–1359 (1981).
18. W. A. Walker, M. Wu, K. J. Bloch. Stimulation by immune complexes of mucus release from goblet cells of the rat small intestine. *Science* 197:370–372 (1977).

19. E. S. Fubara and R. Freter. Protection against enteric bacterial infection by secretory IgA antibodies. *J. Immunol. 111*:395-403 (1973).
20. Z. Itoh and T. Sekiguchi. Interdigestive motor activity in health and disease. *Scand. J. Gastroenterol. Suppl. 82*:121-134 (1983).
21. P. A. Thomas, K. A. Kelly, and V. L. W. Go. Does motilin regulate canine interdigestive gastric motility? *Dig. Dis. Sci. 24*:577-582 (1979).
22. S. F. Phillips and G. J. Devroede. Functions of the large intestine. In *International Review of Physiology Gastrointestinal Physiology III*, vol. 19 (R. K. Crane, ed.), University Park Press, Baltimore, pp. 263-290, (1979).
23. W. S. Nimmo. Drugs, diseases and altered gastric emptying. *Clin. Pharmacokinet. 1*:189-203 (1976).
24. H. W. Davenport. *Physiology of the Digestive Tract*, 4th ed. Year Book Medical Publishers, Chicago, p. 112 (1978).
25. A. Beckett and E. Triggs. Buccal absorption of basic drugs and its application as an in vivo model of passive drug transfer through lipid membranes. *J. Pharm. Pharmac. 19*, suppl, 315-415 (1967).
26. J. Abrams. Nitroglycerin and long-acting nitrates. *N. Engl. J. Med. 302*:1234-1237 (1980).
27. A. Lahiri, T. N. Sonecha, J. W. Crawley, and E. B. Raferty. Efficacy of sustained release buccal nitroglycerin in patients with ischaemic cardiomyopathy. *Clin. Sci. 63*:38 (1982).
28. P. G. Welling. Dosage routes, bioavailability, and clinical efficacy. In *Pharmacokinetics Regulatory, Industrial, Academic Perspectives* (P. G. Welling and F. L. S. Tse, eds.) Marcel Dekker, New York, pp. 97-157 (1988).
29. H. C. Ansel and N. G. Popovich. Aerosols, inhalations and sprays. In *Pharmaceutical Dosage Forms and Drug Delivery Systems*, 5th ed. Lea & Febiger, Malvern, Pa., pp. 390-405 (1990).
30. M. Lippman, D. B. Yeates, and R. E. Albert. Deposition, retention and clearance of inhaled particles. *Br. J. Ind. Med. 37*:337-362 (1980).
31. D. Pavia, J. R. M. Bateman, and S. W. Clarke. Deposition and clearance of inhaled particles. *Bull. Eur. Physiopathol. Respir. 16*:335-366 (1980).
32. D. J. Benford and J. W. Bridges. Xenobiotic metabolism in lung. In *Progress in Drug Metabolism*, vol. 9, (J. W. Bridges and L. F. Chasseaud, eds.) Taylor and Francis, London and Philadelphia, pp. 53-94 (1986).
33. D. Davies. Pharmacokinetic studies with inhaled drugs. *Eur. J. Respir. Dis. 63*:67-72 (1982).
34. N. S. Cherniack. M. G. Altose, and S. G. Kelsen. Organization and mechanics of the respiratory system. In *Physiology*, 2nd ed. (R. M. Berne and M. N. Levy, eds.) C. V. Mosby, St. Louis, pp. 575-597 (1988).
35. H. C. Ansel and N. G. Popovich. Injections, sterile fluids, and products of biotechnology. In *Pharmaceutical Dosage Forms and Drug Delivery Systems*, 5th ed. Lea & Febiger, Malvern, Pa., pp. 255-306 (1990).
36. H. C. Ansel and N. G. Popovich. Transdermal drug delivery systems, ointments, creams, lotions, and other preparations. In *Pharmaceutical Dosage Forms and Drug Delivery Systems*, 5th ed. Lea & Febiger, Malvern, Pa., pp. 307-346 (1990).

37. S. Monash and H. Blank. Location and reformation of the epithelial barrier to water vapour. *AMA Arch. Dermatol. 78*:710-714 (1958).
38. C. R. Behl, G. L. Flynn, T. Kurihara, N. Harper, W. Smith, W. I. Higuchi, N. F. H. Ho, and C. L. Pierson. Hydration and percutaneous absorption 1. Influence of hydration of alkanol permeation through hairless mouse skin. *J. Invest. Dermatol. 75*:346-352 (1980).
39. J. Kao, F. K. Patterson, and J. Hall. Skin penetration and metabolism of topically applied chemicals in six mammalian species, including man: An in vitro study with benzo[a]pyrene and testosterone. *Toxicol. Appl. Pharmacol. 81*:502-516 (1985).
40. M. Hall and P. L. Grover. Stereoselective aspects of the metabolic activation of benzo[a]pyrene by human skin in vitro. *Chem. Biol. Interact. 64*:281-296 (1988).
41. P. H. Van Itallie. The rugged beginning of injection therapy. *Pulse Pharmacy 19*:3-8 (1965).
42. D. R. Luke, L. J. Brunner, and K. Vadiei. Bioavailability assessment of cyclosporine in the rat. *Am. Soc. Pharmacol. Exp. Ther. 18*:158-162 (1990).
43. L. Illum. Drug delivery systems for nasal application. *STP Pharm. 3*:594-598 (1987).
44. S.-F. Chang and Y. W. Chien. Intranasal drug administration for systemic medication. In *Pharmacy International*. Reference ed. Elsevier Science Publishers, Amsterdam, p. 287-288 (1984).
45. M. S. Nolte, C. Taboga, E. Salamon, A. Moses, J. Longenecker, J. Flier, and J. H. Karam. Biological activity of nasally administered insulin in normal subjects. *Horm. Metab. Res. 22*:170-174 (1990).
46. W. A. Ritschel and G. B. Ritschel. Rectal administration of insulin. *Methods Find. Exp. Clin. Pharmacol. 6*:513-529 (1984).
47. M. Rowland and T. N. Tozer. Absorption. In *Clinical Pharmacokinetics Concepts and Applications*. Lea & Febiger, Philadelphia, pp. 16-33, (1980).
48. D. Winne and J. Remischovsky. Intestinal blood flow and absorption of nondissociable substances. *J. Pharm. Pharmacol. 22*:640-641 (1970).
49. K. A. Connors. Aqueous acid-base titrations. In *A Textbook of Pharmaceutical Analysis*. 2nd ed. Wiley-Interscience, New York, pp. 3-44 (1975).
50. M. I. Morasso, R. Pezoa, Y. Villanueva, M. N. Gai, and A. Arancibia. Effect of mixing on the bioavailability of nitrofurantoin capsules. *Il Farmaco 45*:123-130 (1990).
51. T. Dahl, T. Ling, J. Yee, and A. Bormeth. Effects of various granulating systems on the bioavailability of naproxen sodium from polymeric matrix tablets. *J. Pharm. Sci. 79*:389-392 (1990).
52. A. B. Varley. The generic inequivalence of drugs. *JAMA 206*:1745-1748 (1968).
53. P. G. Welling. Effects of gastrointestinal disease on drug absorption. In *Pharmacokinetic Basis for Drug Treatment* (L. Z. Benet, N. Massoud, and J. G. Gambertoglio, eds.) Raven Press, New York, pp. 29-48 (1984).
54. D. B. Williams, W. J O'Reilly, G. Boehm, and M. J. Story. Absorption of doxycycline from a controlled release pellet formulation: The influence of food on bioavailability. *Biopharm. Drug Dispos. 11*:93-105 (1990).
55. M. A. Osman, R. B. Patel, A. Schuna, W. R. Sundstrom, and P. G. Welling. Reduction in oral penicillamine absorption by food, antacid, and ferrous sulfate. *Clin. Pharmacol. Ther. 33*:465-470 (1983).

56. P. G. Welling, H. Huang, P. F. Hewitt, and L. L. Lyons. Bioavailability of erythromycin stearate: Influence of food and fluid volume. *J. Pharm. Sci.* 67:764–766 (1978).
57. T. W. Mischler, A. A. Sugermann, D. A. Willard, L. J. Brannick, and E. S. Neiss. Influence of probenecid and food on the bioavailability of cephradine in normal subjects. *J. Clin. Pharmacol. Ther.* 22:108–112 (1974).
58. P. J. McNamara, R. C. Jewell, B. K. Jenson, and C. J. Brindley. Food increases the bioavailability of acitretin. *J. Clin. Pharmacol.* 28:1051–1055 (1988).
59. P. G. Welling and F. L. S. Tse. Factors contributing to variability in drug pharmacokinetics. I. absorption. *J. Clin. Hosp. Pharm.* 9:163–179 (1984).
60. J. A. Romankiewicz. Effects of antacids on gastrointestinal absorption of drugs. *Primary Care* 3:537–550 (1976).
61. K. F. Ilett, L. B. G. Tee, P. T. Reeves, and R. F. Minchin. Metabolism of drugs and other xenobiotics in the gut lumen and wall. *Pharmacol. Ther.* 46:67–93 (1990).
62. D. J. Back, M. Bates, A. M. Breckenridge, A. Ellis, J. M. Hall, M. Maciver, M. L'E. Orme, and P. H. Rowe. The in vitro metabolism of ethinyloestradiol, mestranol and levonorgestrel by human jejunal mucosa. *Br. J. Clin. Pharmacol.* 11:275–278 (1981).
63. D. J. Back, M. Bates, A. M. Breckenridge, F. Crawford, A. Ellis, J. M. Hall, M. MacIver, M. L'E. Orme, I. Taylor, and P. H. Rowe. In *Drug Metabolism by Gastrointestinal Mucosa: Clinical Aspects* (L. F. Prescott and W. S. Nimmo, eds.) AIDS Press, New York, pp. 80–87 (1981).
64. P. J. Borm, A. C. Frankhuyzen-Sierevogel, E. B. C. Weller, and J. Noordhoek. Absorption and metabolism of hexamethylmelamine and pentamethylmelamine in rat everted perfused gut segments: Correlation with in vivo data. *J. Pharm. Pharmacol.* 37:629–636 (1985).
65. K. F. Ilett and D. S. Davies. In vivo studies of gut wall metabolism. In *Clinical Pharmacology and Therapeutics 1. Presystemic Drug Elimination* (C. F. George, D. G. Shand, and A. G. Renwick, eds.) Butterworths, London, pp. 43–65 (1982).
66. D. M. Pestalozzi, R. Buhler, J. P. von Wartburg, and M. Hess. Immunohistochemical localization of alcohol dehydrogenase in the human gastrointestinal tract. *Gastroenterology* 85:1011–1016 (1983).
67. K. Hartiala. Metabolism of hormones, drugs, and other substances by the gut. *Physiol. Rev.* 53:496–534 (1973).
68. H. Bostrom, D. Bromster, H. Nordenstam, and B. Wengle. On the occurrence of phenol and steroid sulphokinases in the human gastrointestinal tract. *Scand. J. Gastroenterol.* 3:369–375 (1968).
69. P. G. Traber, J. Chianale, R. Florence, K. Kim, E. Wojcik, and J. J. Gumucio. Expression of cytochrome P450b and P450e genes in small intestine mucosa of rats following treatment with phenobarbital, polyhalogenated biphenyls, and organochlorine pesticides. *J. Biol. Chem.* 263:9449–9455 (1988).
70. R. I. Russell, R. MacAllister, and R. Campbell. Relationship of β-glucuronidase activity in gastric juice to the histology of the gastric mucosa. *Gastroenterology* 58:352–357 (1970).
71. S. M. Rogers, D. J. Back, P. J. Stevenson, S. F. M. Grimmer, and M. L'E. Orme. Pharacetamol interaction with oral contraceptive steroids: Increased plasma concentrations of ethinyloestradiol. *Br. J. Clin. Pharmacol.* 23:721–725 (1987).

72. D. J. Back, A. M. Breckenridge, M. MacIver, M. L'E. Orme, H. Purba, and P. H. Rowe. Interaction of ethinyloestradiol with ascorbic acid in man. *Br. Med. J.* 282:1516 (1981).
73. J. H. Moore, R. C. Nobel, W. Steele, and J. W. Czerawski. Differences in the metabolism of esterified and unesterified linoleic acid by rumen microorganisms. *Br. J. Nutr.* 23:869–878 (1969).
74. V. Aries, J. S. Crowther, B. S. Drasar, M. J. Hill, and F. R. Ellis. The effect of a strict vegetarian diet on the faecal flora and faecal steroid concentration. *J. Pathol.* 103:54–56 (1970).
75. V. Aries, J. S. Crowther, B. S. Drasar, M. J. Hill, and R. E. O. Williams. Bacteria and the aetiology of cancer of the large bowel. *Gut* 10:334–335 (1969).
76. B. S. Drasar, P. Goddard, S. Heaton, S. Peach, and B. West. Clostridia isolated from faeces. *J. Med. Microbiol.* 9:63–71 (1976).
77. G. W. Chang, H. E. Fukumoto, C. P. Gyory, A. P. Block, M. J. Kretsch, and D. H. Calloway. Effects of diet on the gut microflora: Fecal enzymes and bacterial metabolites. *Fed. Proc. Fed. Am. Soc. Exp. Biol.* 38:767 (1979).
78. B. R. Goldin, H. Aldercreutz, S. L. Gorbach, J. H. Warram, J. T. Dwyer, L. Swenson, and M. N. Woods. Estrogen excretion patterns and plasma levels in vegetarian and omnivorous women. *N. Engl. J. Med.* 307:1542–1547 (1982).
79. M. A. Peppercorn and P. Goldman. The role of intestinal bacteria in the metabolism of salicylazosulfapyridine. *J. Pharmacol. Exp. Ther.* 181:555–562 (1972).
80. H. Schroder and B. E. Gustafsson. Azo reduction of salicylazosulfapyridine in germfree and conventional rats. *Xenobiotica* 3:225–231 (1973).
81. I. R. Rowland. Factors affecting metabolic activity of the intestinal microflora. In *Drug Metabolism Reviews*. Marcel Dekker, New York, pp. 243–261 (1988).
82. R. S. Goldstein, J. P. Chism, J. M. Sherril, and T. E. Hamm. Influence of dietary pectin on intestinal microfloral metabolism and toxicity of nitrobenzene. *Toxicol. Appl. Pharmacol.* 75:547–553 (1984).
83. D. J. Back, M. C. Breckenridge, M. Challiner, F. E. Crawford, M. L'E. Orme, P. H. Rowe, and E. Smith. The effect of antibiotics on the enterohepatic circulation of ethinylestradiol and norethisterone in the rat. *J. Steroid Biochem.* 9:527–531 (1978).
84. J. Van Eldere, G. Parmentier, J. Robben, and H. Eyssen. Influence of an estrone-desulfating intestinal flora on the enterohepatic circulation of estrone-sulfate in rats. *J. Steroid Biochem.* 26:235–239 (1987).
85. H. Aldercreutz, M. O. Pulkkinen, E. K. Hamalainen, and J. T. Korpela. Studies on the role of intestinal bacteria in metabolism of synthetic and natural steroid hormones. *J. Steroid Biochem.* 20:217–229 (1984).
86. S. L. Gorbach. Estrogens, breast cancer, and intestinal flora. *Rev. Infect. Dis.* 6(Suppl. 1):S85–S90 (1984).
87. K. Norregaard-Hansen, N. A. Klitgaard, and K. E. Pedersen. The significance of the enterohepatic circulation on the metabolism of digoxin in patients with the ability of intestinal conversion of the drug. *Acta Med. Scand.* 220:89–92 (1986).
88. A. N. Alam, J. R. Saha, J. F. Dobkin, and J. Lindenbaum. Interethnic variation in the metabolic inactivation of digoxin by the gut flora. *Gastroenterology* 95:117–123 (1988).

6
The Role of Intestinal Metabolism in Bioavailability

William H. Barr
Virginia Commonwealth University
Richmond, Virginia

INTRODUCTION

There are numerous enzyme systems in various regions of the gastrointestinal tract that are capable of metabolizing a wide variety of drugs. The sequential distribution of these different enzyme systems is a critical variable in the absorption of drugs and, thus, the design and interpretation of bioavailability studies. Both the site and rate of drug release can greatly influence the extent of biotransformation and, therefore, the ultimate amount of unchanged drug available for absorption. An understanding of these metabolizing systems and methods to study them is of value in the systematic design and testing of dosage forms. Unfortunately, due to the complexity of direct studies in humans, much of what we know is from animal models. Nonetheless, a fairly clear picture is emerging on the important role of intestinal metabolism in drug absorption.

When a drug is administered orally, decreased bioavailability may occur due to (1) decreased absorption, or (2) because the drug is metabolized in the gastrointestinal (GI) tract or (3) in the liver. Since the GI tract and liver are anatomically positioned in series, it is not possible to tell which of these mechanisms are operative based only on measurements of unchanged drug in the systemic circulation after oral administration [1]. If additional measurements are made on metabolites in plasma or urine following oral and IV or other routes it may be possible to infer which mechanism, i.e., decreased absorption, hepatic metabolism, or intestinal absorption is involved [2,3].

It is particularly important to know if intestinal metabolism is involved because it is the most sensitive to formulation changes. For example, depending on whether the drug is metabolized by bacterial enzymes in the colon or by mucosal enzymes in the jejunum, the strategy on the design of a controlled release product will change. This information is also critical to the design of studies to assess bioequivalence.

TYPES AND DISTRIBUTION OF ENZYME SYSTEMS

There are several types of enzyme systems capable of metabolizing drugs that are distributed in different regions of the GI tract. These include (1) enzymes in the lumen of the small intestine from mucosal cell secretion and desquamation, (2) luminal enzymes from pancreatic secretions, (3) mucosal cell enzymes located in the brush border, (4) mucosal enzymes located intracellularly (endoplasmic reticulum, mitochondria, cytoplasm) in the columnar epithelial enterocyte, and (5) bacterial enzymes in the distal small intestine and colon.

Thus, distribution of enzyme systems can be viewed from a longitudinal view along the length of the gastrointestinal tract from stomach to duodenum, jejunum, ileum, and colon; and, transversely, from lumen fluid through the brush border of the cell, the cytosolic fluid and organelles of the cell, and to the capillaries in the lamina propria. These systems are illustrated in Figures 1 and 2. These metabolizing systems differ in source, location, and substrate specificity. Examples of enzyme systems that have been shown to be important in affecting the bioavailability of different types of drugs are discussed below, followed by examples of their effect on bioavailability.

Luminal Enzymes

Luminal enzymes include digestive enzymes that are secreted in pancreatic fluid. The pancreas secretes about 700 ml of fluid each day through the common bile duct which drains into the ampulla of Vater in the duodenum. Pancreatic fluid generally contains hydrolyzing enzymes. These enzymes may be involved in the hydrolysis of drug esters that is required prior to their absorption. Glazko et al. [4] showed that pancreatic extract hydrolyzed chloramphenicol esters.

Another class of digestive enzymes are the peptidases which may also split amide linkages and inactivate peptide drugs. This is the major problem in the absorption of polypeptides in the small intestine. This may be a reason for developing dosage forms that deliver drug to the colon, since peptidases may be less prevalent

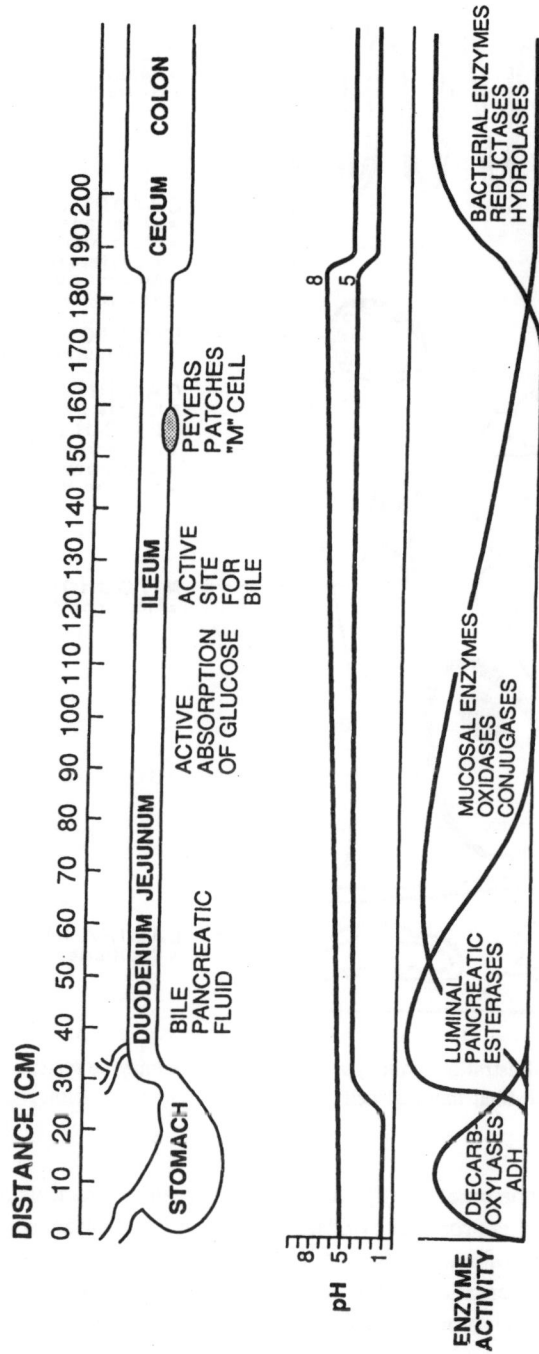

Figure 1 Schematic illustration of the types and locations of enzyme systems distributed longitudinally throughout the GI tract.

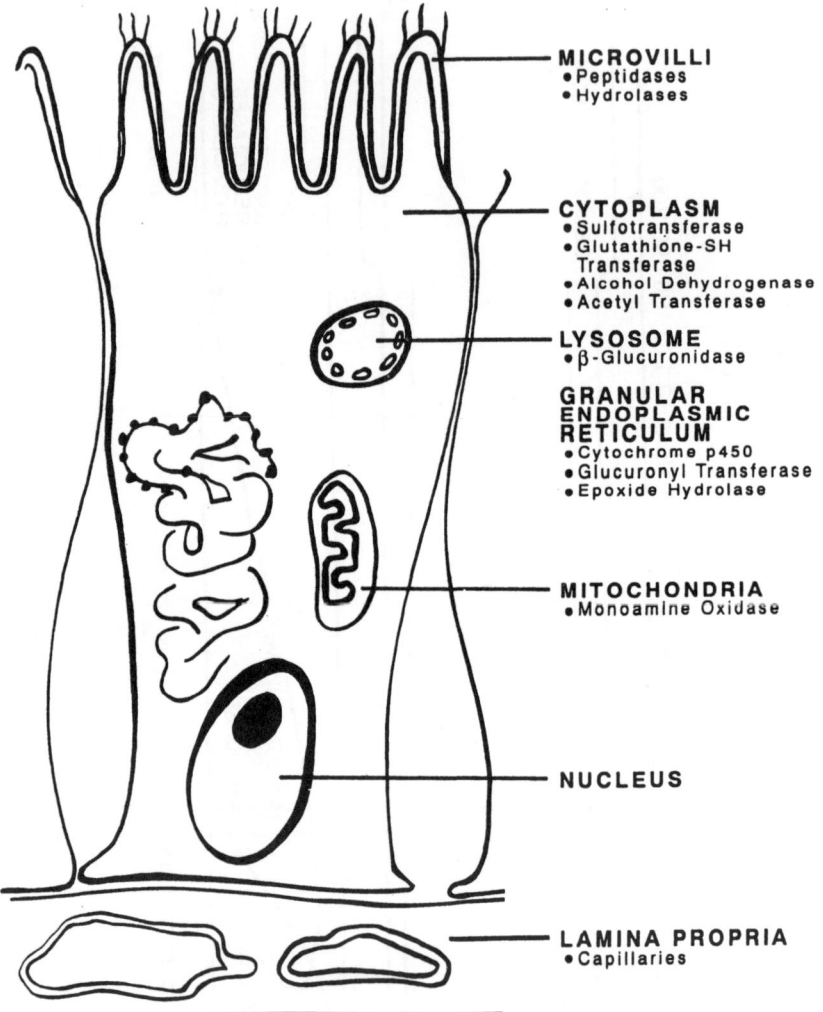

Figure 2 Schematic illustration of the types and locations of enzyme systems distributed transversely in the intestinal mucosal cell.

in this region. Boxenbaum et al. [5] found that pancreatic extract, using similar in vitro conditions to that proposed by Glazko [4], did not hydrolyze isonicotinuric acid, the glycine ester of isnicotinic acid, but incubation with fecal contents did.

Thus, failure of pancreatic extracts to hydrolyze esters or amides would not rule out hydrolysis in vivo because of the presence of mucosal and bacterial enzymes, which can also hydrolyze a variety of esters and amides.

Mucosal Enzymes—Small Intestine

The mucosal columnar epithelial cells contain virtually all of the types of drug-metabolizing enzyme systems normally found in the liver. The mucosal enzymes are of two basic types:

1. Digestive enzymes, which are located primarily in the brush border. They are generally hydrolases capable of splitting esters (fats, carbohydrates) or amides (peptides) and function in normal digestive processes.
2. Xenbiotic biotransformation enzymes, which are generally located in the endoplasmic reticulum (microsomal fraction) or cytoplasm (supernatant fraction) and functionally serve as a first line of defense against entering foreign sustances. This group is further classified into phase I type enzymes that include the monoxygenases (including the P-450 enzyme systems) that are involved in the catalyzation of various oxidation and reduction reactions, alcohol dehydrogenase, monoamine oxidase, epoxide hydrolase, esterases, amidases, and glucuronidases. The phase II enzyme systems include glucuronyltransferase, sulfotransferase, glucuronyltransferase, O-methyltransferase, and glutathione-SH transferase [6-9]. These enzymes are located in various parts of the mucosal cell as illustrated in Figure 2. Examples of the enzyme systems and drug substrates are given in Table 1.

The enzyme activity in the enterocyte is generally less than that of the hepatocyte for a given enzyme system. Often the Km value of the system is the same but Vmax is lower [23]. Thus, because of the lower enzyme capacity—and the fact that after oral dosing the intestinal cell is exposed to a higher concentration of drug than any cell in the body—intestinal enzyme systems are more easily saturated [24].

In general the activities of the phase I enzyme systems are much less in intestine than liver. However, this appears to be greatly dependent upon the amount of xenobiotics in the food ingested. The phase I systems are readily induced [9].

The different regions of the gastrointestinal tract vary greatly in enzyme capacity. For most mucosal enzymes, but not all, the highest activity is found in the proximal small intestine (duodenum and jejunum) with progressively decreasing activity in the distal regions. The stomach and colon generally have significantly less enzyme activity.

There are exceptions to these generalizations, and the capacity and location of these systems are highly dependent upon the species and experimental conditions including availablity of inducing agents [25].

Stomach Mucosa

Recent work in humans [26] has shown that the stomach mucosa is the primary site for first pass metabolism of ethanol by alcohol dehydrogenase (ADH). The AUC of ethanol following oral administration is much less than after IV

Table 1 Examples of Intestinal Mucosal Enzyme Systems

	Enzyme Systems	Substrates	Refs.
PHASE I- (Redox, hydrolysis)			
Hydroxylation	Mixed function oxidase systems (cytochrome p-450 - cytochrome p-450 reductase)	Benzopyrene Benzphetamine	10 11
Oxidation	Alcohol dehydrogenase Monoamine oxidase	Ethanol Tyramine	12 13 14
Reduction	Reductases	Progesterone	15
O-Dealkylation	p-Nitroanisole demethylase Ethoxycoumarin-o-dethylase	p-Nitroanisol Ethoxycoumarine	16
Epoxide hydrolysis	Epoxide hydrolase	Styrene oxide	17
PHASE II (Conjugation)			
Glucuronidation	UDP-glucuronyltransferase	1-Napthol, P-Nitrophenol Estriol, Estrone	18
Sulfation	Sulfokinase	2-Napthol, isoproteranol	19
Glutathione conjugation	Glutathione-S-transferase	Benzo[a]pyrene-4,5 oxide	17
Glycine conjugation	Glycine transferase	Para amino salicylic acid	20
Acetylation	Acetyltransferase	Isoniazid Hydralazine	21 22
Methylation	Calechol-O-methyl transferase	Isoproteranol	19

administration of a small dose of ethanol (0.15 g/kg). Over 80% of an orally administered dose is metabolized by the stomach (i.e., the bioavailability is only 17%). However, when the same amount of ethanol is delivered to the duodenum by nasogastric tube or is given to patients with partial gastrectomies in which the antrum is removed, the first pass effect is completely abolished and the AUC is the same as the IV dose. Therefore, neither the liver nor the intestine contributes significantly to the first pass effect.

This finding appears to validate the anecdote that certain diplomats are taught to coat their stomachs with butter or oil in order to be able to drink more at social functions without getting inebriated. Fats, of course, would slow absorption and decrease gastric emptying, thus increasing the amount of first pass metabolism in the stomach. Also the old adage, "Never drink on an empty stomach," has a physiological basis, since gastric emptying would be more rapid in fasting individuals. Conversely, food decreases gastric emptying and therefore reduces the bioavailability of ethanol [26].

Human gastric ADH and rat gastric ADH appear similar and the rat appears to be a good model. Gastric ADH is non-competitively inhibited by cimetidine and is apparently induced in chronic drinkers [27,26].

Levodopa may also be metabolized by human gastric mucosa as bioavailability is increased by agents that increase gastric emptying (metoclopramide) and decreased by propantheline, which decreases gastric emptying [28,29].

Colon Mucosa

The colon differs from the small intestine, primarily because of the presence of numerous bacteria (10^{11}/gm) that metabolize drugs by several pathways.

However, there is also some nonbacterial enzyme activity in the colonic mucosa, although generally to a lesser extent than in the small intestine. Pacifici et al. [17] compared mucosa from the terminal ileum and proximal colon of six patients undergoing hemicolectomy. They examined phase I metabolism (NADPH cytochrome C reductase*, ethoxycoumarin O-deathylase, microsomal epoxide hydrolase and cytosolic epoxide hydrolase* glutathione reductase, and glutathione peroxidase) and phase II (glutathione transferase*, glucuronyl transferase, acetyl transferase, thioltransferase, glyoxylase*, and sulphotransferase*). Those identified above by (*) were significantly higher in the ileum but the others had about equal activity in the ileum and colon mucosa.

Bacterial Metabolism

The reviews of Scheline [30,31] outline numerous enzymatic drug reactions that are catalyzed by intestinal bacterial enzymes (Table 2). In recent years these metabolic processes have been shown to be a major determinant in the metabolism of some drugs. Interest has also been spurred by the realization that controlled

Table 2 Types of Reactions of Foreign Componds Carried Out by the Gastrointestinal Microflora

1. Hydrolysis of glycosides	13. Reduction of double bonds
a. Glucuronides	14. Reduction of nitro groups
b. Other glycosides	15. Reduction of azo groups
2. Hydrolysis of sulfate esters	16. Reduction of aldehydes
3. Hydrolysis of amides	17. Reduction of ketones
4. Hydrolysis of esters	18. Reduction of alcohols
5. Hydrolysis of sulfamates	19. Reduction of N-oxides
6. Hydrolysis of nitrates	20. Reduction of arsonic acids
7. Dehydroxylation	21. Reduction of sulfoxides
a. C-Hydroxyl compounds	22. Reduction of epoxides to olefins
b. N-Hydroxyl compounds	23. Aromatization
8. Decaboxylation	24. Nitrosamine formation
9. Dealkylation	25. Nitrosamine degradation
a. O-Aklyl compounds	26. Acetylation
b. N-Alkyl compounds	27. Esterifications
c. Other alkyl derivatives	28. Methylation
10. Dehalogenation	29. Ketone formation
11. Deamination	
12. Heterocyclic ring fission	
a. O-Containing ring systems	
b. N-Containing ring systems	

Source: Scheline, [30,31].

release products release significant amounts of drug in the colon where bacterial counts are very high.

There are about 60 types of bacteria in the colon [32]. Contrary to what might be expected, the composition is fairly consistent between individuals, male or female, and in fact, between different races [33].

There is even reasonably good agreement between different animal species. For this reason, the results of studies in animals are often predictive of effects in man. However, because of the largely anaerobic nature of fecal bacteria, sampling and experimental techniques are very critical to obtaining valid results. As with all in vitro studies they may be qualitatively but not quantitatively predictive.

The colon is a targeted site for drug delivery for (1) drugs that specifically act upon the colon and (2) drugs that may be better absorbed from the colon [34].

The antiinflammatory agent, naproxen, was linked by an ester bond to dextran which was enzymatically split off in the colon of rabbits and pigs [35].

5-Aminosalicylic acid (5-ASA) is a commonly used compound for ulcerative colitis or large bowel inflammatory disease [36]. There are a number of drug delivery systems that utilize colonic bacteria to split 5-ASA from ester or azo prodrugs. There are also new dosage forms that have special coatings that are released in the colon due to bacterial enzymes. The definition of bioavailability of these types of products is the rate and extent of release to the site of action which is the lumen of the colon rather thn the systemic circulation. Drug delivery systems that are capable of delivering drugs to the colon are likely to see increasing use with certain poorly absorbed drugs such as polar antibiotics (cephalosporins, aminoglycosides) and macromolecules (peptides, proteins). The colon and rectum are the most sensitive regions of the gastrointestinal tract to absorption enhancers such as fatty acid salts and mixed micelle surfactants [37].

EXPERIMENTAL EVIDENCE FOR INTESTINAL METABOLISM IN HUMANS

Cannulated Mesenteric Vein

The vast majority of work on intestinal metabolism has been done in animals. Some authors have suggested that studies of intestinal metabolism in animals can be used as the primary rationale for development of dosage forms for humans. Because of the great differences between species, it is essential that definitive studies be done in man. Some methods that can be used in man are discussed below. Examples are summarized in Table 3.

The most direct proof of the capability of the intestinal mucosa to metabolize drugs in humans was given by Diczfalusy, et al. [38,18]. During surgical procedures to excise a portion of intestine in six women, they cannulated the mesenteric vein draining a loop of intestine. ^{14}C-estratriol was injected into the lumen of the intestinal loop. The extent of glucuronide conjugation was directly assessed by the amount of unchanged drug and glucuronide in the mesenteric blood. In the upper regions of the small intestine, almost all of the drug in the mesenteric blood was as the glucuronide. Conjugation decreased as distal segments of intestine were used. There was no conjugation in the stomach or colon.

It is unlikely that these studies could be repeated in today's regulatory climate so that this method, while conclusive, is not generally available for use in humans.

Cannulation of Portal Vein

The portal vein can be cannulated via the umbilical vein [42]. Current ethical considerations limit this procedure to patients or individuals requiring the procedure for treatment or diagnosis, since it is a surgical procedure. This procedure has been used to show that pivampicillin is completely hydrolyzed before it reaches the liver [14]. This procedure has also been used to show that flurazepam is extensively conjugated by the intestine [39]. Anderson, et al., [43] have used this procedure to study digoxin administered either orally or intrasigmoidly.

Table 3 Examples of Drugs With Evidence of Intestinal Metabolism in Man

Drug	Type and location	Type of evidence	Reference
Estradiol	Small intestine gut wall glucuronidation	1	18
Estratiol	Small intestine gut wall glucuronidation		18
Estrone	Small intestine gut wall glucuronidation		38
Pivampicillin	Ester hydrolysis	2	14
Flurazepam	N-Desmethylation	2	39
Para aminosalicylic acid	Acetylation	3	21
Para aminosalicylic acid	Acetylation	4	21
Isoniazid	Acetylation	4	21
Equilin sulfate	Hydrolysis of sulfate + reconjugation with sulfate	5	40
Isoproterenol (Isoprenaline)	Sulfation	6	19
Ethanol	Oxidation by ADH	7	26
β-methyl digoxin		8	41

Types of evidence

Direct in vivo
1. Cannulated mesenteric vein
2. Cannulated portal vein (via umbilical)
3. Cannulated collateral vein in cirrhotics

Direct in vitro — incubation of
4. Mucosal tissue/fluid or bacteria

Indirect in vivo
5. Double labeled studies
6. Comparison of drug and metabolite(s) by oral and IV route
7. Comparison of drug and metabolite when drug is administered to different intestinal sites
8. Pharmacokinetics modeling

Cannulation of Peripheral Collateral Veins in Patients With Hepatic Cirrhosis

In individuals with chronic hepatic cirrhosis, collateral venous circulation develops. The veins on the surface of the abdomen can be cannulated which connects with the portal circulation. The major disadvantage of this method is that it can be done only in patients with advanced hepatic disease who may not be representative of the normal population.

This technique was used as early as 1950 [44] to show that the human intestine can acetylate para-aminosalicylic acid (PAS). The concentration of N-acetyl-PAS was much higher in the portal collateral circulation than the peripheral venous circulation in cirrhotic patients given oral PAS.

Direct Sampling of Intestinal Contents

Direct samples of intestinal mucosa, can be obtained during surgery, by biopsy or intubation [45,46]. Samples are incubated with drug under controlled conditions in vitro.

Jenne [22] used intestinal mucosal examples obtained post mortem to confirm the earlier in vivo results (see above) that PAS is acetylated in the human intestine. Similar results were obtained for isoniazid (Jenne [21]).

Although these methods provide direct qualitative evidence for a particular metabolic pathway and drug substrate, they do not provide quantitative information on the extent that the drug is metabolized in vivo.

Use of Radioisotopes — Dual Isotope Labeling

Intestinal hydrolysis of conjugated estrogen was studied using a dual-labeled compound. Equilin sulfate (ES) was studied with a tritiated steroid nucleus (^{3}H-Equilin) and ^{35}S-sulfate [40]. When the dual-labeled equilin sulfate was administered orally as $^3E^{35}S$ it was found that equilin sulfate appeared in the plasma but it was as ^{3}E-S, not $^3E^{35}S$, indicating that the original $^{35}SO_4$ moiety had been cleaved and the sterol was reconjugated in the intestinal tissue or liver before reaching the systemic circulation [40]. Only 10% of the unhydrolyzed sulfate was absorbed and reached the systemic circulation intact. Thus, the assessment of the bioavailability of the administered estrogen sulfate is quite complex.

Comparison of Drug and Metabolite(s) After Oral and IV (or other route) Administration

Often direct evidence is not available and the contribution of the intestine to first pass metabolism is inferred from observations of drug and metabolite levels following oral administration compared to administration by the IV, nasal, or inhalation routes [47]. For example, a change in the type of metabolism is seen in the case of isoproterenol given orally and IV Hepatic metabolism after IV administration results in O-methylation. Sixty percent of the drug is eliminated intact in the urine after IV Only after oral administration does the sulfate occur [19].

Another similar drug, Salbutamol (albuterol), is metabolized to a much greater extent following oral dosing (61%) compared to IV administration (27%) [48].

Alteration of Metabolic Profile by Changes in Intestinal Site of Absorption

All venous effluent from the small intestine and colon leads directly to the liver. Although the liver is reasonably homogenous with respect to enzyme distribution, the intestine is not since both the type of enzyme and amount of enzyme varies depending on intestinal site. Thus, changes in the amount or type of metabolite following changes in the site of absorption provide indirect evidence of intestinal metabolism [49].

It is important in designing these studies that only the site is changed and not the rate of delivery, since the latter could also alter the amount of hepatic metabolism if the process is capacity limited (saturable) [50,51].

The intestinal site may be altered by delivering drug by intestinal intubation to different sites. There are also capsules that can be activated to release drug at different sites in the gastrointestinal tract [52].

A patient with a surgical portocaval anastomosis was used to show that first pass metabolism of propranolol was primarily in the liver for this patient. However, it is interesting that 4-hydroxypropranolol is said to be formed only after oral dosing, not after IV administration [53], which as noted above, provides indirect evidence of gut metabolism. We have observed that propranolol placed in the distal portion of the human intestine by a nasogastric tube consistently produced a 20% increase in AUC compared to drug placed in the proximal intestine or given orally [54]. This may be due to decreased mucosal metabolism in the distal intestine (ileum) compared to duodenum and proximal jejunum.

Pharmacokinetic Inference

Under certain conditions, drug blood levels and urinary excretion data can be used with pharmacokinetic models to show that first pass loss is due to intestinal and/or hepatic metabolism. As with the use of any model, there are certain assumptions that must be considered which have led to a series of refinements on the initial hepatic clearance models of Gibaldi et al. [55] and Rowland [56].

Generally, to use organ extraction methods, one has to have whole blood concentrations rather than plasma concentrations [52]. For example, Hinderling, et al. [40,57] found that the metabolic extraction of β-methyl digoxin was 8% after IV administration but was 20% after oral administration presumably due to gut metabolism.

The use of moment analysis to estimate residence times has also been proposed as a method to evaluate intestinal metabolism [58].

Methods to Study Intestinal Absorption in Animals

Since the primary focus of this review is in the role of intestinal metabolism in human bioavailability, a comprehensive review of animal methodologies will not be given. Studies in animals are important, however, because of the experiment limitations inherent in human studies. Animal studies have been important in (1) confirming the possibility of intestinal pathways that may be important in humans and (2) allowing more detailed information on mechanisms involved in metabolism and transport and physiological factors which influence metabolism [59].

Surgical preparations that allow one to administer drug orally and measure intraportal blood levels and systemic levels have been done primarily in animals, but as noted above could be done in man under certain clinical conditions.

Portocaval shunts that bypass the liver have been used in dogs to show that first pass clearance of salicylamide occurs in liver and intestine, but lidocaine metabolism is primarily in the liver only [60]. The classic work of Harris and Riegelman [13] used surgical preparations in the dog to show the role of the intestine and liver in aspirin first pass metabolism.

A number of animal procedures are available for intestinal metabolism studies [59,61,62]. These include in situ intestinal loops in which the mesentine vein is cannulated [63,64], in vitro everted loops and more recently isolated intestinal cells. The latter have been used to study a large number of substrates and enzyme systems. They have the advantage that the entire cell, including the brush border and endoplasmic reticulum, is intact preserving the structural and spacial integrity of the enzyme systems.

In contrast, some of the cell homogenates such as the microsomal or purified enzyme systems may not preserve important spatial factors or enzymatic cofactors. In some cases, homogenation alters enzymatic properties [65].

ROLE OF THE INTESTINAL METABOLISM IN SYSTEMIC ELIMINATION OF DRUG

It is generally assumed that metabolism by the intestine occurs only when the drug is presented from the luminal side. For example Ilett et al. [66] infused isoproterenol (isoprenaline) into the arterial supply of an intestinal loop of the dog (1980) and found no evidence of sulfate conjugation.

However, Barr et al. [67] found in the rabbit that salicylamide injected directly into the arterial supply was sulfated by the intestinal tissue and glucuronidated by the liver. The salicylamide sulfate was formed in the intestinal tissue after intravenous administration and the metabolite was transported to the mesenteric blood and the lumen of the intestine.

INTERACTION BETWEEN METABOLISM, ABSORPTION VARIABLES AND FORMULATION VARIABLES

An interesting example of the interplay between metabolism and the rate and site of drug release from the dosage form are the conjugated estrogens. The estrogens are administered orally as the sulfate conjugates. This complex process is shown in Figure 3.

The administered conjugated estrogens (sulfates) are deconjugated by luminal sulfatases. Both the sulfate and free estrogen are absorbed but the sulfate is absorbed to a lesser extent.

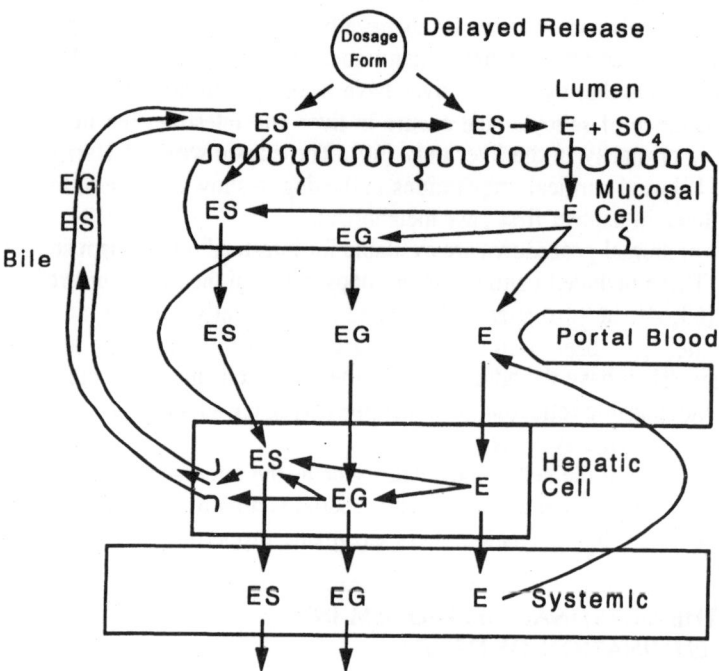

Figure 3 Schematic illustration of the complex metabolic processes involved with absorption of conjugated (sulfate) estrogens (ES) which are hydrolyzed to free (unconjugated) estrogen (E), reconjugated to sulfate (ES) or glucuronide (EG) conjugates in the intestinal and hepatic systems before being delivered to the systemic circulation or being recirculated through the bile. All of these processes will depend on the rate and location of drug delivery from the dosage form.

The free (unconjugated) estrogen is reconjugated to sulfate and glucuronide in the intestinal mucosal cell and liver. This is clearly shown by the double label (^{3}H and ^{35}S) studies of Bhavnani [40].

These processes are probably site specific and saturable. Esterases (sulfatase) are probably present to a greater degree in the distal regions (partly of bacterial origin). Glucuronidation by glucuronyl transferase in the intestinal mucosal cell are probably present to a greater degree in the proximal portion (duodenum and proximal jejunum). Conjugation can occur either in the intestine or liver. Estrogen glucuronide formed at the 3-position (intestine) is not excreted in bile in contrast the conjugates formed in the liver (alcohol glucuronide) which are secreted in bile [68].

All of these processes are influenced by the rate of release of drug from the dosage form.

INTERACTIONS AMONG DRUGS

There is increasing information that interactions among different drugs in the gastrointestinal track may greatly affect intestinal metabolism and thus the availability of drugs. The intestine appears to be highly inducible with respect to phase I-type enzyme systems [9]. Sulfate metabolism is decreased by vitamin C [47] and probably other drugs that compete for the limited sulfate. Cimetidine inhibits the metabolism of some substances in the intestine [69]. Antibiotics can inhibit bacterial metabolism of drugs.

CONCLUSIONS

The drug metabolism systems found in the gastrointestinal (GI) tract have several unique characteristics that are important determinants of the bioavailability of drugs.

First, the GI tract contains a greater variety of enzymes systems that can chemically transform drugs than any other organ or region of the body. The three major classes of systems: (1) luminal enzymes from intestinal and pancreatic secretions, (2) mucosal enzyme systems in the intestinal cell, and (3) bacterial enzyme systems. Each of these have many specific enzyme systems that are capable of phase I type (oxidation, reduction, hydroxylation, deamination, dealkylation) and phase II type (glucuronidation, sulfation, acetylation, reactions).

In addition to the large number and variety of enzymes the GI tract is unique in the sequential distribution of these systems throughout the entire GI tract. Some enzyme systems are primarily in the stomach (e.g., alcohol dehydrogenase) others primarily in the mucosa of the small intestine (e.g., glucuronyl transferase), and still others primarily in the colon (e.g., bacterial reductases).

The third characteristic of intestinal enzyme systems is that they are generally exposed to higher concentrations than other systems (e.g., hepatic). They are therefore more likely to be saturated.

The importance of these characteristics is that the type and degree of metabolism during the absorptive phase (first pass metabolism) is highly dependent at both the rate and site of release. This becomes very critical in the design of controlled release drugs and in the interpretation of bioavailability studies of these products.

Although most of the information we have is from animal studies there is accumulating information that intestinal metabolism may be affected by disease states, age, the presence of other drugs that may act as inducers or inhibitors of intestinal drug metabolism. These physiologic variables may also interact with formulation variables of the dosage form to alter bioavailability in various types of clinical conditions.

There is a need to develop and use methods that will better characterize these variables in clinical studies in man.

REFERENCES

1. A. Venot, E. Walter, Y. LeCourtier, A. Raksanyi, and L. Chauvelot-Woachon. Structural indentification of "First-Pass" models. *J. Pharmacokinet Biopharm* 15:179–188 (1987).
2. C. F. George. Drug metabolism in the gastrointestinal mucosa. *Clin. Pharmacokinet.* 6:259–274 (1981).
3. D. J. Back, M. Bates, A. M. Breckenridge, F. Crawford, A. Ellis, J. M. Hall, M. MacIver, M. L'E. Orme, I. Taylor and P. H. Rowe. *Drug Metabolism by Gastrointestinal Mucosa: Clinical Aspects in Drug Absorption* (Prescott and Nimmo, eds.) ADIS, Sydney, pp. 80–87 (1981).
4. A. J. Glazko, W. A. Dill, L. M. Kazenko, L. M. Wolf, and H. E. Carnes. Physical factors affecting the rate of absorption of chloramphenicol esters. *Antibiot. Chemoth.* 8:517–527 (1958).
5. H. F. Boxenbaum, G. S. Jodhka, A. C. Ferguson, S. Riegelman, and T. R. MacGregor. The influence of bacterial gut hydrolysis on the fate of orally administered isonicotinuric acid in man. *J. Pharmacokinet. Biopharm.* 2:211–234 (1974).
6. K. Hatiala. Metabolism of hormones, drugs and other substances by the gut. *Physiol. Rev.* 53:496–534 (1973).
7. K. Hartiala. Metabolism of foreign compounds in the gastrointestinal tract. In *Handbook of Physiology*, section 9 *Amer. Physiol. Soc.* p. 375 (1977).
8. J. Caldwell. The metabolism of drugs by the gastrointestinal tract. In *Pre-systemic Drug Elimination* (George et al., eds.). Butterworths, London (1981).
9. O. Hänninen. Mucosal biotransformation of toxins in the gut. In receptors and other targets for toxic substances. *Arch. Toxicol. Suppl.* 8:83–86 (1985).
10. R. J. Oshinsky and H. W. Strobel. Drug metabolism in rat colon: Resolution of enzymatic constituents and characterization of activity. *Molec. Cell. Biochem.* 75:51–60 (1987).
11. L. W. Wattenberg, J. L. Leong, and P. J. Strand. Benzpyrene hydroxylase activity in the gastrointestinal tract. *Cancer Res.* 22:1120–1125 (1962).
12. R. J. Levine and A. Sjoerdsma. Estimation of monoamine oxidase activity in man: Techniques and applications. *Annals of the New York Academy of Sciences* 107:966–974 (1963).
13. P. A. Harris, and S. Riegelman. Influence of the route of administration on the area under the plasma concentration-time curve. *J. Pharm. Sci.* 58:71–75 (1969).
14. B. Lund, J. P. Kampmann, F. Lindahl, and J. M. Hansen. Pivampicillin and ampicillin in bile, portal and peripheral blood. *Clin. Pharmacol. Therap.* 19:587–591 (1976).
15. W. Ninstedt and K. Hartiala. Steroid metabolism by the canine intestine I Qualitative experiments with progesterone. *Scand. J. Gastroent* 4:483 (1969).
16. V. Ullrich and P. Weber. A direct test for monoxygenase activity of intact small using surface relectance fluorimetry. *Biochem. Pharmacol.* 23:3309–3315 (1974).
17. G. M. Pacifici, M. Franchi, P. G. Gervasi, V. Longo, P. diSimplicia, A. Tamellini, and L. Givliani. Profile of drug metabolism enzymes in human ileum and colon. *Pharmacol.* 38:137–145 (1989).
18. E. Diczfalusy, C. Franksson, B. P. Lisboa, and B. Martinsen. Formation of estrone glucosiduronate by the human intestinal tract. *Acta Endocrinologica* 40:537–551 (1962).

19. M. E. Conolly, D. S. Davies, C. T. Dollery, C. D. Morgan, J. W. Paterson, and M. Sandler. Metabolism of isoprenaline in dog and man. *Br. J. Pharmacol.* 46:458–472 (1972).
20. N. R. Strahl and W. H. Barr. Intestinal drug absorption and metabolism III. Glycine conjugation and accumulation of benzoic acid in rat intestinal tissue. *J. Pharm. Sci.* 60:278–281.
21. J. W. Jenne. Isoniazid acetylation by human liver and intestinal mucosa. *Federation Proceedings* 22:540 (1963).
22. J. W. Jenne. Partial purification and properties of the isoniazid transacetylase in human liver. Its relationship to the acetylation of p-aminosalicylic acid. *J. Clin. Investig.* 44:1992–2002 (1965).
23. R. S. Shirkey, J. Chakraborty, and J. W. Bridges. Comparison of drug metabolizing ability of rat intestinal mucosal microsomes with that of liver. *Biochem. Pharmacol. 28*, 2835–2839 (1979).
24. W. H. Barr, T. Aceto, M. Chung, and M. Shukur. Dose dependent drug metabolism during the absorptive phase. *Rev. Can. Biol. 32 Suppl.*: 31–42 (1973).
25. P. Wollenberg, and V. Ullrich. The drug monooxygenase system in the small intestine. In *Extra hepatic metabolism of drugs and other foreign compounds* (T.E. Ram, ed.) MTP press, Lancaster, England, pp. 267–276 (1980).
26. J. Caballeria, E. Baraona, M. Rodamilans, and C. S. Lieber. Effets of cimetidine on gastric alcohol dehydrogenase and blood ethanol levels. *Gastroenterol. 96*:388–392 (1989).
27. C. DiPadova, T. M. Worner, R. J. K. Julkunen, and C. S. Lieber. Effects of fasting and chronic alcohol consumption on the first-pass metabolism of ethanol. *Gastroenterol.* 92:1169–1173 (1987).
28. P. T. Mearrick, D. N. Wade, D. J. Birkett, and J. Morris. Metoclopramide, gastric emptying and l-dopa absorption. *Australian & New Zealand J. Med.* 4:144 (1974).
29. M. Sandler, C. R. J. Ruthven, B. L. Goodwin, K. R. Hunter, and G. M. Stern. Variation of levodopa metabolism with gastrointestinal absorption site. *Lancet 1*:238–239 (1974).
30. R. R. Scheline. Metabolism of foreign compounds by gastrointestinal microorganisms. *Pharmacol. Rev.* 25:451–523 (1973).
31. R. R. Scheline. Drug metabolism by gastrointestinal microflora, Cpt 17. In *Extra Heptic Metabolism of Drugs and Foreign Compounds* (T. E. Gram ed.), MTP Press, Lancaster (1980).
32. R. M. Donaldson. Normal bacterial populations of the intestine and their relation to intestinal function. *The New Engl. J. Med.* 270:938–945 (1967).
33. Broitman and Giannelly 1971.
34. J. W. Fara. Colonic drug absorption and metabolism. Proceeding of the 3rd Int. Conf. Drug Absorp., Edinburgh. In *Novel Drug Delivery and its therapeutic application* (L. F. Prescott and W. S. Nimmo, eds.), p. 11 (September 1988).
35. E. Harboe, C. Larsen, and M. Johansen. Dextran pro-drugs provide selective drug delivery to the bowel in rabbits and pigs. *Abstracts*, 3rd Int. Conf. Drug Absorp., Sept. 1988, Edinburgh, pg. 57.
36. K. M. Das and R. Dubin. Clinical pharmacokinetics of sulfasalazine. *Clin. Pharmacokinet 1*:406–425 (1976).

37. S. Muranishi. Absorption barriers and absorption promoters in the intestine. In. *Topics in Pharmaceutical Sciences* D. D. Breimer and P. Speiser, eds.) Elsevier, p. 445 (1987).
38. E. Diczfalusy, C. Franksson, and B. Martinsen. Oestrogen conjugation by the human intestinal tract. *Acta Endocrinologica* 38:59–72 (1961).
39. W. A. Mahon, T. Imaba, and R. M. Stone. Metabolism of flurazepam by the small intestine. *Clin. Pharmacol Therap.* 22:228–233 (1977).
40. B. R. Bhavnani, C. A. Woolever, D. Wallace, and C. C. Pan. Metabolism of [^{3}H] Equilin-[^{35}S] Sulfate and [^{3}H] Equilin sulfate following oral and intravenous administration in normal postmenopausal women and men. Accepted for publication in *J. Clin. Endocrinol. and Metab.* (1989).
41. P. H. Hinderling, E. R. Garrett, and R. C. Webster. Pharmacokinetics of β-methyl digoxin in healthy humans. I. Intravenous studies. *J. Pharm. Sci.* 66:242–253 (1977a).
42. E. B. Christophersen and F. C. Jackson. A technique of transumbilical portal vein catheterization in adults. *Archives of Surgery* 95;960–963 (1967).
43. K. E. Andersson, L. Dencker, and J. Göthlin. Absorption of digoxin in man after oral and intrasigmoid administration studied by portal vein catheterization. *Eur. J. Clin. Pharmacol.* 9, 39–47 (1975).
44. S. H. Blodheim, and H. G. Kunkel. Portal blood in collateral veins of patients with cirrhosis. Acetylation by the intestine. *Proceedings of the Society for Experimental Biology and Medicine* 73:38–41 (1950).
45. H. Boström, D. Brömster, H. Nordenstam, and B. Wengle. On the occurrence of phenol and steroid sulphokinases in the human gastrointestinal tract. *Scand. J. Gastroent.* 3, 369–375 (1968).
46. D. J. Back, M. Bates, A. M. Breckenridge, F. E. Crawfod, A. Ellis, J. M. Hall, M. Maclver, M.L'E. Orme, and P. H. Rowe. The in vitro metabolism of ethinyloestradiol, levonorgestrel and mestranol by human jejunal mucosa. *Br. J. Clin. Pharmacol* 9:281–282 (1980).
47. J. B. Houston, and G. Taylor. Drug metabolite concentration-time profiles: influence of route of drug administration. *Br. J. Clin. Pharmacol.* 385–394 (1984).
48. M. E. Evans, S. R. Walker, R. T. Brittain, and J. W. Paterson. The metabolism of salbutamol in man. *Xenobiotica* 3:113–120 (1973).
49. N. Rietbrock et al. eds. *Drug Absorption at Different Regions of the Human Gastrointestinal Tract: Methods of Investigation and Results.* Vieweg Verlag, Braunschweig-Wiesbaden (1987).
50. J. G. Wagner. Propranatol: pooled michaelis-menton parameters and the effect of an input rate on bioavailability. *Clin. Pharm. Ther.* 37:481–487 (1985).
51. B. G. Woodcock, G. Menke, A. Fischer, Köhne, H. and N. Rietbrock. Drug input rate from the GI tract—Michaelis-Menton kinetics and the bioavailability of slow-release and nifedipine. *Drug Design and Delivery* 2:298–309 (1988).
52. A. H. Staib and B. G. Woodcock. Remote control of gastrointestinal drug diversely in man, Proceedings of the third international conf. on drug absorption, 27-30 Sept. 1988. Edinburg in Prescott, L. F., Novel drug delivery and its therapeutic applications (J. Nimmo, ed.). Wiley, Chichester, pp. 79–88 (1989).
53. P.A. Routledge and D. G. Shand. Presystemic drug elimination. *Ann. Rev. Pharmacol. Toxicol* 19:447–468 (1979).

54. A. Buch and W. H. Barr. (unpublished data).
55. M. Gibaldi, R. N. Boyes, and S. Feldman. Influence of first-pass effect on availability of drugs on oral administration, *J. Pharm. Sci. 60*:1338 (1971).
56. M. Rowland. Influence of route of administration on drug availability, *J. Pharm. Sci. 61*:70 (1972).
57. P. H. Hinderling, E. R. Garrett, and R. C. Webster. Pharmacokinetics of β-methyl digoxin in healthy humans II. Oral studies and bioavailabilty. *J. Pharm. Sci. 66*:314–325 (1977b).
58. D. Brockmeier, and J. Ostrowski, Mean time and first-pass metabolism. *Eur. J. Clin. Pharmacol. 29*:45–48 (1985).
59. W. H. Barr. The use of physical and animal models to assess bioavailability. *Pharmacology 8*, 55–101 (1972).
60. R. Gugler, P. Lain, and P. L. Azarnoft. Effect of portocaval shunt on the disposition of drugs with and without first pass effect. *J. Pharmacol. Exp. Ther. 195*:416–423 (1975).
61. W. H. Barr and S. Riegelman. Intestinal drug absorption and metabolism. I: Comparison of methods and models to study physiological factors of in vitro and in vivo intestinal absorption. *J. Pharm. Sci. 59*:154–163 (1970a).
62. M. Schwenk. *Mucosal Biotransformation Toxicologic Pathology 16*, 138–145 (1988).
63. W. H. Barr, and S. Riegelman. Intestinal drug absorption and metabolism. II: Kinetic aspects of intestinal glucuronide conjugation. *J. Pharm. Sci. 59*:164–168 (1970b).
64. M. Schwenk, C. Scheimenz, V. Lopez del Pinto, and H. Remmer. First-pass biotransformation of ethinylestradiol in rat small intestine in situ. *Naunyn-Schmiedeb. Arch. Pharmacol. 321*:223–225 (1982).
65. A. Koster and J. Noordhoek. Glucerondation in the rat intestinal wall. Comparison of isolated mucosal cells, latent microsomes and activated microsomes. *Biochem. Pharmacol. 32*:895–900 (1983).
66. K. F. Ilett, C. T. Dollery, and D. S. Davies. Isopranaline conjugation—a 'true first-pass effect' in the dog intestine. *J. Pharm. and Pharmacol. 32*:362 (1980).
67. W. H. Barr, Chung, M. and M. Shukur. Intestinal drug metabolism—pre-systemic and systemic mechanisms and implications. In L. Benet, G. Levy, and B. L. Ferraiolo, eds.). *Pharmacokinetics, Modern View*, Plenum Press, N.Y., Communication 7, pp. 426–429 (1984).
68. Johnson, et al., eds. Sex hormones and the intestinal flora. In *Physiology of the Gastrointestinal Tract*, Raven Press, pp. 1373–1374 (1981).
69. J. Caballeria, M. Frezza, C. Hernandez-Munoz, C. DiPadova, M. A. Korsten, E. Bordoana, and C. S. Lieber. Gastric origin of first pass metabolism of ethanol in humans: Effect of gastrectomy. *Gastroenterol. 97*:1702–1709 (1989).

7
Bioavailability of Transdermal and Topical Dosage Forms

Marvin C. Meyer
University of Tennessee
Memphis, Tennessee

INTRODUCTION

The most common type of bioavailability study involves testing of the dosage forms designed to provide drug to the systemic circulation after oral administration. However, there are a wide variety of dosage forms that are intended for nonoral administration. Examples include parenteral products (intramuscular, intravenous), as well as those to be applied to the skin, eye, nasal mucosa, vagina, ear, or rectum. In addition, certain orally administered products act through a local, rather than a systemic effect (e.g., antacids, antidiarrheal preparations, and the antiulcer drug sucralfate). Some type of assessment of the bioavailability of such dosage forms is usually required for approval by the U.S. Food and Drug Administration (FDA), except for dosage forms that are true solutions.

This chapter will focus on those dosage forms that are intended to be applied to the skin, since many of the considerations applicable to this route of administration also apply to other nonoral or locally acting dosage forms. The skin is increasingly being recognized as an important route of drug administration that provides many experimental challenges. This is evidenced by several excellent reviews [1,2] and reference texts [3–8], which provide an in-depth discussion of the progress that has been made in recent years.

Types of Dosage Forms

There are two distinct types of products that are applied to the skin:

1. *Transdermal*: These are designed to provide active drug to the systemic circulation following application to the surface of the skin. Nitroglycerin, clonidine, scopolamine, and estradiol transdermal delivery systems, as well as nitroglycerin ointment, are examples of currently marketed products.
2. *Topical*: These formulations are also designed to be applied to the skin, but are not intended to result in any drug in the systemic circulation. Typical examples include ointments, creams, solutions, lotions, gels, foams, sprays, salves, and medicated bandages. These dosage forms are used for local activity including anti-infective, antipruritic, antimitotic, anti-inflammatory, sunscreen, lubricant, keratolytic, or antihistaminic effects.

When a compound is absorbed into the systemic circulation, the process is also known as *percutaneous absorption*. This may be unintentional, or designed to be minimal, as with topical formulations. In contrast, absorption is the primary goal of transdermal delivery systems.

Evaluation of the bioavailability or bioequivalence of dosage forms applied to the skin is generally done for one of three reasons: (1) the manufacturer wishes to demonstrate that the dosage form proposed for marketing, and produced on a large scale, has an acceptable bioavailability when compared with the dosage form that was employed in the clinical trials conducted to support the New Drug Application (NDA); (2) the manufacturer wishes to demonstrate that a proposed change (e.g., manufacturing process, site of manufacture, new source of raw material, or other) will yield a product that can be expected to perform identically with the dosage form that was approved through the NDA process; or (3) a second manufacturer, through an Abbreviated New Drug application (ANDA), wishes to gain approval to market a product that is a generic version of a product developed by the innovator or holder of the NDA. In each instance, the criteria applied to the determination of bioequivalence should be identical, regardless of the purpose for conducting the study.

A topic that is beyond the scope of this chapter, but is certainly a critical component in the evaluation of any dosage form placed on the skin, is the determination of skin irritation or sensitization. This area has recently been reviewed by Bodde et al. [9].

Characteristics of the Skin

Before discussing the types of studies that may be utilized to evaluate dosage forms designed to be placed on the skin, it is worthwhile to briefly review some of the characteristics of the skin that give it unique properties and that may affect the bioavailability of topically applied drugs.

Barrier Properties

As shown in Figure 1, the uppermost layer of the skin is 10-50 μm thick and is composed of keratinized, unucleated cells. This layer is known as the *stratum corneum* or "horny layer." The next layer is the *epidermis*, 50-100 μm thick, and consists of proliferating cells. The permeability of the stratum corneum to most materials is generally 10-1000 times less than that of the epidermis, and it thus serves as the primary barrier to the absorption of materials into the skin. The deepest layer of the skin is the *dermis*, which contains many capillaries that are involved in the removal of any drug that may have diffused down through the upper layers of the skin [10]. Compounds that permeate through the skin travel through one of several pathways: (1) hair follicles, (2) sweat glands, or (3) stratum corneum, either through the cells (trancellular) or between the cells (intercellular).

The permeability of the skin may change as a function of a variety of factors that must be controlled or accounted for as part of the development of an experimental protocol:

Hydration. The presence of moisture enhances the penetration of almost all agents into the skin by opening the compact structure of the horny layer. Hydration of the skin can be increased by the hydrating components of the vehicle, or by the use of an occlusive dressing or hydrophobic ointment [12].

Age and race. Premature infants may not have a fully developed barrier to percutaneous absorption, resulting in increased bioavailability [13]. However, studies of testosterone in newborn rhesus monkeys [14] did not indicate any differences in absorption, compared with that of adult animals. The stratum corneum of elderly skin is more permeable than that of young adults, probably because of atrophy of the epidermis, or epidermal atrophy, and there is a diminished blood flow. However, the net effect of aging is not predictable, since the flow of interstitial fluid through the connective tissue is also reduced [15]. Roskos et al. [16] have demonstrated that the percutaneous absorption of certain compounds is lower in the elderly (>65 years). They applied radiolabeled compounds to the skin surface and monitored the radioactivity appearing in the urine. The results, shown in Figure 2, indicate that age affected the permeation of hydrocortisone, benzoic acid, aspirin, and caffeine, which are relatively hydrophilic, but the penetration of the more lipophilic testosterone and estradiol were unaffected. Roskos et al. [17] have studied the urinary recovery of testosterone, estradiol,

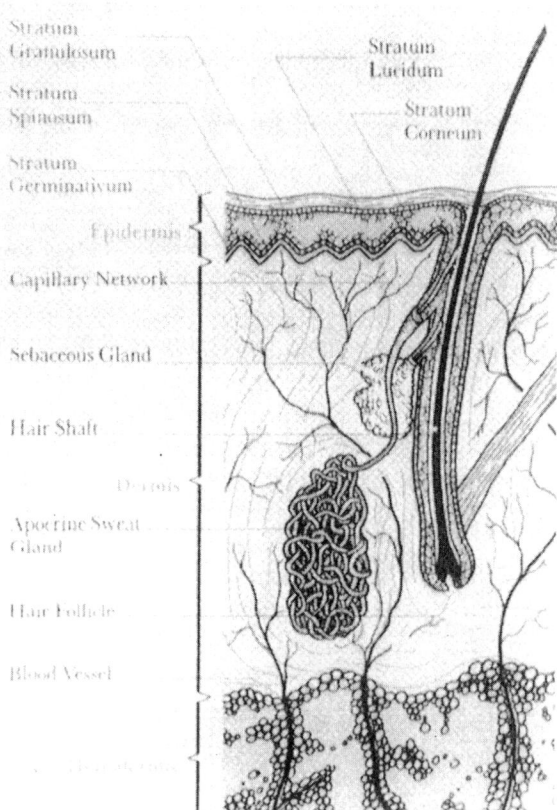

Figure 1 Cross-section of human skin. (From Ref. 11.)

hydrocortisone, and benzoic acid, following topical application to subject populations of 18–35, 65–75, and >75 years of age. There was little difference in the apparent absorption of testosterone and estradiol among the three subject populations. Greater absorption of the more hydrophilic hydrocortisone and benzoic acid was seen in the young, compared with the two older populations. The authors speculate that the aged skin, which has a lower lipid content and is dryer, may result in a decreased dissolution of the more hydrophilic compounds in the skin. In general, the effect of aging on percutaneous absorption has not been evaluated in sufficient detail to permit any generalizations to be made [17]. However, the possibility exists that two topical or transdermal formulations, which appear bioequivalent in young volunteers, may not be equivalent in the elderly or in the newborn. Although there certainly is a potential for age-related effects to result

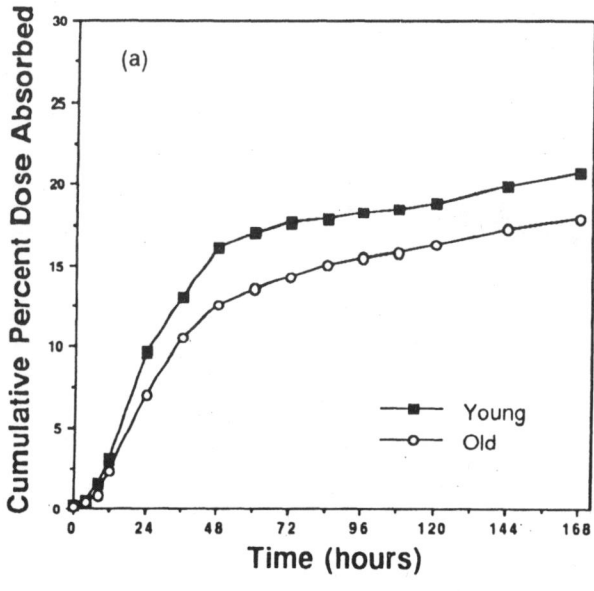

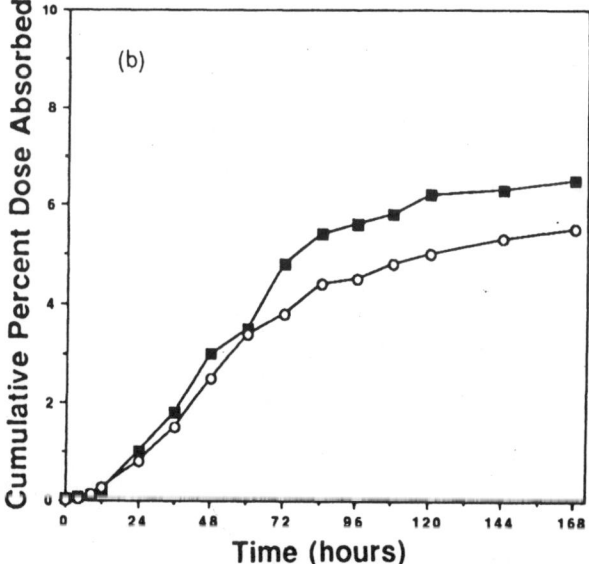

Figure 2 Cumulative percentage of dose absorbed as a function of time after topical administration of (a) testosterone, (b) estradiol, (c) hydrocortisone, (d) benzoic acid, (e) acetylsalicyclic acid, and (f) caffeine. The young subjects (filled symbols) and old subjects (open symbols) are presented on each graph. (From Ref. 16.)

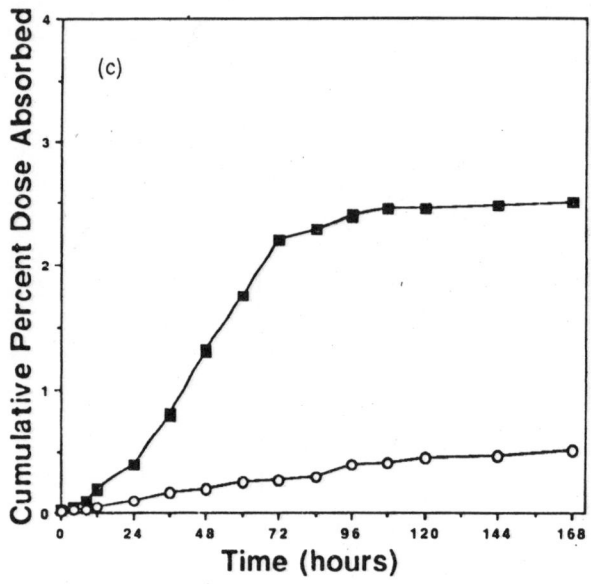

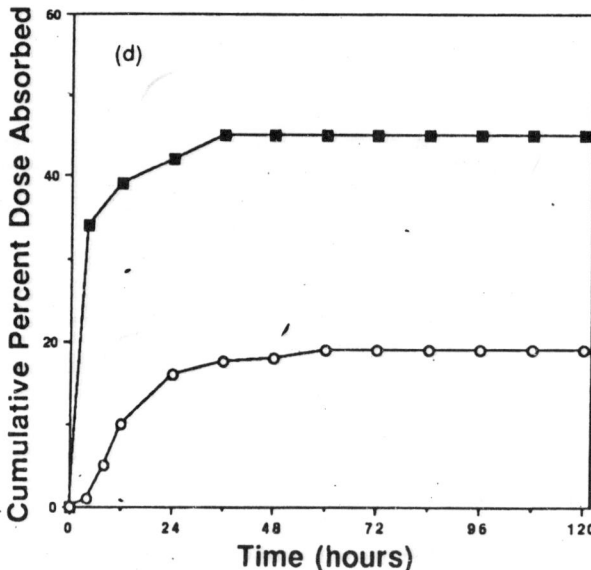

Figure 2 *(Continued)*

Transdermal and Topical Dosage Forms

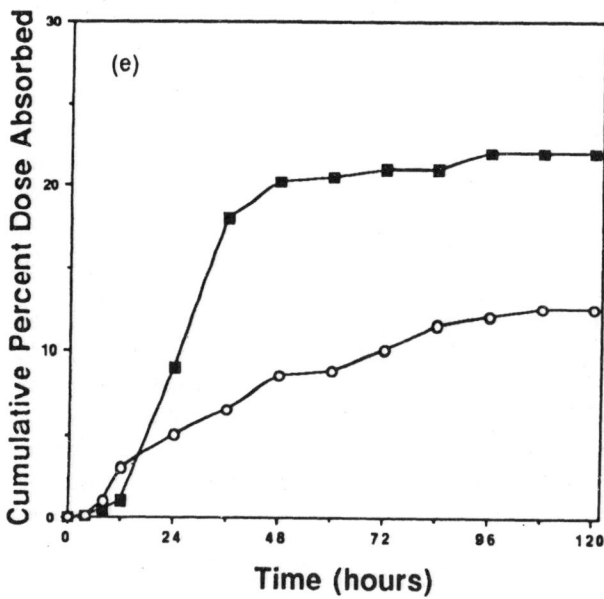

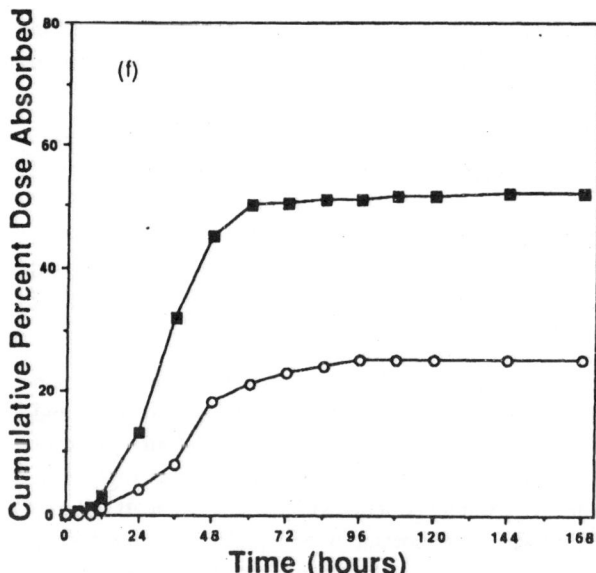

Figure 2 *(Continued)*

in bioinequivalence in the premature infant, newborn, or young child for two formulations that appear equivalent in healthy adults, there is little or no direct evidence of any such occurrences. Given all of the problems and ethical considerations that make testing in children difficult, it now would not appear appropriate to require routine evaluation of the bioequivalence of dosage forms in children, unless their use is primarily directed toward children or unless substantial evidence exists to indicate a need for such studies. More research is also needed into the influence of skin aging on the absorption of drugs, before routine inclusion of the elderly is required for bioavailability tests of drug products applied to the skin.

Considering racial differences, Guy et al. [18] compared the vasodilatation response to topically administered methyl nicotinate in young white, young black, and elderly white subjects. Their measurements utilized laser Doppler velocimetry and photoplethysmography, which are techniques to be described later. The response of the three subject groups was quite similar. Gean et al. [19] determined the cutaneous response to topical methyl nicotinate in black, Oriental, and white subjects. Visual observation of erythema did not reveal any differences among the races. However, the area under the laser Doppler velocimetry response–time curve (AUC) was significantly greater for the blacks and Orientals, compared with whites, at the higher dose levels. Wilson et al. [20] have observed a higher in vitro transepidermal water loss in black skin, and Weigand et al. [21] found the stratum corneum structure of black skin to be more compact than was observed in white skin. Whether or not these differences can result in racial differences in the action of dosage forms applied to the skin remains to be studied.

Skin condition. The condition of the skin can play an important role in percutaneous absorption. Studies in patients with psoriasis, a disease characterized by abnormal keratinization and increased blood flow, have shown greater penetration of corticosteroids into the skin, and increased excretion in the urine [22]. Thus, consideration should be given to conducting studies in both normal and diseased or damaged skin, using techniques such as tape-stripping removal of the stratum corneum.

Site of application. The permeation of a given compound through the skin may or may not be affected by the site of application of the chemical. Moe and Armstrong [23] observed no significant difference in either arterial nitroglycerin concentrations or hemodynamic measurements after application of a nitroglycerin ointment to the arm, chest, or thigh of nine patients with congestive heart failure. Therefore, the site of application was not important in these patients for this dosage form. However, other studies have demonstrated significant differences in the permeability of skin to certain steroids applied to different locations on the body [15,24]. The effect of application site on the performance of a formulation should be part of the evaluation of any new drug product. Whether or not it is also essential for the testing of generic formulations remains to be determined. At the very least, the site of application should be standardized and controlled during any study.

Metabolism by the Skin

Recent reviews [25–29] have summarized many of the enzymatic reactions applicable to topically applied compounds. The reactions and enzymes are as follows:

I. Phase I Reactions
   A. Oxidation
       Enzymes (17β-hydroxysteroid dehydrogenase, mixed function oxidase, monoamine oxidase)
          Examples of oxidative reactions:
             Testosterone to androstene-3,17-dione
             Hydrocortisone to cortisone
             17β-estradiol to estrone
   B. Reduction
       Enzymes (ketoreductase and 5α-reductase)
          Examples of reductive reactions:
             Progesterone to pregnanediol
             Estrone to 17β-estradiol
             Hydrocortisone to allodihydrocortisol
   C. Hydrolysis
       Enzymes (esterases and aryl ester-*O*-dealkylase)
          Examples of hydrolytic reactions:
             Hydrocortisone-17 esters to hydrocortisone
             Hydrocortisone-21 ester to hydrocortisone
             Betamethasone-17-valerate to betamethasone
             Benzoylperoxide to benzoic acid
             Metronidazole esters to metronidazole

II. Phase II Reactions
    Enzymes involved in methylation, glucuronidation and sulfation reactions in the skin have also been reported. Certain disease states have also been shown to be associated with altered skin metabolism:
   1. Reduced aryl-hydrocarbon hydroxylase activity in psoriasis.
   2. Increased metabolism of testosterone to dehydrotestosterone in individuals with acne vulgaris.
   3. Decreased conversion of testosterone to dehydrotestosterone by 5α-reductase in males with testicular feminization syndrome.

Enzyme inhibition and enzyme induction can also occur. For example, coal tar, which is sometimes employed topically, has been demonstrated to induce aryl-hydrocarbon hydroxylase. The conversion of benzoyl peroxide to benzoic acid is an example of the importance of skin metabolism in the degradation of a drug to an inactive compound, before it can reach the systemic circulation. In addition, organisms found on the skin may play a role in the breakdown of certain xenobiotics (e.g., nitroglycerin and betamethasone-17-valerate).

It should be apparent that the skin is not a simple passive barrier that is thoroughly understood. The interaction between the biochemistry and physiology of the skin, the active drug, and the components of the dosage form increase the complexity of evaluating the bioavailability of formulations applied to the skin. As a site for drug administration, the skin may appear to be relatively simple compared with oral administration. However we must be cognizant that delivery of the active drug to the site of action involves many steps (Figure 3). The processes may include (1) dissolution of the drug in its vehicle (some fraction of the dose may be suspended in the vehicle); (2) diffusion of the drug through the vehicle; (3) partitioning of the drug from the vehicle or dosage form into the skin; (4) diffusion of the drug through the stratum corneum, viable epidermis, and upper dermis for the transepidermal path; and (5) diffusion of the drug through the follicle, sebum, viable tissue, and upper dermis for transfollicular route [30]. In addition, we must consider potential effects of the drug or vehicle on the vascular and lymphatic flow, which can effect drug clearance, as well as changes in the composition of the vehicle owing to evaporation or skin uptake. Furthermore, the rate and extent of metabolism may play an important role. Thus, this apparently simple route of administration is clearly not so simple after all.

TRANSDERMAL DELIVERY SYSTEMS

At least in theory, the transdermal system should be easier to study than most topical formulations. Such systems can be applied and removed at precise times, the environment to which the drug is exposed is relatively well controlled owing to the impermeable backing, the release rate is intended to be predictable and relatively constant, and the quantity of drug remaining in the dosage unit can be assayed after removal. The evaluation of dosage forms intended to provide active drug to the systemic circulation after application to the skin follows many of the same principles involved in the determination of the bioavailability or bioequivalence of orally administered formulations. There are a variety of approaches to assess the performance of transdermal delivery systems. In recent years several excellent reviews have been published [7,8,31]. In addition, mathematical models have been developed to describe the kinetics of transdermal drug delivery [32] and percutaneous metabolism [33].

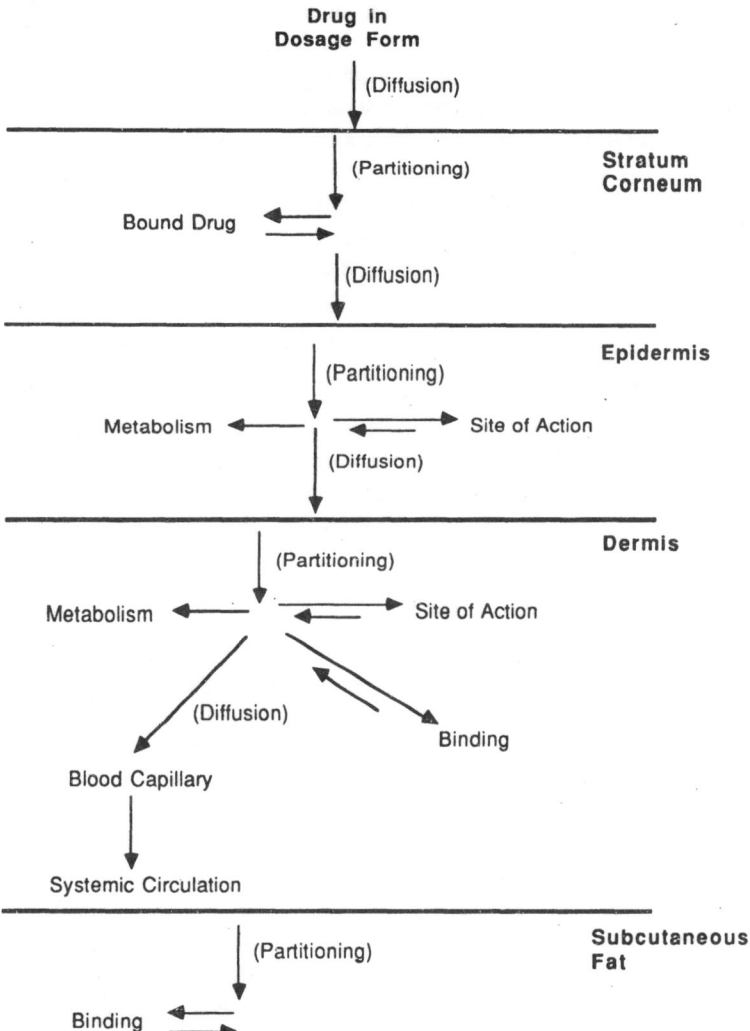

Figure 3 Possible steps involved during the percutaneous absorption of a drug present in a topical dosage form. (Modified from Ref. 30)

In Vivo Human Studies

Studies in which the dosage form is applied to the skin of human volunteers is by far the most common and widely accepted means to evaluate such dosage forms. Bioavailability is usually assessed by determining the concentration of active drug, metabolites, or both, in blood, plasma, or serum after application of the delivery systems. Occasionally (e.g., scopolamine delivery systems), urinary excretion has been employed, since drug concentrations in the blood are too low to quantitate. In general, the development of suitable analytical methods to quantitate blood concentrations of drug are especially challenging, since drugs administered by the transdermal route are typically given at very low doses. The time course of systemically available drug or metabolites should also be followed after removal of the delivery system, to characterize the kinetics of any residual drug that may be retained within the skin. The choice of the reference dosage form for the bioavailability or bioequivalence study will depend on the intent of the study.

New Drug in a Transdermal System

It is conceivable that the first dosage form developed for a new drug could be a transdermal delivery system. If this occurs, then the bioavailability testing of the dosage form will involve the usual types of absorption, distribution, excretion, and metabolic studies required of all new drugs, regardless of the nature of the dosage form.

Existing Drug in a Transdermal System

If the new dosage form is designed to replace a different type of dosage form, then the bioavailability tests should be designed to compare the existing and the new dosage forms. For example, the bioavailability of nitroglycerin transdermal products were evaluated relative to the nitroglycerin plasma concentrations achieved after application of an ointment [34] or the administration of sublingual tablets [35] (Figs. 4 and 5). Similarly, transdermal scopolamine has been tested versus oral, intravenous infusion, and intramuscular injection [35,36]; transdermal clonidine was compared with oral tablets [35]; and transdermal 17β-estradiol was evaluated relative to orally administered conjugated estrogens or oral estradiol tablets [35]. It is obvious that the drug concentration–time profiles for the test and reference products are likely to be, by design, substantially different. It is also important to recognize that a perfectly flat, prolonged plasma concentration–time profile is not necessarily more desirable than a periodic drug-free period, during which time the quantity of drug in the body declines. A systemically absorbed, topical or dermal delivery system can provide for a "smoother" profile, which minimizes peak-to-trough fluctuation. However the relationship between efficacy or toxicity and fluctuations in the plasma drug concentrations is often not well established. Other considerations also come into play, such as plasma concentration–time profiles for metabolites. Transdermal application avoids first-pass metabolism by the liver. This may alter the parent drug/metabolite ratio, when comparing oral and transdermal administration of certain drugs. In addition, as mentioned earlier, the skin is known to have a capacity to metabolize

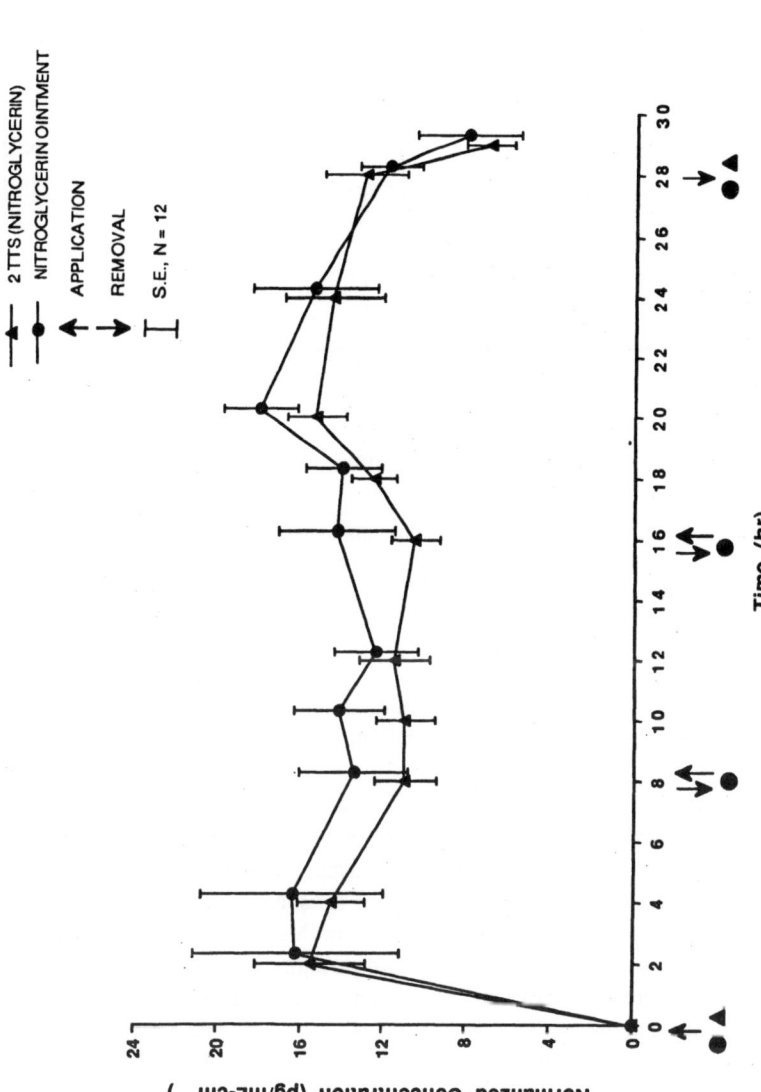

Figure 4 Comparison of mean (±SE) plasma nitroglycerin concentrations (n = 12) after application of a single transdermal patch and an ointment every 8 hr. Data are normalized to equalize the doses. (From Ref. 34.)

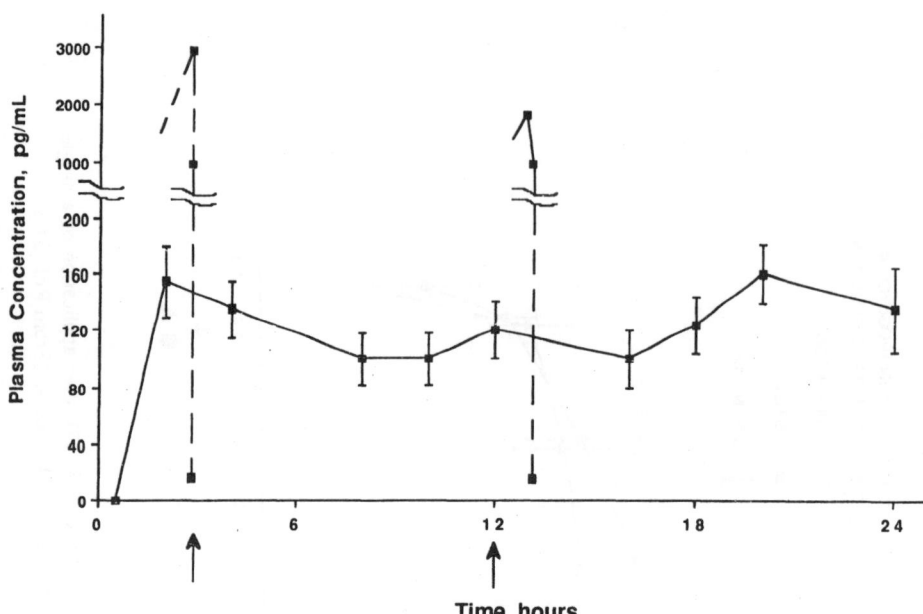

Figure 5 Mean (±SE) nitroglycerin plasma concentrations after administration of 0.3-mg sublingual tablets at 12-hr intervals (- - - ■ - - -) and a single transdermal nitroglycerin patch to 12 subjects (——■——). (From Ref. 35.)

certain chemicals. As a result, the interpretation and evaluation of the data can become complex, since one must decide which, if any, of the metabolites are important.

Because of the various factors that may affect safety and efficacy, some clinical trials should be conducted for transdermal systems designed to replace conventional therapy. Recent studies involving transdermal nitroglycerin systems have clearly indicated the importance of clinical testing for such products. The development of tolerance in patients undergoing long-term therapy could not have been determined with short-term administration, and certainly not from bioavailability studies. It now appears [36-38] that intermittent application of the systems can circumvent the development of tolerance to nitroglycerin. In some instances, long-term clinical trials may be required to establish effectiveness for all therapeutic indications. For example, clinical response with estradiol patches appears similar to oral administration for postmenopausal symptoms [36]. However, demonstration of long-term effectiveness in the prevention of osteoporosis requires more prolonged study. A good example of the clinical evaluation of a transdermal product is for fentanyl. The drug is a potent synthetic opioid agonist, with a short duration of action. Prolonged postoperative analgesia can be achieved by continuous intravenous infusion (i.e., zero-order input), at a rate of about 100 μg/hr. The preliminary study by Plezia et al. [39] used a variety of evaluations in addition to plasma concentrations, including respiratory rate, pulse, oxygen saturation, blood pressure, degree of sedation; patient rating of pain, nausea, and sedation; need for additional analgesics; and itching, erythema, edema, or blisters at the site of application, following removal of the patch. Thus, the development of the transdermal dosage form, to replace the conventional route of administration, requires an assessment of many factors, in addition to the concentration of drug in the blood. For example, parenterally administered fentanyl will immediately be in the systemic circulation, in contrast with the slow absorption from the transdermal formulation. Thus, the lag time for the transdermal to achieve therapeutic concentrations must be determined, particularly for a drug like fentanyl, which is employed to provide analgesia.

Peck and Shah [40] have recently reviewed the types of studies required by the FDA for new transdermal dosage forms. Such formulations are considered "new drugs" and, thus, are subject to full New Drug Application (NDA) requirements. As a result, well-controlled clinical trials must be conducted to demonstrate clinical efficacy, as well as evaluate local and systemic toxicity. Animal toxicity tests may not be required if the toxicity of the active drug is well established. In addition, systemic safety may be established, at least in part, by comparison of the concentrations of drug in the blood achieved with the transdermal system, compared with a conventional dosage form. Studies will need to be conducted to evaluate (1) the in vivo reproducibility of the release and absorption process, in terms of both intersubject and intrasubject variability; (2) the effect of site of application; and (3) the metabolism of the drug during passage through the skin.

Generic Transdermal Formulation

Peck and Shah [40] have also reviewed the requirements of the FDA for approval of generic versions of transdermal products that have already been approved. Unless the drug-release mechanism, adhesive, device materials, or other inactive ingredients are significantly different from the innovator product, extensive safety and efficacy data will not be required. Typically, the objective of bioequivalence studies conducted in support of an Abbreviated New Drug Application (ANDA) is to demonstrate the absence of significant differences between the test and reference dosage forms in terms of drug or metabolite concentrations in vivo. A good example of a bioequivalence study for a transdermal system is shown in Figure 6. The study [41] consisted of a two-way, single-dose crossover study in 24 healthy male volunteers, and involved a comparison of a marketed transdermal nitroglycerin formulation with a newly developed formulation, both

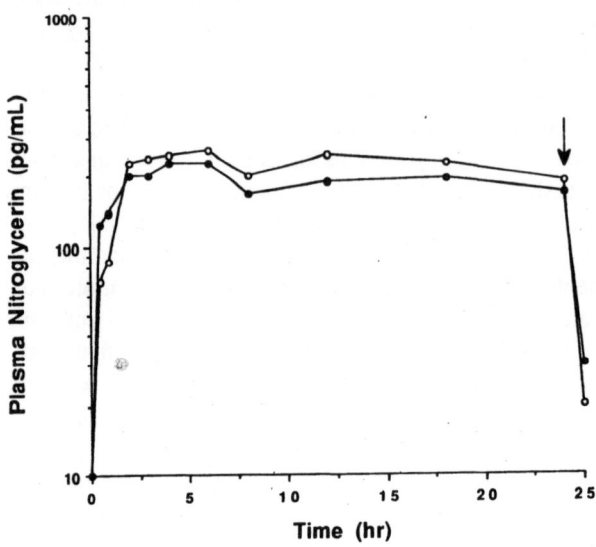

Figure 6 Plasma nitroglycerin concentrations after the administration of two nitroglycerin transdermal formulations. Values represent means (n = 24), with removal of the patches after 24 hr. (From Ref. 41.)

manufactured by the same firm. The same type of protocol could also be applied to the evaluation of a generic formulation and a reference product manufactured by different firms. The following determinations were made as part of the study protocol:

1. *Apparent dose*, as the difference between the mean initial potency of the dosage form and the potency remaining in the device when it was removed 24 hr after application
2. The plasma nitroglycerin concentration–time profile during the 24-hr period of application
3. Changes in subject heart rate and blood pressure
4. Recording of side effects (primarily mild headache)
5. Subjective evaluation of the degree and duration of skin irritation

There is obviously a good correspondence between the mean plasma concentration–time profile for the two formulations (see Fig. 6). Note that other measurements were also made in addition to the quantitation of plasma or drug concentrations. For example, the quantity of drug remaining in the dosage form at the end of the dosing interval is determined as a measure of the release rate of the drug from the formulation. In general, it is also useful to attempt some measurement of pharmacologic activity. Pharmacodynamic measurements should, to the extent possible, be related to the therapeutic use of the dosage form (e.g., heart rate and blood pressure, for transdermal nitroglycerin).

Transdermal systems usually contain a number of components, such as a plastic-backing membrane, reservoir layer, rate-controlling layer or membrane, adhesive layer, plasticizers, and other additives [9]. Each component can vary among the available dosage forms; hence, each type of delivery system can be different in terms of release of drug. It is also important to assess the degree of skin irritation or sensitivity, as well as the degree of adherence of the system to the skin. Obviously, if two formulations are not equally well retained on the skin under normal conditions of use, or if one is more irritating than the other, then differences in clinical effectiveness are possible. Wick et al. [42] have presented a study design that is appropriate to evaluate delivery system adherence. The transdermal system was applied to the skin of human volunteers, and the force required to remove the patches after specified application times during a 24-hr period was determined with a mechanical adhesion tester. In addition, they assessed the percentage of the patch that was not attached, and also examined the skin surface for adhesive residue after removal. In studies of topical formulations, it is also important to carefully control the method of applying the dosage form for thickness of the applied layer and the surface area of the application site. The data in Table 1 [43] illustrate the effect of surface area on the systemic availability of a 2% nitroglycerin ointment, as determined by the area under the plasma concentration–time curve (AUC). There was an approximate proportional increase in AUC with a twofold increase in dose when the surface area was constant. There was also a very large change in the AUC when the same 16-mg dose was applied to two different surface areas. In contrast, Iafrate et al. [44] observed only a 30% increase in AUC, which was not statistically significant, for ten subjects who received the same amount of nitroglycerin ointment spread over either 25 or 50 cm^2. The lack of a proportional change in AUC with increased surface area may, in part, have been due to a lack of control of the thickness of the applied ointment.

In Vivo Animal Studies

Animals are often employed during the developmental phase of a topically applied dosage form. However, animal data are not usually accepted in lieu of human studies. The relevance of animal models in the study of percutaneous absorption has been reviewed by Wester and Noonan [45]. Shaw et al. [35] described the steps involved in developing and testing a transdermal product. Animals may be useful in gaining preliminary information about the percutaneous absorption, skin irritation, and sensitization of a dosage form. However, they are not always

Table 1 Effect of Dose and Surface Area on the Area Under the Plasma Concentration–Time Curve After Application of 2% Nitroglycerin Ointment to Four Volunteers

Method of Application	AUC (ng · mL^{-1} · min^{-1})
16 mg over 25 cm^2	<0.2
16 mg over 100 cm^2	0.40
32 mg over 100 cm^2	0.72

Source: Ref. 43

predictive of a clinical outcome because of differences in drug disposition, skin physiology, and many other factors. For example, animal testing of transdermal clonidine formulations did not indicate the potential for skin sensitization, later found during long-term clinical use [35]. The use of an animal model, the performance of which has been shown to correlate with humans, is an appropriate means to minimize human testing. Unfortunately, very few, if any, examples exist in the literature demonstrating correlations of this type. Certainly, selected drugs, or specific test formulations, may show a similar rank order for humans and laboratory animals, but such correlations do not guarantee the ability to predict how other drugs or formulations will perform. Furthermore, the establishment of such a correlation will require a great deal of effort, since studies will be required in both humans and animals. Consequently, it is generally more expedient to simply conduct the human studies. All of the usual concerns about the extrapolation of results obtained in animals to those anticipated in humans, applies to the use of animals for transdermal dosage form evaluation. Moreover, differences among species in skin characteristics is an added consideration, as discussed later. In addition, there are several experimental variables that must be controlled or accounted for as part of the conduct of in vivo animal studies.

1. Hair removal methods
2. Grading procedures to quantitate response and control of investigator bias
3. Selection of application site
4. Occlusion or protection of site and restraint
5. How samples are applied (area, dose, pressure, application device)
6. Washing or wiping methods
7. Environment (lighting, temperature, humidity)
8. Restraint of animal

Wester et al. [46] have demonstrated the usefulness of the monkey as a model to study the percutaneous absorption of nitroglycerin from an ointment. They administered [^{14}C]nitroglycerin to monkeys as an intravenous injection and as a 2% marketed ointment. They observed an absolute bioavailability, on the basis of total radioactivity, of approximately 75%, and approximately 57% on the basis of unchanged nitroglycerin. These data indicated the extent of alteration of the nitroglycerin to be approximately 20% by metabolism or other breakdown mechanism. Wester et al. [47] also reviewed the use of the rhesus monkey for other compounds, using topically applied ^{14}C-labeled compounds. Benzoic acid, testosterone, and hydrocortisone were each absorbed quite differently, but the data obtained in the monkey were similar to that obtained in man (Fig. 7) [48].

In Vitro Testing

Just as in vitro dissolution testing can be of great assistance in the development of a controlled-release oral dosage form, such testing may also be useful in designing new transdermal or topical formulations. Several types of in vitro methods have been recently reviewed by Abdou [49].

The *United States Pharmacopeia (USP) XXII* [50] has three different types of dissolution methods published for transdermal delivery systems. One method

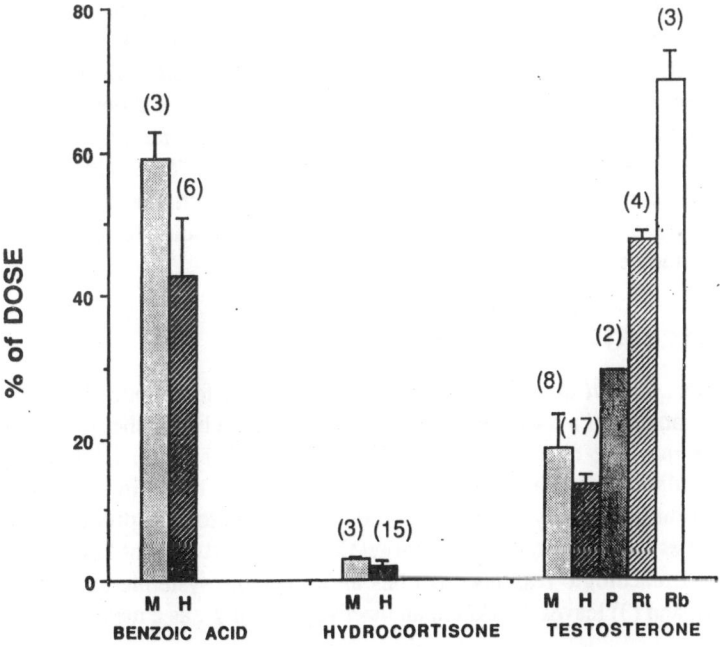

Figure 7 Comparison of the percutaneous absorption of benzoic acid, hydrocortisone, and testosterone in rhesus monkeys (M), humans (H), pig (P), rat (Rt), and rabbit (Rb). (Based on Ref. 48.)

employs the USP paddle, with the delivery system being anchored at the bottom of the dissolution vessel. A second method uses a specially designed cylinder, which replaces the basket and shaft normally used for the USP basket method. The delivery system is attached to the bottom of the rotating cylinder. The third device is based on a reciprocating action, with the delivery system being attached to the bottom of a disk, which is moved with a vertical reciprocating motion.

The *USP XII* does not now contain any monographs for transdermal dosage forms; consequently, no official USP specifications are associated with such products. Furthermore, little work has been published to demonstrate the applicability of any of these methods as a means to assess bioavailability. One may assume that one or more of these methods may be useful for batch-to-batch quality control. However, assurance of the ability of an in vitro test to detect product changes, which may have an effect on in vivo performance, requires some validation of the in vivo–in vitro relationship. For example, Shah and Skelly [51] have conducted dissolution testing of marketed nitroglycerin patches, using a modified FDA paddle method (*USP* apparatus 2), at 50 rpm in water. The patch rested on a watchglass placed at the bottom of the dissolution container, and was held in place with an aluminum wire screen. The release of the nitroglycerin was monitored over a 24-hr period. Their data demonstrated that the release of drug was proportional to the content of each patch. The three marketed products released the drug at distinctly different rates, suggesting the possibility of bioinequivalence. However, since direct comparisons of these products in humans have shown comparable release in vivo, it is obvious that the in vitro results were not predictive of the appearance of the nitroglycerin in the systemic circulation. Thus, although in vitro testing can contribute to the monitoring of batch-to-batch quality and is useful in product development, it does not now appear to be a suitable substitution for in vivo studies.

TOPICAL DOSAGE FORMS

As defined earlier, *topical dosage forms* are those designed for application to the skin for the treatment of a local condition. Some penetration below the stratum corneum may or may not occur, and may or may not be desirable. Unlike a transdermal formulation, topical products are not intended to result in any appreciable absorption into the systemic circulation. The ideal topical product is one that (1) achieves a concentration in the target tissue that is sufficient to result in the desired pharmacologic response; (2) has an acceptable systemic toxicity (preferably none); and (3) leaves the skin in an inactive form (e.g., as a metabolite) [52].

Current regulations for the marketing of topical dosage forms in the United States depend on when the innovator's product was initially marketed. If the original product was approved before 1962, there are currently no requirements for in vivo bioavailability or bioequivalence studies for generic versions of innovator products. Such products need only evaluation of skin irritation, cutaneous toxicity, and contact sensitivity [53]. For post-1962 products, the 1984 Patent Term Restoration Act, or the Waxman-Hatch Amendments, make mandatory a bioequivalence study for all drug products approved through an ANDA. Obviously, this requirement results in somewhat of a dilemma, since classic measurement of drug concentration-time profiles in the systemic circulation are not possible for these types of dosage forms. In fact, some believe that the Waxman-Hatch Amendments do not apply at all to products that are not absorbed, since it is not possible to evaluate either the rate or extent of absorption. However, this point of view is based on legislative and legal arguments, which require resolution in another forum. If we define bioequivalence in its broadest terms, one may state that *two topical products are bioequivalent* if they both result in equivalent clinical effectiveness and equivalent toxicity. This definition leads us to conclude that clinical trials must be conducted for such dosage forms. However, it is also possible that other types of in vivo studies, or perhaps even in vitro methods, could serve as a surrogate for clinical trials, if acceptable correlations can be demonstrated.

If one desires to evaluate the effectiveness of a nonabsorbed topical dosage form, several types of studies may be considered:

1. A well-controlled clinical trial
2. Measurement of a pharmacodynamic effect
3. Measurement of drug penetration into the skin
4. In vitro methods correlated with a clinical endpoint
5. Animal studies
6. Any other method that can be shown to be capable of measuring bioequivalence

General Considerations

In many ways, the evaluation of topical products may be more challenging than for transdermal dosage forms. Often we are not certain of the site of action (i.e., which layer of the skin), the mechanism of action, and the analysis of drug or metabolite concentrations in the skin or systemic circulation may require very sensitive assay methods. Moreover, in general, there is a lack of standardization for how to conduct studies of topical products. During clinical use, topical products may be applied with variable thicknesses, over a variable surface area, and the application site is generally not specified in the labeling. When the applied film is quite thin, the composition of the dosage form can change dramatically as the components evaporate into the atmosphere or are absorbed into the skin, or as fluids of the skin diffuse into the vehicle. The components of the formulation may also precipitate following topical application. If the vehicle is an emulsion it may break or undergo phase inversion. Thus, the thermodynamic activity of the drug can change throughout the period of application, and a formulation that appears satisfactory during initial testing may not be adequate under the conditions employed clinically. Also components of the formulation, such as surfactants or agents that act as penetration enhancers, irritants, or dehydrators could affect the properties of the skin, or could interact with the drug to enhance absorption or inhibit absorption, such as through entrapment within micelles [15,54]. The viscosity of the vehicle can affect the diffusion of the drug. Hence, any bioequivalence comparison of topical formulations should also include an assessment of the physicochemical properties of the products (e.g., rheology). Furthermore, the product may be inadvertently removed from the application site as a result of washing, rubbing by clothing, and such. Consequently, studies involving topical products must be designed to account for as many experimental variables as possible, including the previously described effects of age, race, application site, and skin condition. We must also remember that the objective of topical therapy is to deliver drug to the site of action, while minimizing systemic absorption. It is known, for example, that the percutaneous absorption of topical adrenocorticoids may result in suppression of the hypothalamic–pituitary–adrenal axis, hyperglycemia, glycosuria, and other systemic effects. These effects are more likely when the topical product is applied over a large surface area and with occlusion [55]. Any assessment of a topical formulation should also consider the extent to which unintended systemic absorption may occur. Barry [56] has provided an excellent review of the many factors that may influence the performance of a topically applied dosage form.

It is clear that topical dosage forms may be as subject to bioavailability problems as other dosage forms, given the complexity of topical therapy and topical formulations. Guy et al. [1] have recently published an excellent overview of the methods and pitfalls associated with bioavailability testing of topical dosage forms. They also summarized areas of research that are essential if we are to be able to evaluate such dosage forms with the same degree of rigor that is possible with formulations designed to provide drug to the systemic circulation. There are relatively few publications demonstrating bioavailability differences among various topical products. This, in part, is due to our limited understanding of how to evaluate these dosage forms. Therefore, it is worthwhile to review some of the experimental approaches that have been taken, or are being proposed, in an attempt to better understand this class of dosage forms.

Animal Models

The use of animals in studying percutaneous absorption has recently been reviewed [57]. The primary deficiency involved in the use of animal models to assess topical formulations is that no suitable animal models have been developed for the diseases normally treated by topical dosage forms.

Data obtained in monkeys [47] have been useful to demonstrate the effect of administration site on absorption of testosterone, with the results indicating scalp > cheek = ventral forearm > chest. Studies of testosterone in various animal species has also indicated the ranking of the topically applied steroid to be rabbit > rat > pig > rhesus monkey = human [47]. Other workers have suggested that the hairless guinea pig appears to be the most suitable model for skin studies, and no furry animal skin appears suitable [58].

A particularly elegant animal model is the human skin–sandwich flap [59,60]. Human skin is grafted onto a congentitally athymic (nude) mouse. The mouse is treated with cyclosporine to depress the immune system. The grafted skin has been utilized repeatedly for up to 6 months. Of particular importance is that the surgical procedure results in a model in which the vein exiting the flap can be visualized, and blood samples can be withdrawn to measure systemic absorption of test compounds.

In Vitro Methods

Smith and Haigh [61] have provided an excellent critical review of the types of in vitro diffusion equipment that is available. They also discuss the many experimental variables that must be controlled and the need to demonstrate the validity of any in vitro device. They point out that most in vitro studies involve an infinite-dose, steady-state approach (i.e., the concentration gradient across the barrier remains constant after an initial lag time). However, in clinical practice, the dose is applied to the skin as a finite quantity, which diminishes as absorption proceeds.

If a topically applied drug simply acts by diffusing into the statum corneum, then it might be possible to evaluate bioequivalence solely with an in vitro model. However, given the dynamic characteristics of the skin, the potential for systemic absorption, and the metabolic enzymes present in the skin, it cannot be assumed that the rate and extent of release of active drug from the dosage form can be adequately evaluated with in vitro methods.

Guzek et al. [62] and Potts et al. [63] have demonstrated some of the problems associated with the use of in vitro systems for compounds that are metabolized. They compared the metabolism of a diester derivative of salicylic acid in vitro, using human skin mounted in a diffusion cell, under both sink and nonsink conditions, as well as in vivo with human skin orthotopically grafted to athymic mice. As shown in Figure 8, much greater enzymatic activity was observed in the in vitro system that did not have sink conditions. This was attributed to the prolonged residence of the esters within the skin preparation for the in vitro system, owing to the lack of a blood supply, and possible increased esterase activity from release of enzymes during sample preparation or exposure of the skin to the receiving chamber of the diffusion cell. Therefore, for drugs that can

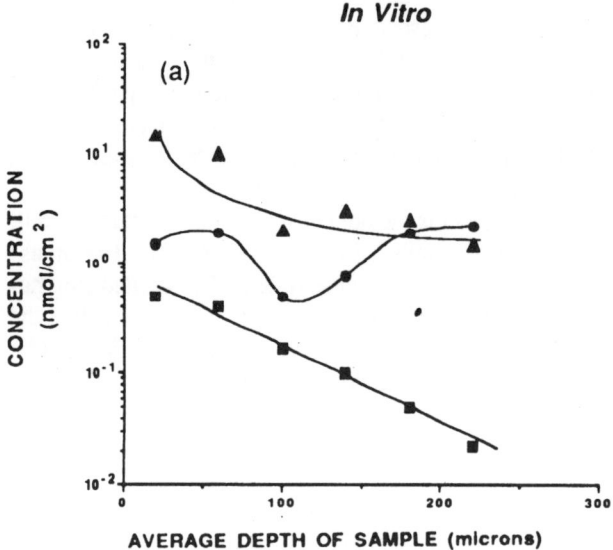

Figure 8 The distribution of salicylic acid (circles), the monoester (squares), and the diester (triangle), as a function of depth in human skin. Studies were conducted (a) in vitro in the absence of sink conditions; (b) in vitro with sink conditions in the receiver chamber, and (c) in vivo using human skin grafted to athymic mice. (From Ref. 63.)

be metabolized during passage through the skin, one may obtain misleading estimates of the extent of metabolism from in vitro results in the absence of sink conditions.

A consensus report has recently been published [64] that was based on a public workshop dealing with the relevance of in vitro percutaneous penetration studies. The conclusions were as follows:

1. Definition
   a. *Percutaneous absorption* may be defined as "permeation of agents through the epidermis and into the deep layers of skin, and general circulation in vivo, a total process that includes transport through the skin and local clearance."
   b. *Skin permeation* is considered to be the initial part of the process, involving only diffusion across the skin.
2. Human skin is preferred for the conduct of in vitro tests. However, research should continue involving animal skin, because of its availability, as well as synthetic membranes, because of their convenience. However Barry has

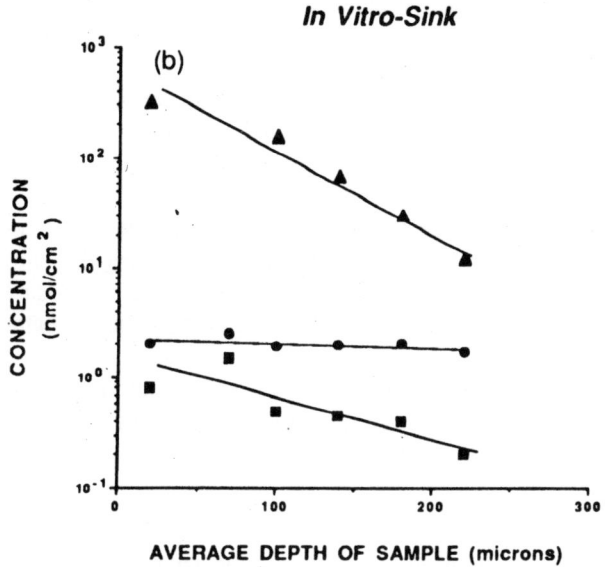

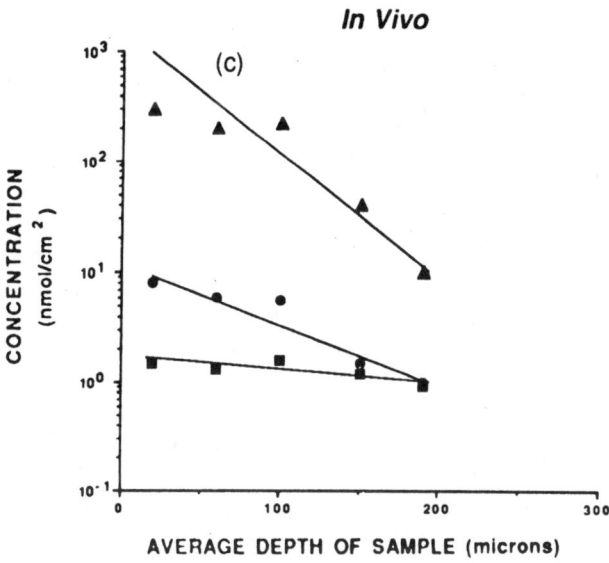

Figure 8 *(Continued)*

recently commented that "If at all possible, investigative problems should not be made more complex by selection of an animal tissue to represent human skin." [65].
3. The report also stated that "minor" modifications in a formulation or manufacturing process could be evaluated using in vitro methods. However, we are not yet at the point where significantly different formulations produced by different firms could be compared by only in vitro methods.
4. The report provided guidance on the characteristics of the human skin membrane, the design of the diffusion cell, the selection of the receptor fluid, the use of a skin surface temperature of 32 °C, the application of the product to the skin surface, the use of occlusion, as well as the analysis and presentation of the data.
5. The report concluded that for topical dosage forms, other than those in true solution, it is desirable to include in vitro release specifications as part of the NDA to assure batch-to-batch drug release equivalence.

Behme et al. [66] have stated:

> The ideal in vitro procedure would be one in which the sample is in direct contact with the receptor phase, because barriers used to isolate the sample from that phase have a potential leveling effect on the rate of appearance of the drug in the receptor phase.

They presented a method that employed the application of samples of a cream into an 80-mesh stainless steel screen. The screen, loaded with the cream, was placed into a thin-layer chromatograph (TLC) developing jar, perpendicular to the bottom of the jar. The receptor phase was stirred with a magnetic bar. However, Shah et al. [67] have pointed out problems with such test methods. The topical dosage form is immersed in a receptor phase, with no rate-influencing barrier, and the method exposes the dosage form to receptor phase on both sides. This may lead to the formation of channels, with entry of the receptor phase and alteration of the release. Furthermore, the method is limited to topicals that are not miscible with the aqueous receptor phase.

Although it is certainly desirable to develop an in vitro test to mimic in vivo performance, there are several reasons why this has not yet been accomplished, including (1) variable dose, amount, and frequency during clinical use; (2) application method (with or without dressing, occluded); (3) skin age and site, as well as skin condition (i.e., damaged, diseased, or normal); and (4) metabolism within the skin. Indeed, there are a host of variables that can have an impact on the development of an in vitro system [68]. For example, metabolic capacity changes as a function of age for benzo[a]pyrene metabolism and epoxide-metabolizing enzyme activity in the skin of rats [69]. In addition, Kao et al. [70] have demonstrated considerable species differences in the metabolism of testosterone and benzo[a]pyrene during penetration through viable, full-thickness skin. Even though there is a general consensus that human skin currently provides the best test model, there is less of a consensus on the best animal skin substitute. Some have suggested that the skin of monkeys and weanling pigs provides the most predictive model for human percutaneous absorption [47]. A variety of membranes have been suggested [71], in increasing order of clinical relevance they are

1. Artificial membrane permeation
2. Permeation through excised animal skin
3. Permeation through human stratum corneum
4. Permeation through excised human skin
5. Permeation through excised human skin—finite dose

There are several sources for human skin, including surgical (face, breast, abdominal), foreskin obtained during circumcision, and fresh cadaver skin. However, there are problems associated with the use of human skin, such as

1. Availability
2. Duration of viability and storage conditions
3. Variability
4. Potential for transmittal of disease from donor to investigator

Chiang et al. [72] have examined the effect of intersubject variability on the assessment of the in vitro release of minoxidil and hydrocortisone from solution and ointment. The flux (mg $\cdot$ cm^{-2} $\cdot$ hr^{-1}) varied over a 25-fold and a 15-fold range for the minoxidil ointment and solution, respectively, using cadaver abdominal skin sections from eight different sources. In contrast, the hydrocortisone flux varied over only a twofold range for the ointment and a 1.4-fold range for the solution, for cadaver skin from four different sources. Clearly, comparisons of different formulations should employ cadaver skin from a single source. In the event skin from different sources must be employed, the flux of each new formulation could be compared with a standard reference formulation using a given section of skin. For example, the data in Table 2 demonstrates a relatively constant ratio for solution/ointment flux for both compounds, independent of the source of the skin section. The authors also point out potential problems with the analysis of in vitro data of this type [72]. The conclusions about formulation differences that are based on flux can depend on the lag time to achieve steady-state flux and whether steady-state flux is actually achieved within a clinically relevant time. Additionally, the use of the cumulative amount of drug delivered within a fixed time can also be misleading, depending on the duration of the lag time.

In view of the problems inherent to the use of human skin, Shah et al. [67] have recently studied the in vitro release from two marketed hydrocortisone

Table 2 Flux of Minoxidil (2%) and Hydrocortisone (Trace) from Solutions and Ointment Vehicles Through Human Cadaver Skin from Various Sources

Cadaver No.	Ointment	Solution	Flux ratio solution/ointment
Flux of minoxidil ($\times 10^5$ mg · cm^{-2} · hr^{-1})			
1	0.51	1.3	2.5
2	0.37	1.3	3.5
3	2.2	7.3	3.4
4	7.8	10.0	1.3
5	1.6	4.4	2.8
6	9.2	18.7	2.0
7	3.8	9.0	2.4
8	4.8	13.6	2.8
		Mean ± SD	2.6 ± 0.7
Flux of hydrocortisone (cpm · cm^{-2} · hr^{-1})			
1	983	946	1.0
2	696	966	1.4
3	1335	1291	1.0
4	991	1166	1.2
		Mean ± SD	1.1 ± 0.2

Source: Ref. 72.

creams, using commercially available synthetic membranes with a Franz diffusion cell. They used six different membranes and tested 0.05 M, pH 5 phosphate buffer; 0.09% sodium chloride, and 0.05 M pH 7.4 phosphate buffer as the recipient media. The method appeared to be reproducible and convenient for the determination of the release characteristics of topical dosage forms (i.e., as a quality control procedure). However, the two test products exhibited similar in vitro release characteristics, and no further work was done to correlate the in vitro data with the in vivo performance of the dosage forms. Consideration should also be given to including in vitro testing as part of any stability program. Quantitation of potency alone may not detect product changes that could affect bioavailability.

Human Testing

The use of in vitro systems and animal models has much appeal as techniques to study drug disposition in dosage forms applied to the skin. They are certainly useful tools to isolate and quantitate variables that may affect drug release from the dosage form. However, at our current state of knowledge, the final evaluation of such dosage forms inevitably ends with studies involving human volunteers or patients. Many of the variables associated with in vivo animal testing also need attention during in vivo human testing (see items 1–7 in the earlier discussion of the use of animals to test transdermal formulations). In addition, several additional variables must be considered:

1. Patient compliance
2. Concomitant use of other medications or cosmetics
3. Skin condition (normal, diseased, sunburn)

Studies with monkeys, for example, have shown, that skin washing between applications of hydrocortisone resulted in increased penetration, but had no effect on the absorption of testosterone [47]. Studies with monkeys have also shown that repeated application of hydrocortisone resulted in a 275% increase in the absorption of hydrocortisone comparing day 1 and day 8. This suggested a possible alteration in the characteristics of the skin with repeated administration [47]. Thus, the use of single or multiple doses may also affect the experimental results.

Several experimental approaches have been described for quantitating the uptake of drug by the skin.

Skin Stripping

Skin stripping is a relatively simple technique in which the layers of the skin are removed by successive application of strips of adhesive tape. Dupuis et al. [73] applied radiolabeled benzoic acid to hairless rats and humans and measured radioactivity in the tape strips and in the urine. They found (1) the quantity of material excreted in the urine and residing in the stratum corneum was twofold greater for the rat; (2) the urinary recovery was proportional to the applied dose in both the rat and human; and (3) there was a good correlation between the quantity of benzoic acid in the stratum corneum after 30 min, and the urinary recovery of radiolabel after 4 days for both species. Rougier et al. [74] have also compared the amount of ^{14}C-labeled benzoic acid, sodium benzoate, caffeine, or aspirin absorbed after the application of each material to the forehead, postauricular, upper outer arm, or abdomen of human volunteers. Absorption was determined by urinary excretion. In addition, in a second study the quantity of material in the stratum corneum was determined by 15 tape strippings, after washing the treated area, 30 min after each application. The ranking for absorption was arm $\leq$ abdomen $<$ postauricular $<$ forehead, with the forehead about twice as permeable as the arm and abdomen for all four compounds. They also found an excellent correlation, $r = 0.97$ ($p < 0.001$) between the mean amount penetrated 4 days after application and the amount of radioactivity in the stratum corneum 30 min after application. The correlation was independent of the compound or site of application. Rougier et al. [75] also applied ten different radiolabeled compounds in ethanol/water solutions to the dorsal skin of hairless rats for 30 min. They found a good correlation between the amount of radioactivity recovered in the urine, feces, skin, and whole animal body after 4 days and the amount of drug recovered by tape-strip removal of the stratum corneum after the 30-min application, $r = 0.998$ ($p < 0.001$). This technique could also be employed with a nonradioactive drug if a sufficiently sensitive assay method is available. Similar studies by Rougier et al. [76], in hairless rats, with theophylline, aspirin, nicotinic acid, and benzoic acid, demonstrated a proportionality between (1) the percutaneous absorption (measured as radioactivity in the urine) and duration of application (0.5, 2, 4, or 6 hr); and (2) the quantity recovered in the stratum corneum by stripping, following a 30-min application, and the quantity of radioactivity recovered in the urine. These workers also noted differences between the relative penetration rates of the four compounds in the rats, in comparison with previous data in humans, suggesting the rat may be a good model for some compounds, but not for all. As a final example, Sheth et al. [77] found a good correlation between the quantity of iododeoxyuridine present in the stratum corneum of the guinea pig treated with different concentrations of drug in aqueous dimethyl sulfoxide (DMSO) solutions, as determined by tape stripping, and the efficacy of the treatment when applied to sites inoculated with herpes simplex virus ($r = 0.97$).

Studies such as these suggest the tape-stripping technique could play a very useful role in assessing bioequivalence. Potential problems include the need to have a sensitive assay to measure amounts of drug on the tape; the uncertainty about whether the method will be applicable to all drugs; the lack of demonstrated correlations between stratum corneum concentrations, urinary excretion, and clinical response; difficulty in assessing rate of penetration; and the inability to estimate the degree of metabolism in the epidermal and dermal layers.

Biopsies

The penetration of a compound into the skin may also be determined by skin sectioning, by taking a punch biopsy (e.g., a cylinder 5-mm diameter × 1-cm deep). The plug is frozen and cut into horizontal sections. One may assay for radioactive or nonradioactive drug, depending on the form of the drug, with the drug and metabolites quantitated separately. Because of the slicing technique, it may not be possible to obtain a precise determination of exactly where the drug is localized. An alternate approach is to take vertical slices, and employ autoradiography to determine where the radioactivity (drug plus metabolites) are located within the skin. The disadvantage to this approach is that one cannot differentiate between drug and metabolites, and the technique is not very quantitative. Biopsy methods are obviously not ideal, since only small samples may be obtained, nonradioactive assays require high sensitivity, and it is difficult to obtain frequent samples. In addition, the methods measure permeation into, and retention within the skin, but do not provide information on systemic availability.

Pharmacodynamic Effects

In 1962, McKenzie and Stoughton [78] published a procedure to measure the percutaneous absorption of corticosteroids following topical application. The method is based on estimates of the extent of blanching or whitening of the skin after exposure to the drug. The procedure involved placing 0.02 ml of an alcoholic solution or suspension of a drug on the flexor aspects of both forearms. After drying, one arm was covered with a perforated aluminum guard and left open to the air. The other arm was covered with an occlusive layer of Saran Wrap. After 16 hr the arms were examined for vasoconstriction, rating the observed blanching as present or absent. Data obtained with this method, or various modifications, are utilized for topical corticosteroid products subject to a NDA in the United States. It is also employed to determine bioequivalence for generic corticosteroid drug products subject to an ANDA.

Since the original publication, numerous other workers have used the method, often with some modification. For example, Jackson et al. [79] studied five different marketed betamethasone valerate 0.1% creams and six different marketed triamcinolone acetonide 0.1% creams, in two groups of 12 subjects. Each subject received five 0.01-ml portions of each cream spread over different skin surface areas to yield doses of 0.02, 0.01, 0.002, 0.001, and 0.0006 mL/cm^2. The area of application was encompassed by a Plexiglas ring open to the air. The creams remained in place for 6 hr. The degree of vasoconstriction was rated on a 0–3 scale, for which 0 was no blanching and 3 was total blanching of the entire area. Statistically significant differences were found among creams containing both drugs, suggesting a lack of bioequivalence. In addition, particularly for the triamcinolone acetonide creams, the largest differences among the six creams were at the lowest dilution (largest application area). This suggests that testing of topicals should not be confined just to a single surface area.

Tur et al. [80] measured the vasodilation resulting from the topical application of methyl nicotinate at various positions on human ventral forearm skin. They used photoplethysmography to monitor vascular effects, and found no difference between lateral and medial sites on the forearms, nor between the left and right arms. However, they did note the peak response was significantly higher for the proximal position than for the distal application, and they warned that the site of application could contribute to variability in the vasoconstrictor assay. Another potential problem is the development of tachyphylaxis with repeated dosing. Barry and Woodford [81] applied several topical corticosteroid creams, three times a day, for 5 days, followed by 2 days of rest. The 5-day application regimen was then repeated. The blanching response initially increased, but then, became less intense during the first 5 days of application. The apparent tachyphylaxis was again observed during the second 5-day treatment period, and the overall response was diminished compared with the initial 5-day treatment period. Burdick [82] also described some of the experimental variables associated with the vasoconstrictor test. He recommended 6 hr of contact, with no occlusion. Scoring of the degree of blanching should be by two trained observers 8, 24, and 32 hr after removal. Burdick noted that occlusion may tend to obscure formulation differences; some individuals may respond more slowly to the drug, and a single measurement at 8 hr may miss the response; and sites within about 4 cm of the wrist or elbow, and sites on the lateral and medial surface of the arm are less responsive to vasoconstrictor action and should be avoided.

In recent years, several reports have been published on the use of the vasoconstrictor test to evaluate marketed corticosteroid formulations. Stoughton [24] has reviewed some of these findings, which clearly demonstrate that one cannot a priori assume equivalence among various formulations. For example, significant differences in vasoconstrictor scores were found among marketed 0.1% triamcinolone acetonide ointments. However, no differences were observed among different strengths (0.025, 0.1, and 0.5%) of triamcinolone acetonide creams from the same manufacturer. Similar results were found for 1 and 2.5% hydrocortisone creams. In contrast, a dose response was observed among 0.01, 0.025, and 0.2% fluocinolone acetonide creams [83]. It would appear that for some drugs the vasoconstrictor response may be saturated over a range of concentrations, whereas for other drugs, a dose-response relationship can be observed. Such results obviously have an influence on the determination of the bioequivalence of comparable formulations. Once the vasoconstrictor response is maximized, differences among formulations will not be discernible. In another study, Stoughton [84] again reported differences in blanching activity among marketed brand and generic creams and ointments. The brand 0.1% triamcinolone acetonide cream and ointment were more active than the generic products. The brand 0.1% betamethasone valerate cream also resulted in greater blanching than the generic creams, but no differences were seen among the brand and generic 0.1% betamethasone valerate ointments. The brand fluocinolone acetonide cream exhibited greater activity than one generic product, but did not differ from four others. Barry and Woodford [85], using a 6-hr occluded blanching test, found significant differences among six commercial hydrocortisone creams. Interestingly, a cream containing 0.1% hydrocortisone resulted in significantly greater blanching than creams containing 1% hydrocortisone.

In an attempt to validate the applicability of the blanching assay to the therapeutic use of corticosteroids, Cornell and Stoughton [86] compared the results obtained by the vasoconstrictor test with those obtained in patients with bilateral, symmetric psoriasis. The studies were conducted over a 10-year period. A total of 23 comparison were made, with two studies involving three different topical formulations and 21 involving a two-formulation comparison. In only 3 of the 23 instances did the vasoconstrictor test fail to predict the results of the clinical trials. The vasoconstrictor test indicated

1. Hydrocortisone valerate cream 0.2% was superior to betamethasone valerate cream 0.1%, but no clinical difference was seen.
2. Alcometasone ointment 0.05% was superior to desonide ointment 0.05%, but no clinical difference was seen.
3. Betamethasone diproprionate ointment 0.05% was superior to alclometasone ointment 0.05% clinically, but no differences were seen in the vasoconstrictor test results.

It is worthwhile to note that for the first two comparisons the vasoconstrictor test would have rejected a clinically acceptable formulation (i.e., the test was too conservative). Only the betamethasone diproprionate ointment–alclometasone ointment comparison would have resulted in clinically inequivalent formulations. Thus it would appear that the use of the vasoconstrictor test for topical steroids intended for the treatment of psoriasis is an appropriate surrogate. Given these data there was a 2:23 chance of rejecting a good product, and a 1:23 chance of accepting an inferior product, which, at least for these products, would appear to represent an acceptable error rate.

The data shown in Tables 3 and 4 are taken from summaries provided by the manufacturers of two products commercially available in the United States. The first study [87] was a comparison of a brand name and a generic topical fluocinonide cream. The creams (0.1 g) were applied to a 4-cm^2 site on the forearms of 20 volunteers. One-half of the subjects had the generic product applied to the left arm and the brand product to the right arm. The other subjects received the products on the opposite arms. The application site was covered with cotton gauze for 24 hr to protect, but not occlude, the site. After the blanching score was assigned, second applications of the creams were made, with a subsequent reading 24-hr later. The mean results were based on a rating scale of 0, 1, 2, or 3. It is not surprising that there was no statistically significant difference between the two creams. With the minimal response and the high variability (CV%), the statistical power was quite low. Accordingly, it would appear to be difficult to be totally assured the two products were bioequivalent, given these

Table 3 Comparison of a Brand Name and Generic 0.05% Fluocinonide Cream Using the Skin Blanching Assay

Product	Mean skin blanching score (CV%)[a]	
	First application	Second application
Brand name	1.05 (78%)	1.00 (86%)
Generic	0.95 (86%)	0.90 (94%)

[a]Scores based on 1, slight blanching to 3, marked blanching.
Source: Ref. 87.

Table 4 Comparison of a Generic and Brand Betamethasone Dipropionate 0.05% Ointment Using the Skin Blanching Assay

	No. subjects with blanching[a]			Mean	
Score:	1.0	0.5	0.0	Score	(CV%)
Reference product	17	5	0	0.89	24%
Generic product	19	3	0	0.93	19%
Vehicle	6	10	6	0.50	76%

[a]Blanching scores based on: 0, no visible blanching; 0.5, very faint blanching; 1.0, distinct blanching.
Source: Ref. 88.

data alone. The study protocol did not require that the vehicle be included as a third treatment phase.

The second study [88] compared two betamethasone dipropionate 0.05% ointments. Approximately 0.02 mL of each ointment was placed into occlusive chambers that were secured to the forearms of 22 male volunteers for 16 hr. The sites were evaluated for vasoconstriction immediately and 1-hr after removal. Blanching was scored as 0, 0.5, or 1.0, with 0 being no change and 1.0 being distinct blanching. The results obtained immediately after removal of the chamber are summarized in Table 4. The conclusions were that both products were superior to the vehicle alone, but were not significantly different from each other. Note that compared with the study summarized in Table 3, this study used occlusion, which may narrow differences between treatments, included a vehicle control, and used a different rating scale. Although these data appear to indicate the bioequivalence of the two products, they were not subjected to any rigorous statistical analysis. These two examples clearly demonstrate the need for some standardization for the testing of such products, including the type of data that should be obtained and how it should be analyzed.

Poulsen et al. [89] described a paired comparison study design to improve visual assessment. A 0.05% fluocinonide cream and a 1% hydrocortisone cream were each applied to eight adjacent sites on the forearm of eight volunteers. The data were analyzed on the basis of three different methods:

1. Total number of sites exhibiting blanching for each formulation. The maximum possible score was 64 (8 sites × 8 subjects).
2. The total intensity score for which the blanching at each site was rated 0–3. The maximum possible score was 192 (8 sites × 8 subjects × a score of 3).
3. The data were also tabulated in terms of the number of times the fluocinonide cream site showed a greater response than the hydrocortisone cream site; the number of times that the hydrocortisone site showed a greater response

than the fluocinonide site; the number of times that the paired sites showed equivalent response; and the number of times that the paired sites showed no response. The maximum possible score for one of these decisions is 64 (8 sites × 8 subjects), and if this should occur, the other three decisions would each have a score of zero. The resulting data for all three methods were statistically analyzed using χ^2 analysis.

Problems associated with the vasoconstrictor test have been noted by several workers [79,90].

1. Occlusion may narrow the differences between two formulations by enhancing the absorption of both.
2. Variability in vasomotor activity or skin characteristics can add variability in the visual reading.
3. Duration of application can affect results, and it may be appropriate to make the observations at several times.
4. Variability may result due to the interpretation of the reader.
5. A flat dose–response curve for blanching may preclude a valid comparison of bioavailability.
6. Vasoconstriction may or may not be related to the therapeutic activity of the drug.
7. The use of single-point determinations may result in some errors in interpretation, particularly when there are differences in the rate at which vasoconstriction is induced by different formulations.

Recent reviews [91,92] have described the control of many of the variables associated with the skin blanching assay, including (1) how to select the volunteers, (2) how to apply the dosage form, (3) where to apply the dosage form, (4) methods of occlusion, (5) duration of occlusion, and (6) interpretation of the results.

One of the concerns over the vasoconstriction test is the somewhat subjective manner in which the degree of blanching is determined. Training is required for consistent scoring by an observer. Usually two or three observers are used, and the results are averaged. In an attempt to eliminate the use of a subjective evaluation and minimize human error, several types of instrumentation have been applied to in vivo studies involving blanching measurements [93–95].

1. *Attenuated total reflectance infrared spectroscopy* (ATR-IR) can quantitate the appearance of drug or vehicle in the skin of human volunteers. However, it will work only for the outer regions of the epidermis, and it requires compounds with an unique infrared (IR) spectrum. A representation of the design of the instrument is shown in Figure 9. For example, ATR-IR has been used to study the effect of oleic acid on the percutaneous absorption of *p*-cyanophenol in vivo [52,96]. An increase in lipid disorder within the stratum corneum was observed with oleic acid, based on an increase in the C-H stretching frequencies

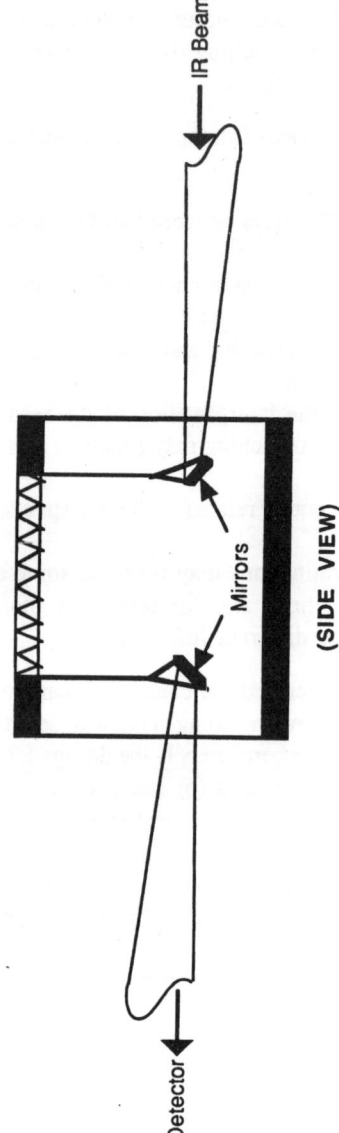

Figure 9 Schematic representation of the attenuated total reflectance infrared spectroscopy (ATR-IR) optical system. (From Ref. 52.)

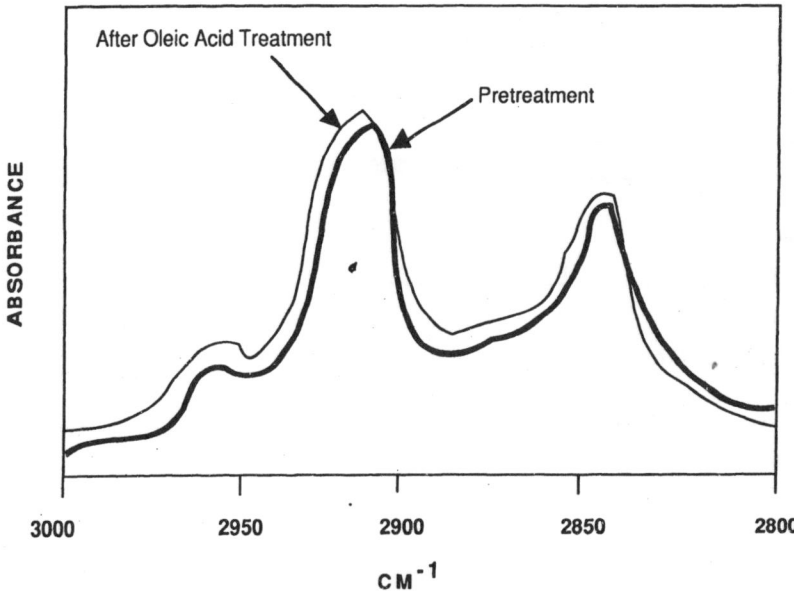

Figure 10 Changes in the IR spectrum of human forearm stratum corneum in the region of the C-H stretching absorbances (3000–2800 cm^{-1}) as a function of the application of oleic acid. (From Ref. 52.)

(Fig. 10). The technique was also employed to quantitate the p-cyanophenol concentration–time profile within the stratum corneum by monitoring the change in the C≡N stretching frequency at 2230 cm^{-1}, which is characteristic for p-cyanophenol.

2. *Laser doppler velocimetry* (LDV). With LDV, light from a helium–neon laser is transmitted to skin by fiber optics. The light is backscattered from the skin components and the erythrocytes in the dermal capillaries, and the reflected light is collected by a second optical fiber. As the light strikes moving erythrocytes, the reflected radiation undergoes a slight shift in frequency (the Doppler effect), and the shift increases with increasing blood flow [97]. The probe holding the fiber optics needs to be in contact with the skin. The resulting electrical output is a measure of peripheral blood flow. The penetration depth is about 1–1.5 mm. Guy et al. [98] have described the use of LDV to monitor vasodilatation resulting from the application of topical methyl nicotinate. Figure 11 illustrates the LDV output following the administration of the vasodilator.

3. *Photopulse Plethysmography* (PPG) utilizes the absorption of infrared

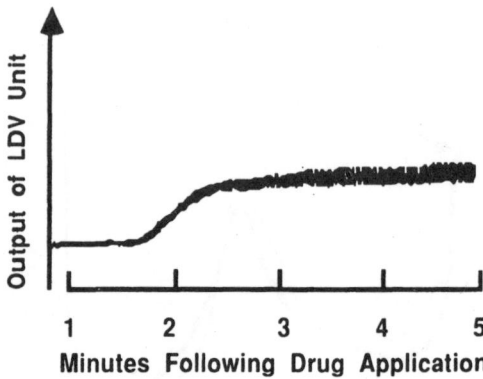

Figure 11 Laser doppler velocimetry response curve after topical application of methyl nicotinate. (From Ref. 98.)

light (800–940 nm) by hemoglobin as a means to detect changes in blood volume in the microcirculation. Penetration is about 1–2 mm. Guy et al. [98] have employed PPG to noninvasively quantitate the percutaneous absorption of methyl nicotinate in humans. Figure 12 illustrates the PPG output following the application of the vasodilator.

4. *Xenon clearance.* Kristensen and Wadskov [99] and Greeson et al. [100] discussed the use of ^{133}Xe washout from human skin as a means to quantitate blood flow changes resulting from corticosteroid treatment. The method involves a determination of ^{133}Xe, which is an inert gas, by a gamma counter following either intracutaneous injection of the gas in normal saline or exposure of the surface of the skin to the gas. Others [101] have shown a good correspondence between the determination of cutaneous blood flow, as determined by LDV and by ^{133}Xe clearance.

5. *Tristimulus reflectance meter* has been used to detect changes in skin color [102]. It simultaneously measures relative brightness (black to white), the color range from green to red, and the color range from blue to yellow.

Berardesca and Maibach [93] have reviewed noninvasive means to objectively quantitate the course of psoriasis. The methods included measurement of transepidermal water loss, which is increased in psoriasis; measurements of changes in blood flow, which is also increased in psoriasis, using methods such as ^{131}Xe washout, LDV, or remittance spectrophotometry; measurements of increased skin thickness using ultrasound; or methods based on changes in the electrophysiology of the skin. The authors conclude that, although it is desirable to have objective, quantitative measurements of changes in the disease to supplement

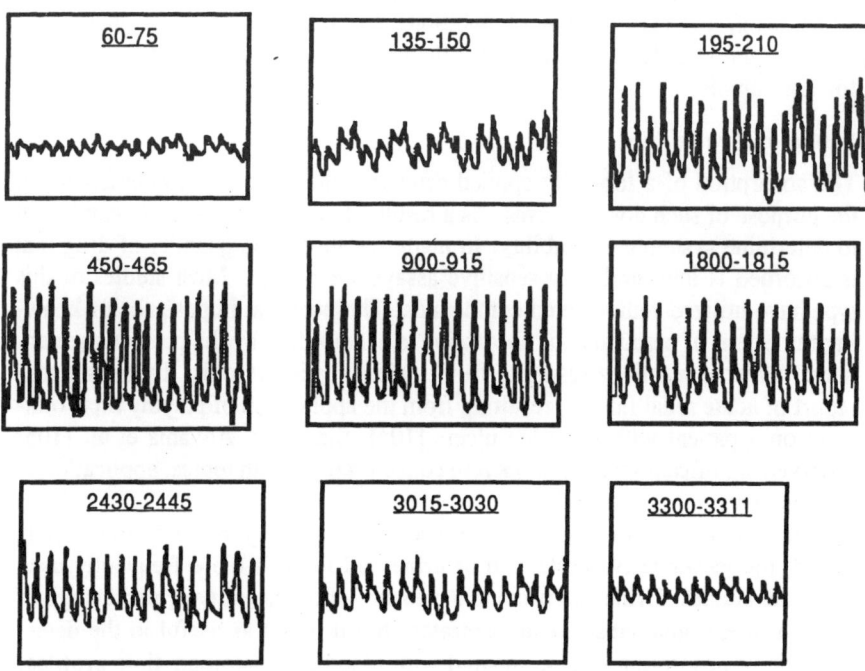

Figure 12 Photopulse plethysmography recording at various times (sec) after a 15-sec topical application of methyl nicotinate. (From Ref. 98.)

clinical observations, these techniques still require extensive documentation and validation before they can be routinely applied to quantitate vasoconstriction. The instrumentation is expensive, commercially available equipment usually requires customization, the necessity that contact be made with the skin can cause blanching, and irregularities in the skin can alter the reading. All things considered, the human eye is still an exceptionally good measuring device, and it is both rapid and inexpensive.

The use of the vasoconstrictor test has been primarily limited to the corticosteroids because their topical application results in blanching. However, Poelman et al. [103] have used the test to study the effect of three different nonsteroidal anti-inflammatory drugs. The agents were applied topically, with occlusion for 1–4 hr. A 0.5% solution of methyl nicotinate was then placed on the application site, and the appearance of vasodilation was determined repeatedly over a 30-min period, using laser Doppler velocimetry. The data were expressed as (1) area under the response–time curve (AUC), which showed significantly greater areas for the vehicles compared with the test formulations containing the active drug; and (2) percentage inhibition, determined as the difference in the AUC for the vehicle and the AUC for the test formulation, divided by the AUC for the vehicle.

Systemic Availability

The absorption of a topically applied drug into the systemic circulation is not the purpose of such dosage forms. As a result, studies are not usually conducted to determine systemic availability. In many instances, the quantity of drug that is absorbed is low, and very sensitive assays are needed. Most studies of this type have utilized radiolabeled compounds. The potential importance of knowing the extent of percutaneous absorption is exemplified by the previously mentioned adverse reactions resulting from topical corticosteroids. There is also a report of acute renal failure, resulting from the application of polymyxin B ointment on a patient with large leg ulcers [104]. Similarly, Aoyama et al. [105] observed significant serum tobramycin concentrations with topical application to burn patients.

Although drug concentrations or amount of radioactivity in blood can be determined, the less-invasive collection of urine and feces is more frequently used in human studies. Urine can provide a measure of the quantity or percentage of dose absorbed, and subsequently excreted, but it is not as useful in the determination of absorption rate, compared with blood concentration–time profiles. A typical study involving a labeled drug was reported by Franz and Lehman [106]. They examined the percutaneous absorption of [^{3}H]sulconazole nitrate, a topical antifungal, in seven humans. The drug was applied as a cream to the abdomen. Two applications, 12-hr apart were used. The site was washed 12, 24, 48, 72, and 96 hr after the second application. Mean total radioactivity, as percentage of dose (range) was 6.7% (3.4–13.2%), 2% (1.5–2.5%), and 34% (13–74%) for urine, feces, and skin washings, respectively.

Bucks et al. [107] have discussed how to perform bioavailability studies in humans using steroids. Acetone solutions of ^{14}C-labeled progesterone, testosterone, estradiol, and hydrocortisone were applied as single and multiple doses, with occlusion or protected without occlusion. They corrected for incomplete elimination by adjusting the urinary excretion data by the fraction of radioactivity excreted after intramuscular or intravenous administration. This assumes the elimination profile for drug and metabolites is the same with both routes of elimination, which may not necessarily be true. In addition, such corrections require intramuscular or intravenous doses of radiolabeled drug. Alternatively, the corrections may be based on literature values in humans or data obtained in animals. Obviously, either of these approaches also depends on the validity of the significant assumptions that are required. They were able to account for 68–100% of the dose of the radioactivity by assaying the urine collected for 7 days (recovery 4-46%), the washings of the application site, and the chamber employed to protect the application site. They also observed that occlusion increased the absorption for estradiol, testosterone, and progesterone, but did not increase absorption for hydrocortisone, which was the least lipophilic steroid. They noted that an earlier study [108] did demonstrate increased absorption of hydrocortisone with occlusion, but that study employed 4 days of continuous occlusion with Saran Wrap. Thus, the absorption could have been increased by the prolonged, and possibly unrealistic, duration of occlusion, as well as the rubbing of the skin by the occlusive protection. These studies illustrate the need to standardize the method of occlusion whenever it is employed. Bucks et al. [109] have designed an application chamber designed to provide protection, but not occlusion, permitting transepidermal water loss. The system consists of a 2.5-cm diameter polypropylene chamber, covered with a semipermeable polytetrafluoroethylene membrane, secured to the application site with an adhesive, transparent dressing. Studies conducted with a series of para-substituted phenols demonstrated a total recovery of 91-102%, with a percentage of dose absorbed ranging from 4 to 31%.

Bucks and co-workers [110] have also conducted multiple-dose studies with [^{14}C]hydrocortisone, testosterone, or estradiol in an acetone vehicle, with application to the ventral forearm skin of human volunteers. A labeled dose was given on days 1 and 8, and unlabeled doses were given on days 2-7 and 9-14. Absorption was determined by assaying radioactivity in urine collected for 7 days. There was no significant difference between the urinary recovery of the three compounds after the first dose or after the eighth dose. These data suggest the absence of buildup of a reservoir of drug in the stratum corneum or alteration of the barrier properties of the skin during multiple-dose administration.

Franz and Lehman [111] have also reported on the use of radiolabeled drug to study percutaneous absorption. They applied [^{14}C]tretinoin (all-*trans* retinoic acid) to the face of eight subjects with mild to moderate facial acne and made comparisons with results obtained in monkeys. The recovery was 1.1% in urine when applied to normal human skin and 1.5% through dermatitic skin which had been damaged by repeated applications of the drug. If one assumes that the fraction of the dose excreted in the urine of humans is the same as for monkeys, the fraction of the dose absorbed was estimated to be 5% for the normal skin and 7% for the dermatitic skin. About 50% of the dose was recovered in the wash employed 10 hr after application. The monkey appeared to be more sensitive (and, hence, not a good model) to repeated applications of tretinoin. About 10% of the dose was recovered in the urine when the application was to normal skin, but 48% for dermatitic skin. These workers also noted that the applied dose will not necessarily all be available as such for absorption, since some tretinoin may be converted to 13-*cis*-retinoic acid, and possibly other isomers or breakdown products. Thus, the assessment of the absorption of this material is relatively complex.

Finally, we should note a potential problem with the use of formulations containing radiolabeled drug [112–115]. If the labeled drug is simply extemporaneously incorporated into a formulation containing the therapeutic dose of unlabeled drug, the addition of the labeled drug must result in a homogenous mixture and must not alter the characteristics of the formulation. To be strictly correct, all drug (labeled and unlabeled) should be added at the time the dosage form is produced.

Eller et al. [116] used nonradioactive minoxidil in determining the percutaneous absorption of the drug. A radioimmunoassay was used that was capable of quantitating picogram per milliliter concentrations of drug in serum and higher concentrations in urine. The authors reported low nanograms per milliliter serum concentrations and microgram amounts excreted in the urine after multiple applications to the chest or the scalp of a fixed solution administered 2, 4, 6, or 8 times a day. These data demonstrate the need for sensitive assays to determine the percutaneous absorption of topical formulations that are not designed to result in systemic availability. Other work [117] has indicated an apparent bioavailability of approximately 1% following topical administration of doses that are clinically relevant. The absorption of the drug appeared to be independent of the number of doses administered each day. This was attributed to the fact that the drug was being administered faster than it was being absorbed from the skin. In essence, the skin was saturated with drug. Consequently, studies designed to determine the systemic availability may not be capable of discerning differences in formulations after the stratum corneum becomes saturated. If the stratum corneum is the rate-limiting step, the differences in formulations are likely to be noted only in terms of a lag time for the appearance of the drug in the systemic circulation, or differences in the falloff curves following partial depletion of the reservoir of drug in the stratum corneum. The absorption of minoxidil was also observed to approximately double when applied to shaved heads, compared with bald subjects [118].

Clinical Trials

Clinical trials are the least accurate, least sensitive, and least reproducible of the general approaches for measurement of bioavailability or bioequivalence. In general, clinical trials are not acceptable for formulations intended for systemic availability if analytical methods are available to measure systemic concentrations. However, clinical trials may be the only means to determine the bioavailability or bioequivalence of dosage forms intended to deliver the active moiety locally. Examples include topical preparations for the skin, eye, and mucous membranes; oral dosage forms not intended to be absorbed (e.g., an antacid or radiopaque medium); and bronchodilators administered by inhalation if the onset and duration of pharmacologic activity are defined [119]. Although corticosteroid products have been subject to the vasoconstrictor test, in some instances, the corticosteroids have also been evaluated in clinical trials, using patients with eczema or psoriasis. For example, Scholtz and Dumas [120] have determined the relative potencies of several topical steroids by applying the agents, using occlusion, to psoriasis plaques on stabilized patients. Assessment of efficacy was done on the basis of a rating of unchanged or normal appearance. Data may also be presented as log-dose versus percentage return to normal.

In other cases, a pharmacologic effect can be measured in healthy volunteers, using a response that is known to be related to the intended use of the formulation. For example, Woolfson et al. [121] studied the effectiveness of a local anesthetic in three different vehicles and six concentrations, using a pinprick method with 20 human volunteers. Both time of onset and duration of anesthesia were determined. Once at least 90% of the subjects experience anesthesia, further increases in the concentration of drug in the vehicle did not reduce the time of onset. However, the duration of anesthesia did exhibit a trend toward longer times as drug concentration was increased. Other methods for evaluating local anesthesia induced by topically applied dosage forms have been reviewed by Woolfson and McCafferty [122]. To provide some background into the approaches that have been suggested to evaluate the bioequivalence for certain topical products, we will focus on three types of drugs: (1) antifungal products; (2) tretinoin, a drug employed in acne; and (3) minoxidil, a drug employed topically to stimulate hair growth.

Antifungal products. During the course of developing a new antifungal drug, a minimum of two well-controlled clinical trials are required to show the product is superior to the vehicle control. For a generic product, a single randomized, double-blind, three-way parallel group study has been proposed [123], comparing the test drug to the innovator, as well as to the vehicle used for the generic product. The vehicle control helps to eliminate investigator bias and permits a better measure of the effectiveness of the generic product.

If the reference product is approved for tinea pedis (a fungal disease of the foot), the patients should have the disease, as confirmed by clinical examination and mycological testing. If the clinical efficacy is confirmed, then the generic product may be utilized for all of the conditions of use specified for the innovator product. The evaluation is to be conducted 4 weeks after initiating treatment, at the time treatment is discontinued, and then 2 weeks later. This last evaluation is the most important in determining bioequivalence.

Assuming the test and reference product have identical success rates of 50%, it is estimated that at least 108 evaluable patients will be needed for the test and reference products, and 60 patients will suffice for the vehicle dose, since it should be easier to show a difference between active product and vehicle than between active and active. The more the test differs from the reference, the larger the number of patients who will be needed. Bioequivalence is demonstrated if the 90% confidence interval for the success rate of the test product is within ±20% of the success rate for the reference product.

The requirements for studying solutions may be waived, as long as the formulation is essentially the same as the innovator. Differences in solution composition could result in a lack of efficacy owing to certain properties (e.g., low viscosity causing runoff of the solution after application). However, if the solvent is the same, and there are no excipients in one of the formulations that could alter bioavailability, then it seems reasonable to omit requirements for clinical testing of generic solutions.

A good example of the types of studies that are appropriate in evaluating new formulations, is the work of Aly et al. [124] involving bioequivalence studies of a lotion and cream form of the antifungal drug ciclopirox. During the development of the products, in vitro studies were carried out using human cadaver and domestic pig skin treated with the two formulations. They measured the penetration of the drug into various layers of the skin by determining the inhibition of fungal growth after inoculation of the skin with spores of two different dermatophytes. Second, guinea pigs were inoculated dorsally with *Trichophyton mentagrophytes*, and after 3 weeks, the resulting lesions were treated with the lotion, cream, and the two vehicles. They then proceeded to human studies involving inoculation of four sites on the forearms of human volunteers with *T. mentagrophytes*. Each site was treated with the lotion, cream, or the two vehicles. After 15 days of treatment the sites were examined clinically and mycologically. Finally, a multicenter, double-blind, parallel-group clinical trial was conducted comparing the lotion to the vehicle in patients with plantar, interdigital, or vesicular tinea pedis. The patients were evaluated after 15 days of treatment, at the end of the treatment (29 days), and again 2 weeks later (day 43). Assessment was based on the absence of all signs and symptoms (clinical cure) and negative culture and KOH test. Figures 13 and 14 summarize the results of the clinical trial. Figure 13 illustrates that the lotion was significantly more effective than the vehicle control, based on clinical observation and mycological testing ($p < 0.001$). Figure 14 demonstrates the greater effectiveness ($p < 0.001$) of the lotion after 43 days in patients with interdigital tinea pedis, compared with the subgroup who had plantar tinea pedis, which is more resistant to treatment, and requires longer than 43 days of treatment.

Tretinoin. As of April 1990, the FDA was working on a guidance for tretinoin products [125]. The following study design is based on preliminary discussion held during a recent FDA-sponsored workshop [126]. A potential bioequivalence study design may require a double-blind, 12-week, multicenter, parallel study, including brand, generic, and vehicle, in patients with grade 2

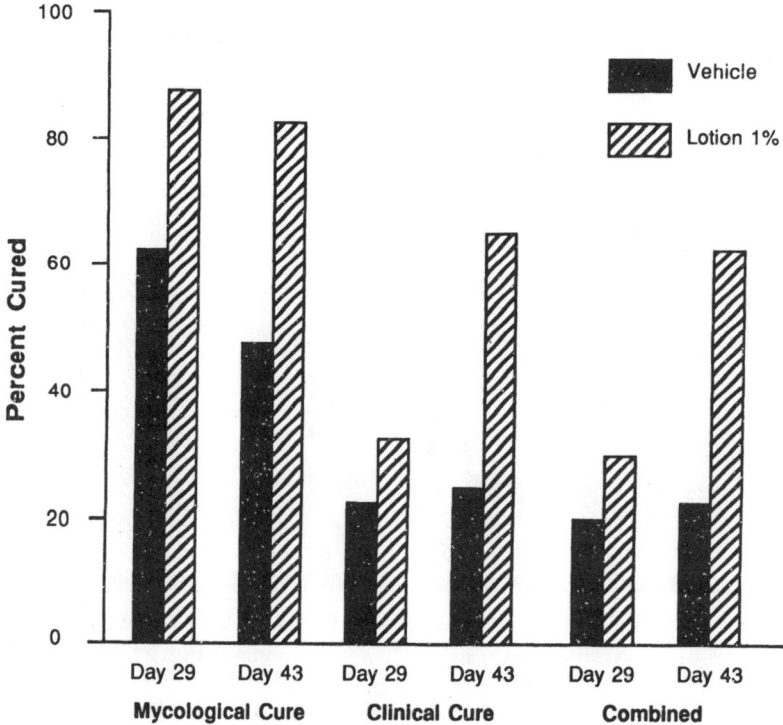

Figure 13 Mycological cures (negative KOH and culture), clinical cures (absence of all signs and symptoms of disease), and combined outcome (clinical and mycological cures) of treatment with ciclopirox illumine lotion 1% or the lotion vehicle in patients with tinea pedis. (From Ref. 124).

and grade 3 acne (mild to moderate). The primary endpoint will be lesion counts (inflammatory and noninflammatory) and a global evaluation by the investigator. Patients may be evaluated at baseline and at 1, 2, 4, 8, and 12 weeks. Irritation and sensitization rates will also be determined.

Complicating factors include the need to thoroughly instruct the patients on the use of the drug; the assessment of patient compliance (e.g., by periodically weighing the residue in the container); the influence of the menstrual cycle in the course of acne; and the high placebo rate associated with acne treatment. In addition, it has been reported that tretinoin may isomerize to isotretinoin, with exposure to light following topical application [127,128].

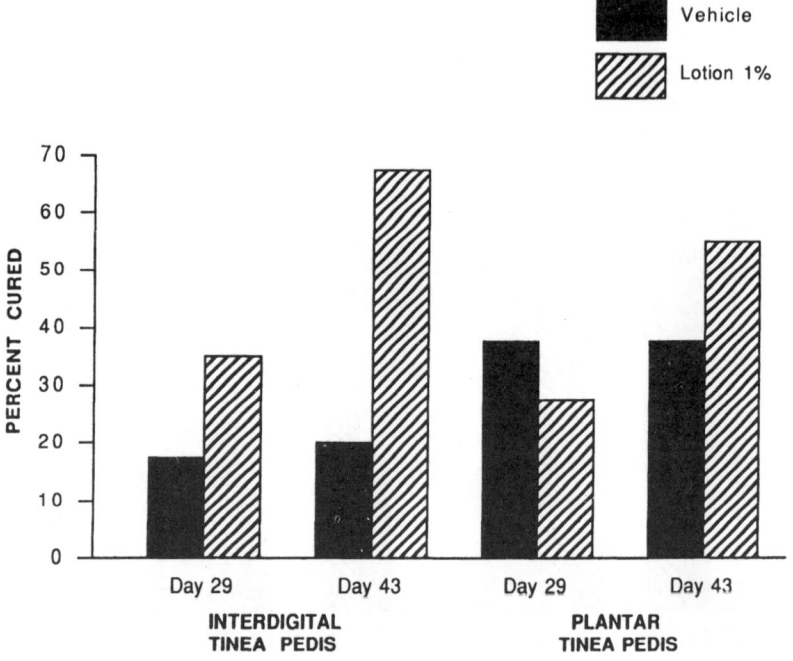

Figure 14 Percentage of patients with resolution of signs and symptoms of disease and negative KOH and culture results in patients with interdigital or plantar tinea pedis. (From Ref. 124).

Minoxidil. The quantiative assessment of hair growth stimulation also presents some challenges [129]. Noninvasive means include manual counting of actual hairs, or computerized analysis of expanded photographs. Alternatively, samples of hair may be cut and weighed. An animal model, the postadolescent stump-tailed macaque, which exhibits frontal alopecia, has also been used to study the action of topical minoxidil [130].

Headington and Novak [131] evaluated the effect of minoxidil on hair growth in subjects with male-pattern baldness. Methods included subjective assessment of hair growth by investigator and subject; measurement of length of hairs (expressed as the difference between baseline and posttreatment maximum and minimum length); histological examination of a few hairs; and microscopic examination of punch biopsies.

Wester et al. [132] studied cutaneous blood flow in human balding scalps using both LDV and PPG. They tested the effect of 0, 1, 3, and 5% solutions of minoxidil. Only the 5% solution resulted in significant differences in instrument readings. However, these authors correctly cautioned that a correlation has not been established between vasodilatation and increased hair growth. Furthermore, since the noninvasive measurements applied only to the first 1–1.5 mm of skin, it could not be determined what effect minoxidil had on the germinal part of the hair follicle that is present 4–6 mm below the surface. The LDV appeared to be more sensitive to changes in blood flow, and the authors concluded it was more suitable. They also recommended the use of ^{133}Xe washout method in combination with LDV, as a means to simultaneously measure changes in subcutaneous, as well as cutaneous, blood flow rates.

SUMMARY

From the discussion presented in this chapter, it should be clear that we have made considerable progress in understanding dosage forms designed to be applied to the skin. However, there still is much to learn. In the context of determining the bioavailability or bioequivalence of such products, some of the experimental variables requiring control and some of the experimental pitfalls have been described. The following represent some of the issues or areas of research that still require discussion and experimentation.

The use of the vasoconstrictor test appears to be a useful tool to assess the bioavailability of topical corticosteroids. However, work is needed to establish the exact mechanism of action to determine to what extent skin blanching is actually related to the therapeutic use of such drug products.

Clinical trials appear to be the only means to assess bioavailability–bioequivalence of topical dosage forms for the foreseeable future. However there are still several issues that need further consideration.

1. What should be done to evaluate multiple strengths of a given product? The conduct of a full clinical trial for each strength, using hundreds of patients, would seem excessive. However to assume equivalence of all strengths, based on data for a single strength, might be incorrect. Perhaps this is an area for which some form of in vitro testing could be particularly useful.

2. Bioequivalence is based on equivalent rate and extent of absorption. What if the test product exhibits a faster cure rate or a greater percentage of patient recovery, compared with the reference product during clinical trials? Such findings could result in a conclusion that the test product is bioinequivalent to the reference. It may seem inappropriate to reject a formulation that results in a more rapid cure rate. However, what if the faster cure was due to greater percutaneous absorption, leading to higher systemic availability or differences in metabolite formation? The 1984 amendments to the U.S. Food, Drug and Cosmetic Act require that a generic product be equivalent to the reference for both rate and extent. Unless it can be demonstrated that differences in clinical response

are not the result of differences in rate or extent of absorption, there does not seem to be an alternative to rejecting such formulations under current federal regulations.

3. How should bioequivalence be interpreted relative to toxicity, dermal irritation, and such? If a test product cannot exhibit any less toxicity or irritation than the reference for topical products, does it follow that a test transdermal formulation that is less irritating than a reference transdermal should also be rejected? To what extent does irritation also alter permeation? What is causing the irritation, a component of the dosage form, the release rate of the drug, or is it a result of a drug–component interaction? Should the test product be rejected as bioinequivalent if, for example, clinical trials show 30% of the patients receiving the reference, 10% of the test, and 5% of the vehicle control exhibit a dermal reaction?

4. What are the ethics involved in requiring a placebo–vehicle control? Since the anticipated conclusion is equivalence, patients participating in clinical trials of generic products do not stand to benefit beyond what they could expect if they were simply prescribed the reference product. This is unlike the testing of a new drug product, when the patient may have at least some probability of receiving a drug that is superior to the accepted reference. Basically, the use of the placebo requires that some fraction of the test patient population will not receive a known effective treatment for some period (e.g., at least 4 weeks for a topical antifungal). What must be considered is the balance between causing some patients to go without effective treatment for some period, against the risk of declaring two formulations equivalent, based on faulty data generated in the absence of the use of a proper vehicle control. Since the latter error could ultimately affect a larger population of subjects, the inconvenience to the relatively small group of patients who initially receive the placebo is probably justified.

Experimental design can also be problematic. For example, if the clinical use of a topical product results in application of the medication to various sties on the body, should the testing of the product include the use of multiple sites? Since the permeability of diseased skin can be different than healthy skin, are we making an error by only testing formulations, such as the corticosteroids, on healthy subjects? Should human testing automatically include different age groups and races?

Should a determination of the extent of systemic availability be required for all bioequivalence studies of topical formulations? What if the test and reference formulations are excreted 1.0 and 1.5% in the urine, does this 50% difference indicate bioinequivalence?

Issues such as these suggest that much work remains to be accomplished in developing appropriate experimental approaches and standards for the evaluation of dosage forms designed to be applied to the skin.

REFERENCES

1. R. H. Guy, A. H. Guy, H. I. Maibach, and V. P. Shah. *Pharm. Res.* 3:253-261 (1986).
2. H. Loth. *Methods Find. Exp. Clin. Pharmacol.* 11:155-164 (1989).
3. H. Schaefer, A. Zesch, and G. Stuttgen. *Skin Permeability*. Springer-Verlag, New York (1982).
4. R. L. Bronaugh and H. I. Maibach. *Percutaneous Absorption*, 2nd ed. Marcel Dekker, New York (1989).
5. B. W. Barry. *Dermatological Formulations*. Marcel Dekker, New York (1983).
6. R. C. Scott, R. H. Guy, and J. Hadgraft, eds. *Prediction of Percutaneous Penetration*. IBC Technical Services, Great Britain (1990).
7. Y. W. Chien. *Transdermal Controlled Systemic Medications*. Marcel Dekker, New York (1987).
8. J. Hadgraft and R. Guy. *Transdermal Drug Delivery*. Marcel Dekker, New York (1989).
9. H. E. Bodde, J. Verhoeven, and L. M. J. van Driel. *Crit. Rev. Ther. Drug Carr. Syst.* 6:87-115 (1989).
10. G. E. Parry, A. L. Bunge, G. D. Silcox, L. K. Pershing, and D. W. Pershing. *Pharm. Res.* 7:230-236 (1990).
11. P. Zanowiak and M. R. Jacobs. Topical anti-infective products. In *Handbook of Nonprescription Drugs*, 7th ed. (S. C. Laitin, ed.) American Pharmaceutical Association, Washington, D.C., pp. 525-529 (1982).
12. B. W. Barry. *Topical Therapeutic Products Workshop Notes*. Sponsored by the AAPS and FDA, March 26-28, 1990, Arlington, Va., pp. 55-58.
13. J. B. Besunder, M. D. Reed, and J. L. Blumer. *Clin. Pharmacokinet.* 14:189-216 (1988).
14. R. C. Wester, P. K. Noonan, M. P. Cole, and H. I. Maibach. *Pediatr. Res.* 11:737-739 (1977).
15. J. W. Wiechers. *Pharm. Weekbl. Sci. Ed.* 11:185-198 (1989).
16. K. V. Roskos, H. I. Maibach, and R. H. Guy. *J. Pharmacokinet. Biopharm.* 17:617-663 (1989).
17. K. V. Roskos, R. H. Guy, and H. I. Maibach. *Dermatol. Clin.* 4:455-465 (1986).
18. R. H. Guy, E. Tur, S. Bjerke, and H. I. Maibach. *J. Am. Acad. Dermatol.* 12:100-106 (1985).
19. C. J. Gean, E. Tur, H. I. Maibach, and R. H. Guy. *Arch. Dermatol.* 281:95-98 (1989).
20. D. Wilson, E. Berardesca, and H. I. Maibach. *Br. J. Dermatol.* 119:647-652 (1988).
21. D. A. Weigand, C. Haygood, and G. R. Gaylor. *J. Invest. Dermatol.* 62:563-568 (1974).
22. A. Zesch and H. Schaefer. *Arch. Dermatol. Res.* 252:245-256 (1975).
23. G. Moe and P. W. Armstrong. *Am. J. Med.* 81:786-770 (1986).
24. R. B. Stoughton. *Annu. Rev. Pharmacol. Toxicol.* 29:55-69 (1989).
25. R. J. Martin, S. P. Denyer, and J. Hadgraft. *Int. J. Pharm.* 39:23-32 (1987).
26. R. H. Guy, J. Hadgraft, and D. A. W. Bucks. *Xenobiotics* 17:325-343 (1987).

27. P. K. Noonan and R. C. Wester. In *Percutaneous Absorption*, 2nd ed. (R. L. Bronaugh and H. I. Maibach, eds.) Marcel Dekker, New York, pp. 53-76 (1989).
28. J. Kao. In *Percutaneous Absorption*, 2nd ed. (R. L. Bronaugh and H. I. Maibach, eds.), Marcel Dekker, New York, pp. 259-282 (1989).
29. D. R. Bickers. *Current Concepts in Cutaneous Toxicity*. Academic Press, New York, pp. 95-126 (1980).
30. B. W. Barry. *Dermatological Formulations*. Marcel Dekker, New York, pp. 127-233 (1983).
31. Y. W. Chien. In *Controlled Drug Delivery Fundamentals and Applications*, 2nd ed. (J. R. Robinson and V. H. L. Lee, eds.) Marcel Dekker, New York, pp. 523-552 (1987).
32. R. H. Guy and J. Hadgraft. *J. Controlled Release 1*:177-182 (1985).
33. R. H. Guy and J. Hadgraft. *Int. J. Pharm. 11*:187-197 (1982).
34. L. Chu, R. M. Gale, L. G. Schmitt, and J. E. Shaw. *Angiology 35*:545-552 (1984).
35. J. E. Shaw, M. E. Prevo, and A. A. Amkraut. *Arch. Dermtaol. 123*:1548-1556 (1987).
36. G. Ridout, G. Santus, and R. H. Guy. *Clin. Pharmacokin. 15*:114-131 (1988).
37. W. Rudolph, J. Dirschinger, D. Hall, G. Reiniger, and A. Bayeric. *Eur. Heart J. 10*(Suppl. A):50-55 (1989).
38. H. DeMots and S. P. Glasser. *J. Am. Coll. Cardiol. 13*:786-793 (1989).
39. P. M. Plezia, T. H. Kramer, J. Linford, and S. R. Hameroff. *Pharmacotherapy 9*:2-9 (1989).
40. C. C. Peck and V. P. Shah. In *Prediction of Percutaneous Penetration, Methods, Measurements, Modelling* (R. C. Scott, R. H. Guy, and J. Hadgraft, eds.) IBC Technical Services, Great Britain, pp. 286-289 (1990).
41. P. K. Noonan, M. A. Gonzalez, D. Ruggirello, J. Tomlinson, E. Babcock-Atkinson, M. Ray, A. Golub, and A. Cohen. *J. Pharm. Sci. 75*:688-691 (1986).
42. K. A. Wick, S. M. Wick, and R. W. Hawkinson. *Clin. Ther. 11*:417-424 (1989).
43. S. Sved, W. M. McLean, and I. J. McGilveray. *J. Pharm. Sci. 70*:1368 (1981).
44. R. P. Iafrate, R. L. Yost, S. H. Curry, V. P. Gotz, and G. J. Caranasos. *Pharmacotherapy 3*:118 (1983).
45. R. C. Wester and P. K. Noonan. *Int. J. Pharm. 7*:99-110 (1980).
46. R. C. Wester, P. K. Noonan, S. Smeach, and L. Kosobud. *J. Pharm. Sci. 72*:745-748 (1983).
47. R. C. Wester and P. K. Noonan. *J. Soc. Cosmet. Chem. 30*:297-307 (1979).
48. R. C. Wester and H. I. Maibach. *Toxicol. Appl. Pharmacol. 32*:394-398 (1975).
49. H. M. Abdou. *Dissolution, Bioavailability and Bioequivalence*. Mack Publishing Co., Easton, Pa., pp. 189-203; 252-257 (1989).
50. United States Pharmacopeial Convention, Inc. *United States Phamacopeia XXII*. Rockville, Md., pp. 1580-1583 (1989).
51. V. P. Shah, J. P. Skelly. In *Transdermal Controlled Systemic Medications*. (Y. W. Chien, ed.) Marcel Dekker, New York, pp. 399-410 (1987).
52. R. O. Potts. In *Topical Therapeutic Products Workshop Notes*. Sponsored by the AAPS and FDA, March 26-28, 1990, Arlington, Va., pp. 34-39.

53. V. P. Shah. Presentation in the *Topical Therapeutic Products Workshop*. Sponsored by the AAPS and FDA, March 26-28, 1990, Arlington, Va.
54. R. Woodford and B. W. Barry. *J. Invest. Dermatol. 79*:388-391 (1982).
55. *USP DI*, Vol. IA. United States Pharmacopeial Convention, Inc., Rockville, Md., p. 66 (1990).
56. B. W. Barry. *Dermatological Formulations*. Marcel Dekker, New York, pp. 127-233 (1983).
57. R. C. Wester and H. I. Maibach. In *Percutaneous Absorption*, 2nd ed. (R. L. Bronaugh and H. I. Maibach, ed.) Marcel Dekker, New York, pp. 221-238 (1989).
58. C. R. Behl. In *Topical Therapeutic Products Workshop Notes*. Sponsored by the AAPS and FDA, March 26-28, 1990, Arlington, Va., pp. 18-31.
59. Z. Wojciechowski, L. K. Pershing, S. Huether, L. Leonard, S. A. Burton, W. I. Higuchi, and G. G. Krueger. *J. Invest. Dermatol. 88*:439-446 (1987).
60. L. K. Pershing and G. G. Krueger. In *Percutaneous Absorption*, 2nd ed. (R. L. Bronaugh and H. I. Maibach, eds.) Marcel Dekker, New York, pp. 397-414 (1989).
61. E. W. Smith and J. M. Haigh. In *Percutaneous Absorption*, 2nd ed. (R. L. Bronaugh and H. I. Maibach, eds.) Marcel Dekker, New York, pp. 465-510 (1989).
62. D. B. Guzek, A. H. Kennedy, S. C. McNeill, E. Wakshull, and R. O. Potts. *Pharm. Res. 6*:33-39 (1989).
63. R. O. Potts, S. C. McNeill, C. R. Desbonnet, E. Wakshull. *Pharm. Res. 6*:119-124 (1989).
64. J. P. Skelly, V. P. Shah, H. I. Maibach, R. H. Guy, R. C. Wester, G. Flynn, and A. Yacobi. *Pharm. Res. 4*:265-267 (1987).
65. B. W. Barry. In *Prediction of Percutaneous Penetration, Methods, Measurements, Modelling* (R. C. Scott, R. H. Guy, and J. Hadgraft, eds.) IBC Technical Services, Great Britain, p. 212 (1990).
66. R. J. Behme, T. T. Kensler, and D. Brooke. *J. Pharm. Sci. 71*:1303-1305 (1982).
67. V. P. Shah, J. Elkins, S. Lam, and J. Skelly. *Int. J. Pharm. 53*:53-59 (1989).
68. B. J. Poulsen. Presented at the *Topical Therapeutic Products Workshop*. Sponsored by the AAPS and FDA, March 26-28, 1990, Arlington, Va.
69. H. Mukhtar and D. R. Bickers. *Drug Metab. Disp. 11*:562-567 (1983).
70. J. Kao, F. K. Patterson, and J. Hall. *Toxicol. Appl. Pharmacol. 81*:502-516 (1985).
71. AAPS/FDA/AAD/SPS/USAEHA Workshop. In Vivo Percutaneous Penetration/Absorption, May 1-3, 1989, Washington, D.C.
72. C. Chiang, G. L. Flynn, N. D. Weiner, and G. J. Szpunar. *Int. J. Pharm. 50*:21-26 (1989).
73. D. Dupuis, A. Rougier, R. Roguet, C. Lotte, and G. Kalopissis. *J. Invest. Dermatol. 82*:353-356 (1984).
74. A. Rougier, C. Lott, and H. I. Maibach. *J. Pharm. Sci. 76*:451-454 (1987).
75. A. Rougier, D. Dupuis, C. Lotte, R. Roguet, and H. Schaefer. *J. Invest. Dermatol. 81*:275-278 (1983).
76. A. Rougier, D. Dupuis, C. Lotte, and R. Roguet. *J. Invest. Dermatol. 84*:66-68 (1985).
77. N. V. Sheth, M. B. McKeough, and S. L. Spruance. *J. Invest. ermatol. 89*:598-602 (1987).

78. A. W. McKenzie and R. B. Stoughton. *Arch. Dermatol.* 86:608–610 (1962).
79. D. B. Jackson, C. Thompson, J. R. McCormack, and J. D. Guin. *J. Am. Acad. Dermatol.* 20(Part I):791–796 (1989).
80. E. Tur, H. I. Maibach, and R. H. Guy. *Br. J. Dermatol.* 11:197–203 (1985).
81. B. W. Barry and R. Woodford. *Br. J. Dermatol.* 97:555–560 (1977).
82. K. H. Burdick. *Arch. Dermatol.* 110:238–242 (1974).
83. R. B. Stoughton and K. Wullich. *Arch. Dermatol.* 125:1509–1511 (1989).
84. R. B. Stoughton. *Arch. Dermatol.* 123:1312–1314 (1987).
85. B. W. Barry and R. Woodford. *Br. J. Dermatol.* 95:423–425 (1976).
86. R. C. Cornell and R. B. Stoughton. *Arch. Dermatol.* 121:63–67 (1985).
87. H. Schein, Personal communication, Thames Pharmacal, Ronkonkoma, N.Y. (1990).
88. M. A. Goshko, Personal communication. Lemmon Company, Sellersville, Pa. (1990).
89. B. J. Poulsen, K. Burdick, and S. Bessler. *Arch. Dermatol.* 109:367–371 (1974).
90. V. P. Shah, C. C. Peck, and J. P. Skelly. *Arch. Dermatol.* 125:1558–1561 (1989).
91. E. W. Smith, E. Meyer, J. M. Haign, and H. I. Maibach. In *Percutaneous Absorption*, 2nd ed. (R. L. Bronaugh and H. I. Maibach, eds.), Marcel Dekker, New York, pp. 443–460 (1989).
92. J. M. Haigh and I. Kanfer. *Int. J. Pharm.* 19:245–262 (1984).
93. E. Berardesca and H. I. Maibach. *Int. J. Dermatol.* 28:157–160 (1989).
94. R. O. Potts. *J. Soc. Cosmet. Chem.* 37:9–33 (1986).
95. D. P. Conner. Presented at the *Topical Therapeutic Products Workshop*, Sponsored by the AAPS and FDA, March 26–28, 1990, Arlington, Va.
96. V. H. W. Mak, R. O. Potts, and R. H. Guy. *Pharm. Res.* 5:S129 (1988).
97. R. H. Guy, E. Tur, and H. I. Maibach. *Int. J. Dermatol.* 24:88–94 (1985).
98. R. H. Guy, R. C. Wester, E. Tur, and H. I. Maibach. *J. Pharm. Sci.* 72:1077–1078 (1983).
99. J. K. Kristensen and S. Wadskov. *J. Invest. Dermatol.* 68:196–200 (1977).
100. T. P. Greeson, N. E. Levan, R. I. Freedman, and W. H. Wong. *J. Invest. Dermatol.* 61:242–244 (1973).
101. G. A. Holloway, Jr. and D. W. Watkins. *J. Invest. Dermatol.* 69:306–309 (1977).
102. K. P. Wilhelm, C. Surber, and H. I. Maibach. *Arch. Dermatol. Res.* 281:293–295 (1989).
103. M. C. Poelman, B. Piot, F. Guyon, M. Deroni, and J. L. Leveque. *J. Pharm. Pharmacol.* 41:720–722 (1989).
104. R. S. Pedersen, L. Lonka, and H. E. Hansen. *Scand. J. Urol. Nephrol.* 21:153–154 (1987).
105. H. Aoyama, A. Nishizaki, Y. Aoki, Y. Izawa. *Burns* 10:290–299 (1984).
106. T. J. Franz and P. Lehman. *J. Pharm. Sci.* 77:489–491 (1988).
107. D. A. W. Bucks, and J. R. McMaster, H. I. Maibach, and R. H. Guy. *J. Invest. Dermatol.* 90:29–33 (1988).
108. R. J. Feldman and H. I. Maibach. *Arch. Dermatol.* 91:661–666 (1965).
109. D. A. W. Bucks, H. I. Maibach, and R. H. Guy. *Pharm. Res.* 5:313–315 (1988).
110. D. A. W. Bucks, H. I. Maibach, and R. H. Guy. *J. Pharm. Sci.* 74:1337–1339 (1985).

111. T. J. Franz and P. A. Lehman. Presented at the AAPS/FDA/AAD/USAEHA Workshop, In Vivo Percutaneous Penetration/Absorption, May 1-3, 1989, Washington, D.C.
112. P. J. W. Ayres and G. Hooper. *Br. J. Dermatol.* 99:307 (1978).
113. M. Whitefield. *Br. J. Dermatol.* 99:736 (1978).
114. N. A. Orr, J. F. Smith, and E. A. Hill. *Br. J. Dermatol.* 99:737 (1978).
115. P. J. Ayres and G. Hooper. *Br. J. Dermatol.* 99:737-738 (1978).
116. M. G. Eller, G. J. Szpunar, and A. A. Della-Coletta. *Clin. Pharmacol. Ther.* 45:396-402 (1989).
117. G. J. Szpunar, E. P. Dalm, and K. S. Albert. *Pharm. Res.* 3(Suppl.):114S, #61 (1986).
118. G. J. Szpunar, E. P. Dalm, and K. S. Albert. *Pharm. Res.* 3(Suppl.):114S, #62 (1986).
119. *Fed. Reg.* 54:28941 (1989).
120. Schotz, J. R. and Dumas, R. J. *Proceeding 13th International Congress Dermatolog.* vol. 2. Springer-Verlag, New York, p. 179.
121. A. D. Woolfson, D. F. McCafferty, K. H. McClelland, and V. Boston. *Br. J. Anaesth.* 61:589-592 (1988).
122. A. D. Woolfson and D. F. McCafferty. *J. Clin. Pharm. Ther.* 14:103-109 (1989).
123. C. Evans. *Draft Guidance for the Performance of a Bioequivalence Study for Topical Antifungal Products.* U.S. Food and Drug Administration, Rockville, Md., (Feb. 12, 1990).
124. R. Aly, H. I. Maibach, F. K. Bagatell, W. Dittmar, H. Hanel, V. Falanga, J. J. Leyden, H. L. roth, R. B. Stoughton, I. Willis, B. B. Abrams, and M. Lakshminarayanan. *Clin. Ther.* 11:290-303 (1989).
125. *F-D-C Reports.* T&G-11 (Apr. 2, 1990).
126. Topical Antifungal and Acne Drug Product Bioequivalence Workshop, Nov. 16, 1989, Food and Drug Administration, Rockville, Md.
127. P. A. Lehman and A. M. Malany. *J. Invest. Dermatol.* 93:595-599 (1989).
128. P. A. Lehman, J. T. Slattery, and T. Franz. *J. Invest. Dermatol.* 91:56-61 (1988).
129. V. H. Price. *Clin. Dermatol.* 6:218-227 (1988).
130. H. Uno, A. Cappas, and P. Brigham. *J. Am. Acad. Dermatol.* 16:657-668 (1987).
131. J. T. Headington and E. Novak. *Curr. Ther. Res.* 36:1098 (1984).
132. R. C. Wester, H. I. Maibach, R. H. Guy, and E. Novak. *J. Invest. Dermatol.* 82:515-517 (1984).

8
In Vitro Methods to Determine Bioavailability: In Vitro–In Vivo Correlations

Peter G. Welling
Parke-Davis Pharmaceutical Research Division
Warner-Lambert Company
Ann Arbor, Michigan

INTRODUCTION

During the last 25 years there has been considerable interest within the pharmaceutical industry, academia, and regulatory sectors in the in vitro–in vivo relationships of oral dosage forms. In vitro specifications such as physical and chemical properties, stability, water content, disintegration, solubility, and the rate and extent of dissolution are routinely used as quality and process controls in dosage form manufacturing. These characteristics are well established, and it is tempting to consider that one or more of them may be useful to predict behavior of the dosage form in the gastrointestinal (GI) tract and its overall absorption characteristics. More specifically, it is desirable to establish some form of correlation so that in vivo bioavailability may be accurately predicted from in vitro data.

The advantages of establishing such a relationship are to be measured in terms of cost, time, and safety. For an in vitro test to be useful in this context, it must predict in vivo behavior to such an extent that an in vivo bioavailability test becomes redundant. This statement will be addressed in more detail later. However, one assumes, for the moment, that this can be achieved, then the need for in vivo bioavailability tests would be drastically reduced, and they would not be needed at all in many cases. The combined costs of both clinical and analytical components of a bioavailability study in normal volunteers may range from 10,000 to 100,000 dollars, depending on the drug, formulation, and the type of study. The duration of a bioavailability study, again considering both clinical and analytical portions, may vary from a few weeks to several months, involving up to 1 or more years of total resources. In vivo bioavailability studies also involve those safety issues that normally accompany administration of drugs to healthy subjects or to patients. It would be nice, very nice indeed, if inexpensive in vitro tests could be substituted for in vivo bioavailability tests, in whole or in part. Considering just the foregoing cost factors—and other associated, peripheral cost factors have not been considered here—the savings to the pharmaceutical industry and, hence, the public would run into many millions of dollars annually.

Achievement of this goal, to establish accurate and robust in vitro–in vivo bioavailability correlations, has driven the hearts and minds of those who concern themselves with this type of thing for the last 25 years. In 1965, Dr. Gerhard Levy alluded to the possibility of ". . . relatively generalized [in vitro] test procedures suitable for development and control purposes, and for inclusion in official compendia as a test of physiologic availability" [1].

The goal appeared reasonable, at first. One simply had to establish some in vitro characteristic, match it with in vivo behavior, and the problem is solved. In fact, it has turned out to be not that simple. There have been many attempts to establish in vitro–in vivo correlations and many publications debating the issue. It is not my intent to provide detailed lists of the many various studies, nor of the many arguments for and against, but rather, to consider the problem involved in establishing in vitro–in vivo relationships, the awesome dimensions of the task, and the apparent futility of its application in general and specific cases.

COMPARISON OF IN VITRO AND IN VIVO ENVIRONMENTS

In vitro disintegration or dissolution tests are generally carried out under carefully controlled conditions, which are necessary for any type of quality control. Release of drug is determined in one or, perhaps sequentially, two solvents under sink or nonsink conditions at controlled temperatures. The GI tract, on the other hand, presents a complex environment. As described by Davis [2] and many others, the GI tract provides a continuously changing environment for pH, enzyme secretions, motility, presence of other substances, absorption surfaces, and absorption routes. The manner in which these various factors influence drug bioavailability depends on the drug, the dosage form, the dosage regimen, the dose level, and patient or subject characteristics. In vivo absorption may, or may not, be dissolution rate-limited. The drug, the dosage form, or both, may have variable stability in the presence of GI secretions and other GI components. A controlled-release dosage form may have entirely different stability and absorption characteristics from a conventional-release dosage form.

To these factors must be added other complicating factors, such as drug-drug interactions, food effects, age effects, and special patient populations. These factors may have an unpredictable effect on the rate and extent of drug absorption [3].

In vivo bioavailability is thus influenced by many factors in an environment that is far more complex, variable and unpredictable than any in vitro test environment. The need to predict the behavior of a drug dosage form in a complex environment, based on an artificial in vitro environment, is the essence of the problem that has plagued researchers in this area.

WHAT PARAMETERS SHOULD BE USED IN VITRO–IN VIVO CORRELATIONS?

The earlier literature on in vitro–in vivo relationships focused on disintegration as the most pertinent in vitro parameter. More recently, dissolution rate has been used as a manufacturing process standard and is generally considered to be the in vitro parameter most likely to correlate with in vivo bioavailability.

In vivo bioavailability is described in terms of the rate and extent of drug absorption. Rate of absorption is reflected in peak drug concentrations in plasma (C_{max}) and the times at which they occur (t_{max}). Other methods may be used to describe absorption rate profile, for example, deconvolution [4–6] and statistical moment theory [7]. However, use of these approaches does not detract from the basic relationships between absorption rate, C_{max}, and t_{max}. Extent of absorption is reflected in C_{max} and also the area under the plasma drug curve (AUC).

Therefore, one has the quandary as to which term(s) to select in seeking an in vitro–in vivo relationship. Accurate correlation, if it is achievable, will depend on accurate selection of the in vitro parameter that has the greatest intrinsic effect on drug absorption characteristics. Usually, the in vivo parameters C_{max} and AUC are compared with in vitro dissolution rate. However, both of these in vivo parameters are functions of both the rate and extent of absorption; consequently, they may be influenced as much by solubility as by dissolution rate. Thus, depending on the site(s) at which drug is absorbed from the GI tract, solubility and dissolution rate may have varying effects on the drug-absorption profile. Similarly, saturable presystemic metabolism may affect the extent of drug absorption from different dose levels. This would not be predicted from an in vitro test.

GUIDELINES FOR TESTS TO DETERMINE IN VITRO–IN VIVO RELATIONSHIPS

There have been several attempts to establish guidelines to examine relationships between in vitro dissolution and in vivo bioavailability, both for conventional and controlled-release oral dosage forms [8–11]. These attempts have been controversial and have given rise to considerable debate in the literature [12,13]. In 1985, the Pharmaceutical Manufacturers Association (PMA) published a position paper discussing the complex relationship that exist between in vitro dissolution and in vivo bioavailability [13].

The characteristics of controlled-release oral dosage forms present additional complications. These dosage forms are designed to release drugs slowly in the GI tract. A variety of mechanisms have been used to achieve that goal (e.g., coating, wax matrices, osmotic pump devices, and others). Because each of these dosage forms is unique, it would not be expected that a single dissolution test could accurately predict drug absorption from these dosage forms in the complex environment of the GI tract.

One suggestion for a controlled-release dosage form is that a variety of formulations, with varying dissolution characteristics, be prepared for each product. Bioavailability studies should then be conducted to establish in vitro–in vivo relationships.

But what range of dissolution rates should be tested to establish this relationship? What if the dissolution rate of a particular test product falls outside that range? Given our current knowledge, establishing a meaningful correlation between in vitro dissolution and in vivo absorption would require the manufacturer to prepare many formulations with dissolution characteristics that are faster or slower than the "optimal" rate. It would also require development of many different dissolution protocols and the conducting of a great number of in vivo bioavailability comparisons, also using different protocols. Preparations of numerous formulations, conduct of dissolution tests, and comparison with in vivo parameters are monumental tasks that would greatly increase the cost of drug products and would be of doubtful usefulness.

ATTEMPTS TO ESTABLISH IN VITRO–IN VIVO CORRELATIONS

Many attempts have been made to establish in vitro–in vivo correlations for a variety of drugs. Some of these are summarized in Table 1. The table describes studies on a variety of dosage forms for a broad spectrum of therapeutic indications, and provides a brief comment on the results obtained.

Of all the studies reported in this table, and they represent a reasonable cross-sectional sample of endeavors in seven therapeutic areas, good correlations that may be of clinical value were reported only for digoxin products. Although

Table 1 Investigations of In Vitro Dissolution and In Vivo Bioavailability Relationships

Drug	Test Formulations	Comments	Ref.
Antibacterials and Antifungals			
Doxycycline	Three 100-mg capsules compared with a suspension and a solution	Rank order correlation between dissolution rates and absorption rate constants, but no statistically significant difference in bioavailability of the three capsule products.	14
Griseofulvin	Four 125-mg tablets compared in dog and humans	Good in vitro–in vivo correlation using specific sink condition dissolution method. Low in vivo correlation between dog and human.	15
Nitrofurantoin	Fourteen 50- and 100-mg products	No useful correlation between extent of urinary excretion and either disintegration or dissolution.	16
Nitrofurantoin	Nineteen 100-mg products	Neither disintegration nor dissolution accurately reflected absorption.	17
Nitrofurantoin	Six formulations with widely divergent dissolution rates	Good correlation obtained, but two different dissolution methods were required for tablets and capsules.	18
Cardiovascular			
Digoxin	Two 0.25-mg tablets	Equivocal results. The products were bioequivalent despite statistical differences in dissolution rate within 1 hr.	19
Digoxin	Five 0.25-mg experimental tablets	Significant correlation between dissolution and urinary excretion.	20
Digoxin	Twelve tablets from eight companies	Excellent correlation between dissolution rate and bioavailability.	21
Digoxin	Seven 0.25-mg tablets	Close correlation between dissolution rate and bioavailability.	22
Isosorbide dinitrate	Two experimental 40-mg tablets	Products were bioequivalent despite different in vitro release rates.	23

Continued

Table 1 *(Continued)*

Drug	Test Formulations	Comments	Ref.
Chlorothiazide	Three 250-mg tablets and two 500-mg tablets	Products were bioequivalent despite differences in in vitro dissolution rates. Dissolution test was modified to agree with in vivo data.	24
Diltiazem	60-mg and 120-mg tablets	Rate of absorption related to dissolution for these two products. Surface area may be a factor.	25
Quinidine gluconate	Two 648-mg controlled-release tablets	Products were bioinequivalent, despite identical dissolution. Dissolution test modified to discriminate products.	26
Central Nervous System Drugs			
Promethazine	Two 50-mg tablets, one 25-mg tablet, and a solution	Nondiscriminatory. No significant differences among products in in vitro or in vivo data.	27
Steroids and Hormones			
Prednisone	5-mg and 50-mg tablets	Bioequivalent despite 25-fold difference in dissolution rate.	28
Prednisone	Five 20-mg tablets	Nondiscriminatory. No difference in in vitro dissolution or in vivo bioavailability among products.	29
Prednisone	5-mg and 50-mg tablets	In vitro dissolution rate not predictive of overall bioavailability.	30
Prednisolone	Five 5-mg tablets	Products were bioequivalent despite difference in in vitro dissolution. Dissolution test modified to agree with in vivo data.	31
Hydrocortisone	Four 20-mg tablets	No correlation between dissolution and bioavailability.	32
Norethisterone	Three 0.05-mg tablets and a solution	No correlation between in vitro and in vivo data. In vitro data similar between products.	33

Continued

Table 1 *(Continued)*

Drug	Test Formulations	Comments	Ref.
Respiratory Tract			
Theophylline	Two 100-mg tablets	Absorption rate of one product same as in vitro rate. Absorption rate of other product 2.7-fold greater than in vitro rate.	34
Theophylline	Four experimental controlled-release formulations	Correlations obtained between in vitro and in vivo data.	35, 36
Anti-inflammatory and Analgesic Agents			
Aspirin	One commercial and four experimental formulations	All preparations were bioequivalent, despite different dissolution rate of one preparation.	37
Aspirin	Four 300-mg tablets	No in vitro–in vivo correlation.	38
Indomethacin	Two 75-mg controlled-release capsules and one 25-mg conventional-release capsule	Rank order correlation between in vitro and in vivo data.	39
Indomethacin	Four indomethacin preparations	All preparations were bioequivalent, despite different dissolution rate of one preparation.	40
Ketoprofen	50-mg conventional capsules and two 200-mg sustained-release (SR) capsules	Slower absorption and reduced systemic bioavailability from slower-dissolving SR capsule.	41
Hypoglycemic Agents			
Glyburide (glybenclaide)	Four marketed preparations	Two dissolution tests yielded different rank orders of dissolution rates. Neither test correlated with in vivo data.	42

these studies were able to establish recommendations for a lower level for dissolution rate for acceptability [20,21], they were unable to establish upper dissolution rate limits [22].

Most studies have resulted either in poor in vitro–in vivo correlations, or moderate or rank order correlations that are based on very few formulations.

To the writer's knowledge, there have been no studies that have accurately correlated in vitro and in vivo data to the point that the use of upper and lower limits for in vitro dissolution parameters can be confidently used to predict in vivo behavior and, therefore, to replace in vivo testing. Good in vitro–in vivo correlations were recently reported for the oral osmotic pump dosage form [43]. Although no details were presented for particular drugs, this may represent a good example of how such correlations may be achieved for a dosage form the release rate of which is essentially independent of the environment. Some tests have shown that all products tested in a given study met compendial dissolution criteria and were also bioequivalent. However, these studies are not relevant to the problem, as neither test is discriminatory. For quinidine gluconate, an in vitro dissolution test failed to discriminate between two controlled-release products that were bioinequivalent in vivo [26]. A new, discriminating procedure was developed and was used to formulate a new product that was bioequivalent to the innovator [44].

Thus, although it is clearly desirable to establish dissolution tests that accurately predict in vivo behavior, this has been an elusive goal. This is partially the result of the cost of conducting appropriate studies in order to test for correlations and, partially, the result of the complex nature of the problem. Correlation of such diverse phenomena may be impossible to achieve in most cases.

As the in vivo environment cannot be changed, one might consider further refinement of in vitro tests to more accurately reflect the in vivo system. This might involve setting up a battery of in vitro tests, with their associated costs, or by conducting in vitro tests under conditions more similar to those in the GI tract [45]. Such approaches have been described, but with varying success, as indicated by the results described in Table 1.

CONCLUSIONS

Many attempts have been made to establish in vitro–in vivo correlations for both conventional and controlled-release oral dosage forms. Most of these have been unsuccessful. Notably, the *United States Pharmacopeia* does not currently present standards for in vitro–in vivo correlations, and the United States Food and Drug Administration (FDA) and other regulatory agencies worldwide require in vivo bioavailability or bioequivalence data in all New Drug Application (NDA) and Abbreviated New Drug Application (ANDA) submissions, or their overseas equivalents.

It is clear that a complex relationship exists between in vitro dissolution and in vivo bioavailability. While it is desirable to use product dissolution to predict in vivo behavior, many years of investigation have shown that this goal cannot be achieved with our current knowledge. Indeed, the assumption of such a relationship could be potentially dangerous.

Dissolution testing is essential as a quality control to ensure process and batch consistency in the manufacturing process. It has failed, however, to predict differences among products that are poorly available in vivo or those that are super-bioavailable relative to existing standards.

In vitro data may be used as a guide to assist in the development of oral dosage forms. However, the ultimate assessment of the dosage form and its behavior under the variety of conditions to be expected in therapy, must be made in vivo in healthy volunteers, and in appropriate patient populations.

REFERENCES

1. G. Levy, J. R. Leonards, and J. A. Procknal. *J. Pharm. Sci.* 54:1719 (1965).
2. S. S. Davis. *J. Controlled Release* 2:27 (1985).
3. P. G. Welling. Clinical factors affecting drug absorption. In *Pharmacokinetics, Processes and Mathematics. ACS Monogr.* p. 59 (1986).
4. J. G. Wagner. *J. Pharmacokinet. Biopharm.* 3:457 (1975).
5. D. J. Cutler. *J. Pharmacokinet. Biopharm.* 6:227 (1978).
6. P. V. Pedersen. *J. Pharm. Sci.* 69:298 (1980).
7. S. Riegelman and P. Collier. *J. Pharmacokinet. Biopharm.* 8:509 (1980).
8. M. K. T. Yau and M. C. Meyer. *J. Pharm. Sci.* 70:1017 (1981).
9. J. P. Skelly, W. H. Barr, L. Z. Benet, J. T. Doluisio, A. H. Goldberg, G. Levy, D. T. Lowenthal, J. R. Robinson, V. P. Shah, R. J. Temple, and A. Yacobi. *Pharm. Res.* 4:75 (1987).
10. J. P. Skelly, G. L. Amidon, W. H. Barr, L. Z. Benet, J. E. Carter, J. R. Robinson, V. P. Shah, and A. Yacobi. Report of the workshop on in vitro and in vivo testing and correlation for oral controlled/modified release dosage forms, Washington, D.C. (Dec. 1988).
11. Stimuli to the Revision Process. In vitro/in vivo correlation for extended release oral dosage forms. *Pharmacopeial Forum*, July–August, p. 4160 (1988).
12. PMA Joint Committee on Bioavailability. The role of dissolution testing in drug quality, bioavailability, and bioequivalence testing. *Pharm. Technol.* 9:62 (1985).
13. PMA Comments on *USP* Stimuli to the Revision Process. In vitro–in vivo correlation for extended release oral dosage forms. Dec. 1988.
14. E. J. Antal, J. M. Jaffe, R. I. Poust, and J. L. Colaizzi. *J. Pharm. Sci.* 64:2015 (1975).
15. N. Aoyagi, H. Ogata, N. Kaniwa, M. Koibuchi, T. Shibazaki, A. Ejima, N. Tamaki, H. Kamimura, Y. Katougi, and Y. Omi. *J. Pharm. Sci.* 71:1169 (1982).
16. M. C. Meyer, G. W. A. Slywka, R. E. Dann, and P. L. Whyatt. *J. Pharm. Sci.* 63:1693 (1974).
17. G. L. Máttok, R. D. Hossie, and I. J. McGilveray. *Can. J. Pharm. Sci.* 7:84 (1972).
18. R. W. Mendes, S. Z. Masih, and R. R. Kanumuri. *J. Pharm. Sci.* 67:1616 (1978).
19. J. H. G. Jonkman, C. F. Gusdorf, W. J. V. van der Boon, G. Grasmeijer, and J. N. Jedema. *Arnzeim. Forsch.* 37:62 (1987).
20. B. F. Johnson, H. Greer, J. McCrerie, C. Bye, and A. Fowle. *Lancet 1*:1473 (1973).
21. J. Lindenbaum, V. P. Butler, J. E. Murphy, and R. M. Cresswell. *Lancet 1*:1215 (1973).

22. T.R.D. Shaw, K. Raymond, M.R. Howard, and J. Hamer. *Br. Med. J.* 4:763 (1973).
23. L. F. Chasseaud, T. Taylor, R. M. Major, I. W. Taylor, V. Luckow, A. Darragh, and R. F. Lambe. *Arzneim. Forsch.* 33:1298 (1983).
24. V. P. Shah, P. Knight, V. K. Prasad, and B. E. Cabana. *J. Pharm. Sci.* 71:822 (1982).
25. G. Campistron, M. Rostin, Y. Coulais, C. Caillard, G. Zarrouk, J. Frances, J. F. Thiercellin, J. L. Montastruc, and G. Houin. *Fundam. Clin. Pharmacol.* 1:67 (1987).
26. V. K. Prasad, V. P. Shah, P. Knight, H. J. Malinowski, B. E. Cabana, and M. C. Meyer. *Int. J. Pharm.* 13:1 (1983).
27. R. Zaman, I. L. Honigberg, G. E. Francisco, J. A. Kotzan, J. T. Stewart, W. J. Brown, V. P. Shah, and F. R. Pelsor. *Biopharm. Drug Dispos.* 7:281 (1986).
28. S. S. Stubbs. *Transplantation Proc.* 7:11 (1975).
29. G. E. Francisco, J. L. Honigberg, J. T. Stewart, J. A. Kotzan, and W. J. Brown. *Biopharm. Drug Dispos.* 5:335 (1984).
30. A. R. DiSanto and K. A. DeSante. *J. Pharm. Sci.* 64:109 (1975).
31. T. J. Sullivan, R. G. Stoll, E. Sakmar, D. C. Blair, and J. G. Wagner. *J. Pharmacokinet. Biopharm.* 2:29 (1974).
32. R. B. Patel, M. C. Rogge, A. Selen, T. J. Goehl, V. P. Shah, V. K. Prasad, and P. G. Welling. *J. Pharm. Sci.* 73:964 (1984).
33. C. W. Vose, J. K. Butler, B. M. Williams, J. E. H. Stafford, J. R. Shelton, D. A. Rose, R. F. Palmer, A. M. Breckenridge, M.L'E. Orme, and M. J. Serlin. *Contraception* 19:119 (1979).
34. N. Ohmori, N. Inotsume, M. Matsukura, A. Higashi, R. Iwaoku, Y. Tobino, M. Nakano, and I. Matsuda. *Int. J. Clin. Pharm.* 24:148 (1986).
35. R. Dietrich, R. Brausse, G. Benedikt, and V. W. Steinijans. *Arzneim. Forsch.* 38:1229 (1988).
36. G. Benedikt, V. W. Steinijans, and R. Dietrich. *Arzneim. Forsch.* 38:1203 (1988).
37. M. Nieder, J. Rasper, W. Gielsdorf, D. Russmann, and H. Jaeger. *Arzneim. Forsch.* 33:439 (1983).
38. P. K. Karogo and D. G. Sixsmith. *East Afr. Med. J.* 59:509 (1982).
39. H. Bechgaard, R. R. Brodie, L. F. Chasseaud, P. Houmoller, J. O. Hunter, P. Siklos, and T. Taylor. *Eur. J. Clin. Pharmacol.* 21:511 (1982).
40. J. A. Settlage, W. Gielsdorf, M. Nieder, J. Rasper, and H. Jaeger. *Arzneim. Forsch.* 33:885 (1983).
41. G. W. Houghton, M. J. Dennis, E. D. Rigler, R. L. Parsons. *Eur. J. Drug Metab.* 9:201 (1984).
42. J. B. Chalk, M. Patterson, M. T. Smith, and M. J. Eadie. *Eur. J. Clin. Pharmacol.* 31:177 (1986).
43. L. J. Leeson. In vitro/in vivo correlation: Release characteristics independent of environment. Workshop on In Vitro and In Vivo Testing and Correlation for Oral Controlled/Modified Release Dosage Forms. American Association of Pharmaceutical Scientists and U.S. Food and Drug Administration, Washington, D.C. December 14–16 (1980).
44. J. P. Skelly and W. H. Barr. Regulatory assessment. In *Controlled Drug Delivery, Fundamentals and Applications* (J. R. Robinson and V. H. L. Lee, eds). Marcel Dekker., New York, p. 309 (1987).
45. P. Finholt and S. Solvang. *J. Pharm. Sci.* 57:1322 (1968).

Part Two
Species Differences, Pharmacodynamic Models

Part Two

9
Animal Models for Oral Drug Absorption

Jennifer B. Dressman
The University of Michigan
Ann Arbor, Michigan

Kenji Yamada
Taisho Pharmaceutical Company
Saitama, Japan

Animal models for oral drug absorption are used for several purposes. These include determining the main site of absorption within the gastrointestinal (GI) tract, identifying the mechanism of absorption, determining how efficient the absorption process is, and testing new formulations for their ability to deliver the drug in a timely and effective manner. Results in animals can be used to aid in selection of the most appropriate oral formulation and as a guide in the design of controlled-release dosage forms. To make the best use of animal models, it is necessary to be familiar with both the similarities and differences between the anatomy and physiology of the GI tracts of the various species available and that of the human GI tract.

This chapter focuses on the gross features of gastrointestinal physiology that affect dosage form performance and drug absorption, and how these features vary among species commonly used to evaluate human-scale dosage forms. Key aspects of oral dosage form performance include ability to release the drug from the dosage form, the residence time of both the dosage form and the released drug at the sites of absorption, and the ability of the mucosa to absorb the drug. These all depend on the anatomical arrangement of the GI tract and its gross physiological features. In this chapter, the ability of species commonly used in absorption studies to provide a good model for the environment experienced by drugs and dosage forms as they move through the human GI tract is evaluated by the foregoing criteria. In addition, some practical matters relating to availability and handling of the animals are considered.

A list of specific characteristics for evaluating animal models starts with the anatomical dimensions of the GI tract, both on an absolute and on a relative basis. First, the gut must be able to accommodate a human-scale dosage form without inducing any abnormal physiological responses, such as altered motility (cramping, delayed transit), or responses secondary to trauma to the mucosa caused by the dosage form. Second, it is desirable that the *ratio* of sizes of the various compartments within the GI tract approximate those of humans, so that residence times and volumes of lumenal contents at the various locations will be similar, at least in a relative way, to what might be expected in humans. For example, if the stomach is twice as large, but the small intestine is half as long, in the model species as in the human, one would expect to get skewed results for the absorption profile just because the environment to which the dosage form is exposed would be so different as a function of time in the two species.

As well as being anatomically similar, it would be desirable to have similar physiological characteristics. One important area of consideration is the gastrointestinal mucosa; in terms of its morphological characteristics, the location of the main absorbing mucosa, and the availability and importance of the various transport mechanisms, including passive diffusion, paracellular diffusion, and active transport systems. In addition to affecting the relative importance of the various mechanisms of absorption, differences in the enzyme distribution in the brush border of the small intestine could potentially affect the gut wall metabolism of drugs.

A second important consideration is the arrangement of the blood and lymph supply to the gut, which may affect the extent of first-pass metabolism and, thereby, the efficiency of delivery to the drug's target site.

Third, secretory levels of gastric and pancreatic juices are important, since they establish the pH profile of the upper GI tract. The pancreatic secretions are also the major source of enzymes that can potentially catalyze decomposition of proteins, peptides, fats, and carbohydrates (pepsin in the stomach and brush border enzymes are additional important sources of peptidase activity). Bile composition and secretion levels are important because, as the main source of surfactant in the GI tract, the bile is an important determinant of the degree to which the fluid in the small intestine can solubilize the drug. As well as the levels of acid, bicarbonate, enzymes, and bile secreted under basal conditions, it is also worthwhile to have an appreciation of the various stimuli for secretion and the degree to which these stimuli elevate the levels secreted. Another influence on the composition of the lumenal fluids is the microbial population. Although this is very small in the upper GI tract under normal circumstances, the colon contains large numbers of organisms that are capable of metabolizing residual foodstuffs and also some drugs. As a result of the dense microbial population, the pH in this region is affected by fermentation as well as the pH of the chyme entering from the ileocecal valve. The pH in the proximal human colon has been measured by Brown et al. [1] as pH 6 (range 5.5–7.5), whereas in the lower colon, a mean value of pH 7.5 (range 6.8–8.4) was recorded.

Finally, it would be desirable to have an interdigestive motility pattern that is similar to the 2-hour cycle existing in humans [2], and this cycle should be interrupted by feeding. This would facilitate the interpretation of fed- versus fasted-state tests done in the animal.

Some of the species that have been used in bioavailability studies include primates, dogs, pigs, and rabbits. Humans are naturally the species of choice, followed by animals that are close in terms of evolution, such as the lower primates, or those that have reasonably similar body size and digestive habits, such as dogs and swine. In addition to these species, some smaller animals have been used because of convenience in terms of laboratory space required, cost, and handling. Of these, only rabbits will be discussed in this chapter. Although rats, mice, and other small rodents are useful in elucidating transport mechanisms and for doing preliminary oral absorption screens, human-scale dosage forms cannot usually be tested in these species owing to the small dimensions of their GI tracts.

Tables 1, 2, and 3 summarize the anatomical and physiological features relevant to drug absorption of the GI tracts of humans, dogs, monkeys, and swine. It must be noted that all values for swine given in the tables are for domestic swine. Minipig strains are more often used as models for drug absorption in humans, and the values listed may overestimate the anatomical dimensions for these strains. Data for monkeys refer to rhesus monkeys unless otherwise stated.

Table 1 shows anatomical and physiological data for the stomach in the species considered. Monkeys, swine, and dogs have several gastric features in common with humans. All possess a simple stomach; that is, there is only one major compartment. Another point of commonality is that all of these species produce a pepsin enzyme, which is most active under acidic conditions. Furthermore, the stomach is lined with a glandular mucosa that secretes substantial quantities of gastric acid, so the stomach tends to have an acidic pH. The amount of glandular and aglandular mucosa in the stomachs of five species [25] is compared in Figure 1.

The fundus and pyloric regions, which contain the parietal cells responsible for secretion of gastric acid, are much more extensive in humans than in the pig and the horse, while being fairly similar between human and dog. Ruminants are not suitable as models for human bioavailability because of the tremendous differences in the structure and function of the upper GI tract.

Table 8 Composition of Bile in Several Species

	Flow (μl/min/kg)	Na+	K+	Ca2+	Mg2+	Cl−	HCO3−	Bile acids (mm)
				(mEq/L)				
Human	1.5–15.4	132–165	4.2–5.6	1.2–4.8	1.4–3.0	96–126	17–55	3–45
Dog	10	141–230	4.5–11.9	3.1–13.8	2.2–5.5	31–107	14–61	16–187
Sheep	9.4	159.6	5.3			95	21.2	42.5
Rabbit	90	148–156	3.6–6.7	2.7–6.7	0.3–0.7	77–99	40–63	6–24
Rat	30–150	157–166	5.8–6.4			94–98	22–26	8–25
Guinea pig	115.9	175	6.3			69	49–65	
Turkey	10	161–223	4.4–6.8			85–110	18–54	74
Dogfish shark	1.2	227	5.0	18.0	9.0	224	5.8	21

Numbers indicate range or means of published values.
Source: From Ref. 49.

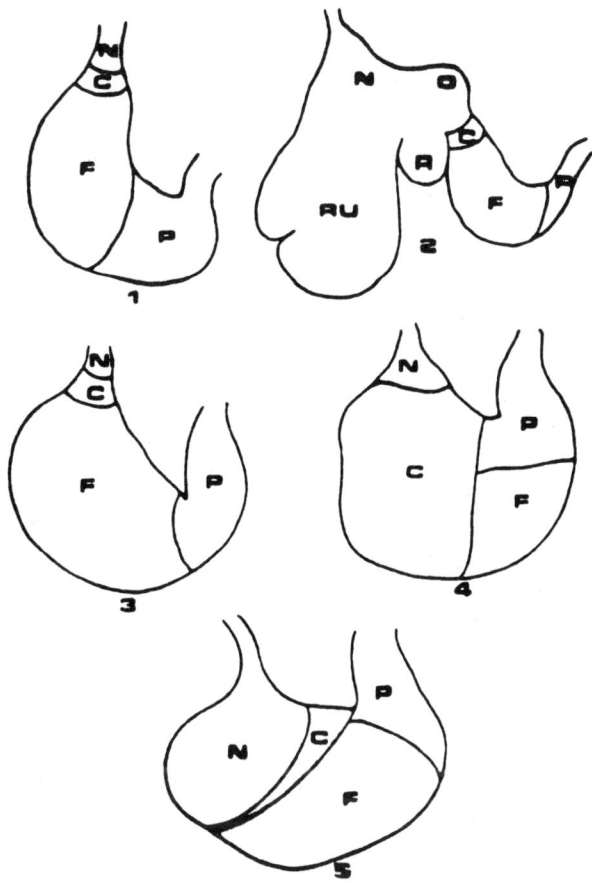

Figure 1 Comparison of regional distributions of gastric mucosa in five species: (1) human, (2) ruminant, (3) dog, (4) pig, (5) horse. N corresponds to nonglandular mucosa, C to the cardiac region, F to the fundic region, P to the pyloric region, R to the reticulum and RU to the rumen. (From Ref. 25.)

Gastric volumes vary considerably, with that of monkey being smallest and that of swine largest. Gastric acid output is considerably lower in the fasted state than in the fed state in all these species, although the fasting gastric pH is usually in the acid region. In humans, meals initially tend to buffer the gastric pH to higher levels, then as gastric acid is secreted, the pH gradually returns to its fasted-state value. In dogs and swine, the initial elevation in gastric pH is not

Table 2 Comparison of Anatomical and Physiological Data for the Small Intestine of Humans, Dogs, Swine, and Rhesus Monkeys

Parameter	Human	Dog	Swine	Monkey
Dimensions				
Length (autopsy) (m)	7	4	15–20	5 cm (duod)
(in vivo) (m)	3	1.5		
Duodenal diameter (cm)	3–4	2–2.5	2.5–3.5	1.5–2
Villi: length	0.5–1.5	Long, slender	0.5–1	
shape	Filamentous			Ridges, leaflike
Peyer's patches: location	Ileum	Duodenum, jejunum, ileum	Jejunum, ileum, colon	Ileum
Secretions				
Bile: major acid	Cholic	Cholic	Hyocholic	
concn by gallbladder	×5	×8–10	×2	
flow rate (L/day)	0.8–1	0.1–0.4		
Pancreatic juice flow rate (mL/min)	1	2–3	1	
Intestinal pH: fasted	6.1 [5.6–6.4][a]	6.5–7.5	7.2 (duodenum)	7–9; 5.5–6.0
fed	5.4 [5.0–5.8][a]	6.5–6.9		

[a]Lower duodenum.
Source: Data from Refs. 6, 8, 24, 26.

as clear as in humans, but the pH response has not been directly compared using identical meals.

The dimensions of the small intestine are listed in Table 2. One problem with interpretation of these lengths is that the intestine loses tone when the subject dies, resulting, for example, in a small intestinal length in humans, reported as 7 m in *Gray's Anatomy* [27], but more like 300 cm in intestinal intubation studies in conscious humans [28]. However, the values in the literature for animals most likely refer to autopsy values and should probably be compared with the 7-m value for humans. The small intestine, but not other regions of the GI tract, is lined with villi and, although these may differ in terms of size and morphology among species, they always serve the purpose of dramatically increasing the surface area available for absorption of nutrients and drugs. Thus, the small intestine is the major site of nutrient absorption in each of these species as well as in humans.

Each of these species secretes a pancreatic juice rich in enzymes and bicarbonate. As a result of the balance between gastric acid and pancreatic secretions, intestinal pH is close to neutral for these species, with a slight tendency to more basic values in the monkey, and a slight tendency toward more acidic values in humans. Each of these species also possesses a gallbladder, from which bile is secreted into the proximal part of the small intestine (note that some other species, such as horses and rats, lack a gallbladder). The bile salt composition is a little different in pigs and dogs than in humans and, furthermore, the ability of the gallbladder to concentrate the bile is lower in pigs than the other species.

Each of these species also possesses a cecum and colon, although the relative size and function varies somewhat (Table 3). In humans, the colon consists of three parts, namely, an ascending colon, a transverse, and a descending colon, for a total length of about 1–1.5 m. The ascending colon, which only occupies about 20 cm of the total colonic length, is currently thought to be the main location for absorption from this region. In swine, the colon overall and, in particular, the ascending colon has a much greater length, while in dogs and monkeys the colon is relatively short. Microbial metabolism occurs in the colon as well as the cecum, but its contribution to the overall assimilation of foodstuffs is of little importance in these species, with the possible exception of swine.

The final aspect of GI physiology that one is interested in comparing among species is the motility pattern. A very important feature of upper GI motor activity relative to dosage form transit is the interdigestive migrating motility complex (IMMC). This strong pattern of contractions that occurs periodically in the fasted state [2] is thought to be responsible for clearance of large, nondisintegrating dosage forms from the stomach. The basic motility patterns, in terms of an interdigestive migrating motility complex which can be interrupted by feeding, appear to be present in all the species considered here.

The remainder of this chapter is devoted to a discussion of rabbits, monkeys,

Table 3 Comparison of Anatomical and Physiological Data for the Cecum and Colon of Humans, Dogs, Swine, and Rhesus Monkeys

Parameter	Human	Dog	Swine	Monkey
Cecum:				
length (cm)	7	12–15	20–30	5–6
diameter (cm)	6		8–10	
volume (L)	about 1	0.25	1.5–2.2	
Colon:				
length, overall (m)	0.9–1.5	0.6–0.75	4–4.5	0.4–0.5
length, asc. colon (cm)	20		Long, coiled	10
diameter (cm)	6	Similar to SI	8–10	
haustrae	Present	Absent	Present	Present
Microbial metabolism, colon	Volatile fatty acids Vitamins	Very minor	Volatile fatty acids Vitamins	
pH, colon	6 (upper) 7.5 (lower)			

swine, and dogs, on an individual species basis, relative to their usefulness as models for studying performance of oral formulations designed for human use.

RABBITS

Although rabbits are readily available, relatively inexpensive, and easy to house and handle, there are several physiological and anatomical differences from humans that limit their use as a model for oral absorption.

The major problem with rabbits, as an animal model, is their size. Depending on the dosage form being studied, rabbits may be borderline or too small to be useful in terms of GI dimensions. In a study by Aoyagi et al. [31] (Fig. 2), enteric-coated aspirin tablets, diameter 11 mm, did not produce significant salicylate levels, although 1-mm enteric-coated granules produced salicylate levels within 1 hr of administration. These results highlight the limitations of the rabbit's gastric dimensions, as salicylate levels were quickly achieved in humans and dogs after administration of either the tablet or the pellet formulation.

Subsequent gastric-emptying studies (Fig. 3) showed that there is no emptying of 11-mm enteric-coated tablets from the rabbit stomach within 24 hr of administration and that even the emptying of 1-mm particles ranged between 20 and 100% in the 24-hr period.

A second departure from human physiology is that the cecum assumes much

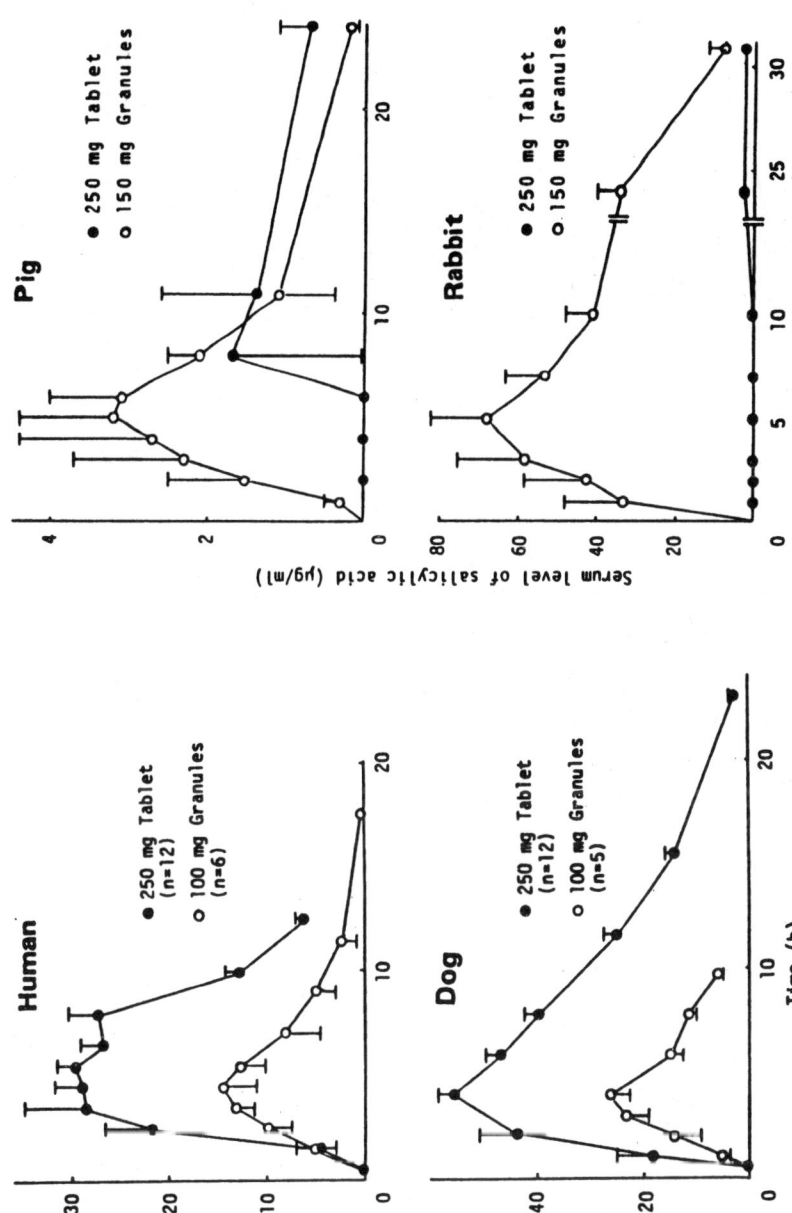

Figure 2 Salicylate levels, expressed as total salicylic acid urinary excretion rate or mean serum levels, after administration of enteric coated tablets (diameter 11 mm) or granules (diameter 1 mm) to humans, swine, dogs, and rabbits. In all experiments, the subjects were fasted overnight. Vertical bars show standard errors. (From Ref. 31.)

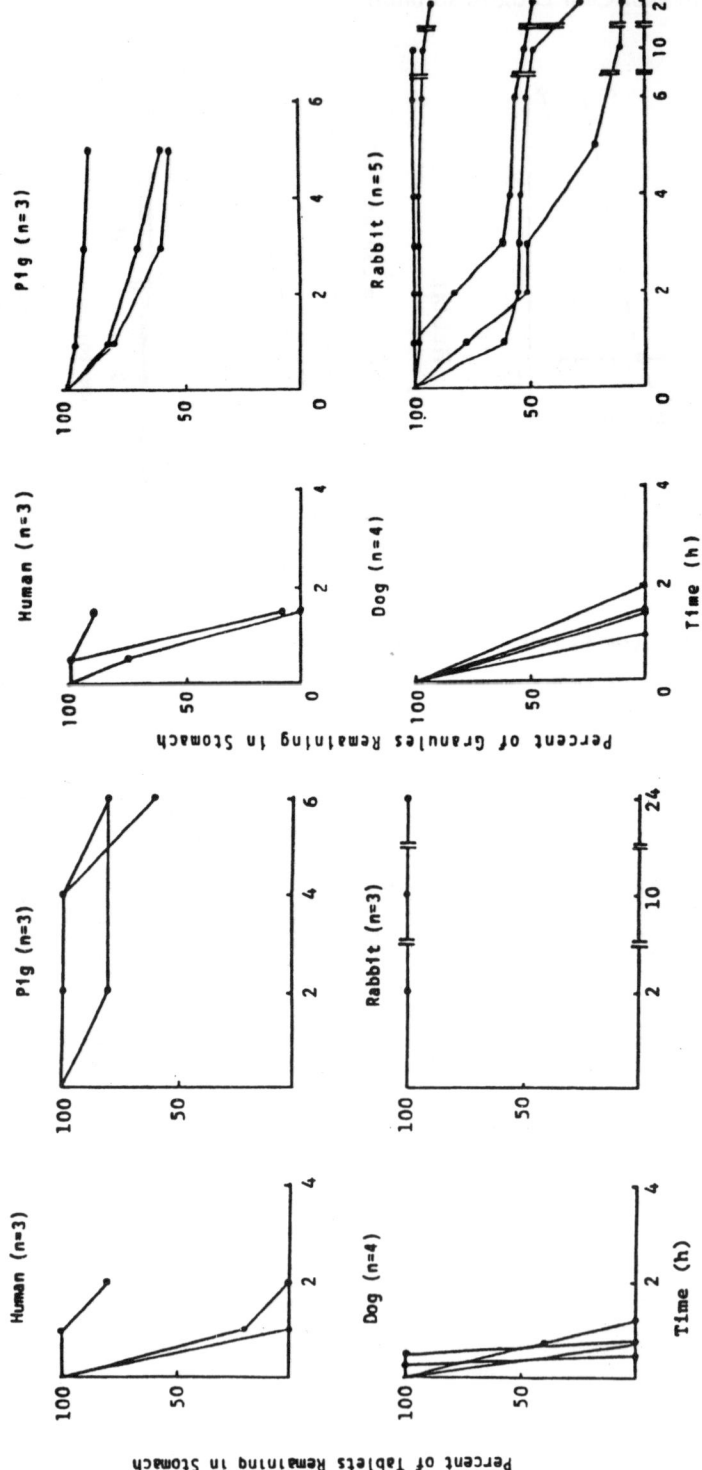

Figure 3 Gastric emptying of enteric-coated barium sulfate tablets 11 mm in diameter (left panels) and barium sulfate granules 1 mm in diameter (right panels) in humans, swine, dogs, and rabbits. Five tablets were given to humans, dogs, and pigs, and two tablets to rabbits. Fifty granules were administered to humans and animals. In all experiments, subjects were fasted overnight before the study. (From Ref. 31.)

Animal Models for Oral Drug Absorption

greater importance in the rabbit. Not only is it anatomically larger in relationship to the rest of the GI tract, but the contribution of microbial metabolism to assimilation of foodstuffs is much greater than in the human. Products of cecal fermentation include volatile fatty acids and vitamins. In fact, reingestion of the soft feces (coprophagia) is required for maintenance of an adequate nutritional status [32]. Therefore, if one wishes to study rabbits in the fasted state, they must be temporarily maintained in cages that prevent access to the feces.

These anatomical and physiological disparities probably contribute to the lack of correlation between bioavailability in rabbits and in humans, observed even for immediate-release dosage forms. Modification of the gastric-emptying characteristics in rabbits can attenuate the differences from humans to some extent. For example, Aoyagi et al. [33] studied the bioavailability of four griseofulvin formulations in humans and rabbits. These rabbits were modified by the method of Maeda et al. [34] to compensate for the tendency of rabbits to empty slowly from the stomach and, under these circumstances, there was some success in correlating the results with those observed in humans (Fig. 4).

MONKEYS

The main attraction of using monkeys is that they are closest to humans in terms of evolutionary development and, therefore, might be expected to respond to drugs more similarly than lower species. In higher primates, there are several major concerns associated with use in the laboratory [35,36]. The first is their availability. Many of the higher primates are now protected species and, furthermore, supplies of many other types of primates are dwindling. Because of the lack of availability, monkeys are difficult and expensive to procure, compared with most other species used for bioavailability testing. One solution is to maintain a self-perpetuating colony, but this requires a lot of specialized expertise.

A second concern is that monkeys require specialized handling and housing procedures. Housing requirements range considerably; some types of monkey can be housed collectively, whereas others are very territorial and must be housed singly or as pairs. As higher mammals, the intelligence level of monkeys should not be overlooked; they will not thrive if they become bored by their surroundings. Some types, such as howler monkeys, are not suited at all for captivity and may die within a fairly short period in a laboratory setting [36]. It should also be noted that keeping monkeys in a laboratory setting poses risks for the technical staff. This was exemplified dramatically in 1989 by the death of a technician at a company in Michigan after being bitten by a monkey and contracting a viral disease.

On top of these considerations, there is the ethical dilemma associated with studying the higher primates in a laboratory setting. Therefore, despite the attractiveness of using species that are phylogenetically close to humans, it is

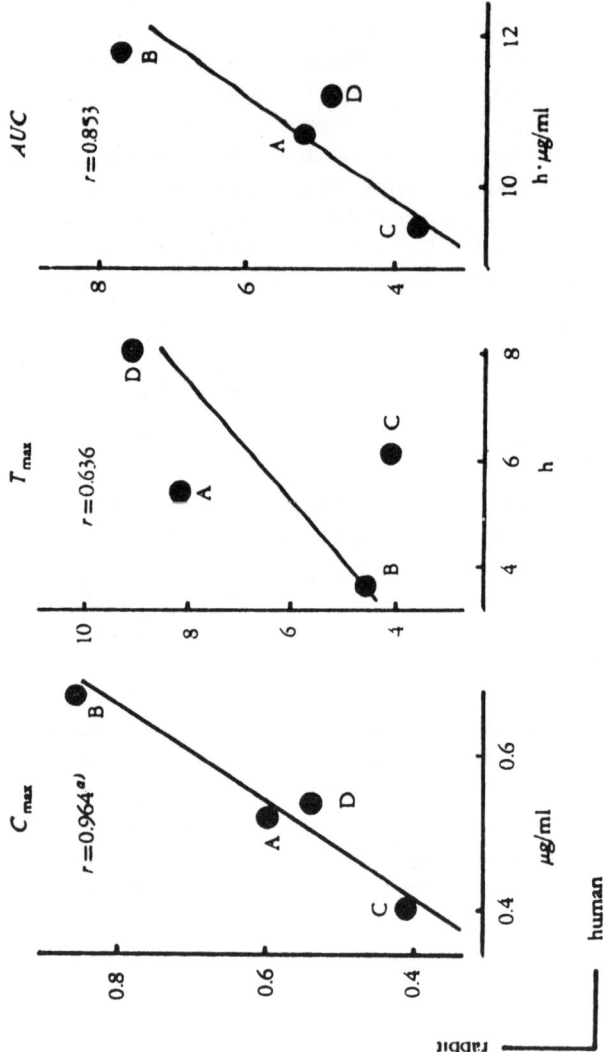

Figure 4 Correlation of pharmacokinetic parameters for griseofulvin after oral administration in humans and gastric-emptying-controlled rabbits. Solid lines show the regression equations ($p < 0.05$). (From Ref. 33.)

extremely unlikely that the higher primates (chimpanzees in particular) will be used extensively in drug research in the future.

A list of primates commonly used in research in 1973 [37] is given in Table 4. Of these, most published studies of drug absorption have utilized macaques such as rhesus or cynomolgus monkeys.

Figure 5 shows a male rhesus monkey. These monkeys are quite small compared with humans, the average head and body length being somewhat less than 0.5 m and the body weight only a few kilograms. Their small size makes them

Table 4 List of Primates Commonly Used in Research in 1973

Prosimians	
Tree shrews	*Tupaia glis*
Galagos	*Galago* spp.
New World monkeys	
Capuchins	*Cebus* spp.
Marmosets	*Callithrix* spp.
Owl monkeys	*Aotus trivirgatus*
Spider monkeys	*Ateles* spp.
Squirrel monkeys	*Saimiri sciureus*
Tamarins	*Saguinus* spp.
Woolly monkeys	*Lagothrix* spp.
African monkeys	
Guenons	*Cercopithecus* spp.
Green monkeys	*Cercopithecus aethiops*
Mangabeys	*Cercocebus* spp.
Patas monkeys	*Erythrocebus patas*
Talapoins	*Miopithecus talapoin*
Baboons	
Savanna baboons	*Papio cynocephalus*
Hamadryad baboons	*Papio hamadryas*
Asian macaques	
Celebes black ape	*Macaca nigra*
Cynomolgus	*Macaca fascicularis*
Japanese macaque	*Macaca fuscata*
Pigtailed macaque	*Macaca nemistrina*
Rhesus	*Macaca mulatta*
Stumptailed macaque	*Macaca arctoides*
Apes	
Chimpanzees	*Pan troglotydes*
Gibbons	*Hylobates* spp.

Source: From Ref. 37.

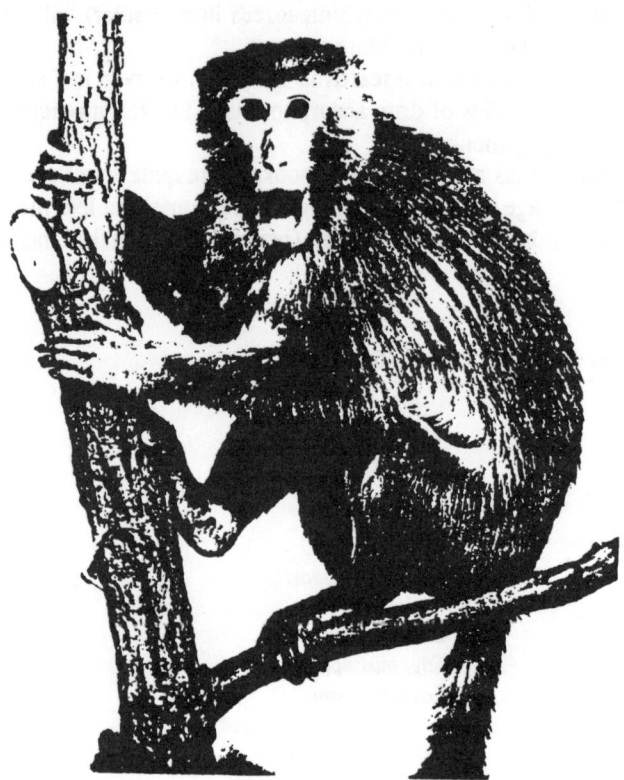

Figure 5 *Macaca mulatta (Rhesus mulatta)*, the rhesus or bandar monkey. This large group with many subspecies ranges across most of Asia. It is the nonhuman primate most commonly used in research. The figure shows a male rhesus monkey, weighing 9 kg. (From Ref. 37.)

attractive for laboratory housing and studies, even though they tend to be less docile than the larger pigtail and stumptail macaques.

Their lack of size is not necessarily a drawback from an anatomical viewpoint because, like most smaller animals, the GI tract is proportionately larger than that of humans. As a result, the GI dimensions of the rhesus monkeys are readily able to accomodate most human-scale dosage forms.

Across the primate family, there is a huge variation in the dietary habits, from insectivores, through omnivores, to types that survive on vegetarian or fruit and nut diets [38]. This naturally leads to a range of structural arrangements and relative dimensions within the GI tract. For example, some types of monkeys that live on a totally herbivorous diet, such as the leaf eater monkey, have multicompartment stomachs. For the commonly used primates, like the rhesus monkey, the stomach is simple, with a gastric size of about 100 mL (see Table 1).

When monkeys are allowed to range freely, their gastric acid production is similar to humans [21]. Under restraint conditions, however, the gastric acid response changes. It has been observed that in Old World monkeys, including the macaque family, the secretion of gastric acid is almost completely shut down when the animal is restrained, and the pH of the gastric contents may be neutral and sometimes even slightly alkaline. In addition, the quantities of gastric juice secreted are also reduced, and GI motility appears to be inhibited. New World monkeys, by contrast, appear to secrete greater amounts of acid when restrained than when allowed to range freely. These contrasting responses illustrate the need to choose the type of monkey carefully, depending on the aims of the experimental protocol.

Of course, changes in the physiological status also occur for other species when they are placed in a stressful environment, but perhaps because of the high intelligence level, stress effects on the physiology appear to be quite pronounced in monkeys, and there have even been reports in the literature of baboons, spider, and woolly monkeys dying while under restraint [21]. Since it is usually recommended that monkeys over 10 kg be restrained for all procedures, the larger monkeys do not appear to be particularly suitable for testing oral dosage forms because of the likelihood of stress-induced changes in physiology.

The rhesus monkey has a duodenal length of about 5 cm, much shorter than the 25- to 30-cm length in humans, so by extrapolation, the overall length of the small intestine is most likely somewhat shorter. The diameter in rhesus monkeys is a little larger than would be expected from the overall size of the animal: the duodenum has a diameter of 1.5–2 cm, and the jejunum and ileum around 2 cm. This may compensate, to some extent, for the shorter length in terms of absorptive capacity. Also, villi in the rhesus monkey tend to be broad and leaf shaped, as opposed to the filamentous appearance of human villi. Taken together, the dimensional comparisons and villous morphology suggest that the absorptive capacity of the small intestine in the rhesus monkey may be lower than in man.

With respect to enzyme distributions along the small intestine, the enzymes in the brush border are qualitatively similar in the rhesus monkey and in humans. For example, there is a concentration in the upper small intestine of phosphatases and esterases, whereas leucine aminopeptidase is found mainly in the jejunum and proximal ileum in the rhesus monkey [21].

The pancreatic juice contains both digestive enzymes and bicarbonate and appears to be secreted at fairly similar rates. In monkeys, the intestinal juice pH has been reported to be between 7 and 9, quite alkaline relative to man.

The distribution of Peyer's patches, the lymphoid tissue of the gut that is thought to be involved in mediating immunological responses, is distributed in rhesus monkeys similarly to in man, with the largest concentration in the ileum.

The last area of comparison is the colon. Carnivores and insectivores, such as talapoin monkeys, in general tend to have short colons, whereas both the stomach and cecum tend to be relatively large in herbivores, with omnivores, like humans, having intermediate relative dimensions [38]. Consideration of the dietary habits is, therefore, of great importance in the selection of the type of monkey to be used in an oral drug study, since these habits influence both the type and size of stomach and the relative length of the colon. In the rhesus monkey, the overall length of the colon is about 40–50 cm, or about one-third that of the human colon. Of the three regions (proximal, transverse, and descending), the transverse colon is disproportionately long. However, in section, the colon of the rhesus monkey is virtually indistinguishable from that of humans.

As far as the motility in the large bowel is concerned, both monkeys and humans exhibit mass movements in the aborad direction. Like humans, monkeys have strips of longitudinal muscle running along the outside of the colon, which pucker the colon into saccules called haustrae. Haustral mixing and shuttling patterns can therefore be observed in monkeys as well as in humans.

It is difficult to evaluate the usefulness of monkeys for bioavailability screening because the open literature contains relatively few studies that have directly compared absorption of drugs in monkeys versus humans. Nadolol, methyldopa, and acyclovir [39–41] are three examples of drugs that are incompletely absorbed and yet are absorbed to similar extents in monkeys and man (Table 5). Although these results are encouraging, it would be rather naive to assume that monkeys are a good general model for drug absorption. In particular, there is no evidence in the open literature to evaluate the usefulness of macaque monkeys as animal models for testing controlled- or sustained-release dosage forms. And even if the correlation in bioavailability with humans were excellent, the multitude of problems associated with their use, ranging from risks to personnel to the ethical issues, will probably all serve to limit the use of primates in oral drug absorption studies in the future.

Table 5 Bioavailability of Methyldopa, Nadolol and Acyclovir in Humans, Macaque monkeys, and Dogs

Drug	Bioavailability (%)		
	Dog	Human	Monkey
Nadolol	88–104	20–33	12–44
Acyclovir	75	18	4
Methyldopa	92, 83 (intact)	25, 29 (intact)	18 (intact)

Source: Data from Refs. 39–41.

SWINE

As with monkeys, the lack of published studies makes it difficult to assess, on a general basis, how well correlated drug absorption in swine is with humans.

The stomach of swine is much larger than that of humans, on the order of several liters. This is probably partly due to the larger body size, but also may be partly attributed to dietary preferences. Although officially an omnivorous species, domestic pigs are predominantly herbivorous and, as a result, the gastric chamber is somewhat modified. For example, there is a diverticulum or pouch at the top of the stomach which is probably a site for microbial metabolism of ingesta (Fig. 6) and the percentage of parietal cell-containing mucosa is smaller than in humans (see Fig. 1).

The data for acid output in swine are rather confusing. Basal volume production is similar to man, whereas basal acid output has been reported as 1.4 μg/15 min. One study in over 20 swine indicate that the fasted gastric pH lies between 3.75 and 4.0 [6], with a second, smaller study indicating a mean pH of 2.67 3-hr postprandially [5], suggesting that the stomach pH is higher than in humans. However, a third study reported values of pH 1.6–1.8 in two groups of young healthy animals, with a range of 0.8–3.0 [7].

Peak acid outputs of about 1.25 μg $\times$ kg^{-1} $\times$ hr^{-1} have been measured in pigs [22]. Studies [7] in 4-week-old pigs indicated that 1 hr after a protein meal the gastric pH was between 2.6 and 6, but that by 8 weeks of age the pH 1 hr after the same type of meal was between 1.3 and 3.3. Taken together, these results suggest that the postprandial acid output may be higher in pigs than in humans.

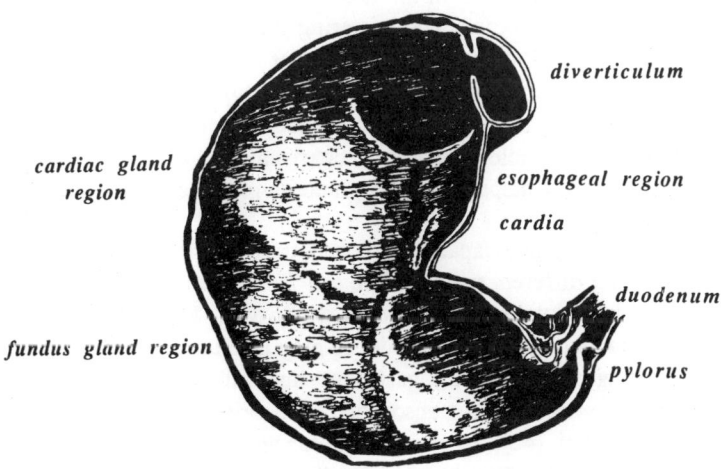

Figure 6 Stomach of swine showing proximal diverticulum. (Redrawn from Ref. 23.)

Another relevant aspect of gastric physiology in swine lies in their susceptibility to gastric ulcers. Many studies have been conducted in ordinary domestic swine, with the incidence of gastric ulcers reported between 5 and 50% of the general pig population [22], with usual incidence of about 20% [24]. Swine restricted to a laboratory setting are often administered cimetidine on a routine basis because of this propensity to ulcers, reducing their suitability as a model for oral drug absorption.

There appear to be some important differences in GI transit between pigs and humans. Pigs exhibit the migrating myoelectric complex when fasted, but the fed-state behavior for gastric emptying is different from that in humans. In pigs, the emptying of food from the stomach is bimodal, with about 30–40% of contents emptying in the first 15 min, followed by a more sustained emptying about 1 hr later [22]. Emptying also appears to be incomplete, so there may be food present in the stomach 24 hr a day. The ability to retain food in the stomach for such a long period may lead to the false assumption that one is studying the pig in the fasted state, when, in fact, there is still food present.

The lack of complete emptying may explain the retention of the enteric-coated dosage forms by minipigs that had been restricted from food overnight. In a comparative study using 11-mm and 1-mm diameter particles rendered radiopaque gy barium sulfate (see Fig. 3), Aoyagi et al. [31] found that most were emptied within 2 hr in dog and man, but less than 50% of the granules and even fewer tablets were emptied within 2 hr by the miniswine stomach. Similar effects were later observed by following salicylate serum levels after administration of enteric-coated tablets (see Fig. 2). Onset of levels was observed within 1 hr in dogs and humans, but not for 8 hr after administration to miniswine. Therefore, to ensure that one is studying drug absorption in the fasted state, it may be advisable to evacuate the swine's stomach before administering the dosage form.

In swine, the small intestine is about twice as long as in humans. The diameter of the small intestine in swine is about 2.5–3.5 cm, which is very similar to that of humans. As an omnivore, the villi would be expected to be fairly similar to those in man in terms of morphology. These comparisons lead to the expectation that the surface area of the principal absorptive mucosa in the pig is greater than that in humans.

The pig has substantially less capacity to concentrate bile in the gallbladder and also manufactures a different primary bile salt from man. Bile salts in the pig are derived from hyocholic acid rather than cholic acid. The differences in both bile concentration and type of bile produced may lead to differences in the solubilizing and wetting capacity of the gastrointestinal milieu and, perhaps as a result, may lead to differences in drug absorption for poorly soluble compounds.

In a study by Aoyagi et al. [42], for example, Gottingen minipigs demonstrated consistently longer t_{max} values than humans for three out of four griseofulvin tablet formulations (Fig. 7). The t_{max} in humans followed the rank order from

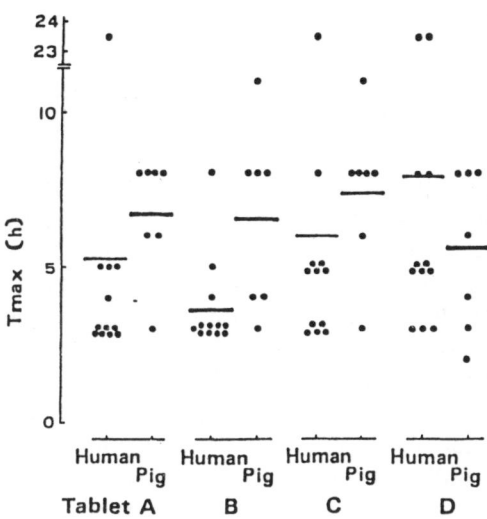

Figure 7 Times for peak blood levels of griseofulvin in humans and swine, after administration of four different tablet formulations to humans (n = 12) and minipigs (n = 7). (Adapted from Ref. 42.)

the dissolution tests, from 3.5 to 8 hr, whereas in pigs all t_{max} were long, at least 5.5 hr. An alternative explanation for these observations, though, would be prolonged gastric emptying [43].

The pancreatic juice contains both digestive enzymes and bicarbonate in pig and humans and appears to be secreted at fairly similar rates. The duodenal pH in the fasted state is a 0.5–1 pH unit higher in swine than in humans. Less is known about the intestinal pH in the fed state—the only data readily available in the literature is that the pH of chyme entering the small intestine is between 3 and 4, a figure that is more reflective of gastric than small intestinal pH.

Peyer's patches are more widely distributed in swine than in humans, being located throughout the small intestine and often being found in the colon.

Another difference in intestinal physiology is that the cecum of the pig is several times larger than in humans, and there is significant production of volatile fatty acids from carbohydrates in this region [29,30] along with catabolism of amino acids and synthesis of B vitamins [22], although the contribution to the nutritional status is not to the same extent as, for example, the horse. In other wrods, the pig leans toward herbivore anatomy, whereas the human leans toward carnivore, although both are intermediate. The pig also has a very long colon and, of special note, is the coiled structure and relative predominance of the ascending colon. The transverse colon, however, is relatively short in the pig. Like humans, pig colon features haustrae, and thus the motility patterns in the colon are likely to be similar.

A comparison of total transit times (Table 6) is useful for designing controlled-release delivery systems. In swine, reports vary from similar to somewhat longer transit times for food. Hill [45] reported total transit times of 15-25 hr in humans, compared with 17-50 hr in swine. Other studies [7] suggest that the total transit time in very young (4-week-old) pigs is shorter, about 12-24 hr, than in slightly older (10-week) pigs, in which the mean transit time was found to be 35 hr.

To summarize for swine, the most important differences seem to relate to gastric motility and the anatomy of the large bowel. Also, one must acclimatize the pig to the laboratory setting to minimize stress-related changes in gastric acid secretion and avoid having to administer cimetidine if possible. A greater difficulty may lie in the fact that gastric emptying of food appears to be incomplete, and unless the stomach is evacuated before administration of the dosage form, one cannot be sure the animal is truly in the fasted state. The residence time in the small intestine may be longer than in humans, owing to the greater length of this segment of the GI tract. The less-concentrated bile may result in a lower capacity to solubilize poorly soluble drugs, and the higher intestinal pH may also affect release, dissolution, and absorption of some compounds. Last, the comparatively much longer length of the ascending colon and the greater importance of the cecum as a site of fermentation and absorption of nutrients may result in a greater role for this region in drug absorption for the pig than for other species.

For monkeys and dogs, breed or subspecies selection is an important consideration. One gets the sense from talking to those involved with minipigs that there is some variation in tractability in these animals among strains.

The differences in scale of regions in the GI tract may be overcome to some extent by the use of minipigs, rather than regular domestic swine. Since the minipigs were bred to be merely a smaller version of regular swine, differences related to anatomical arrangement, secretory levels, and motility patterns are expected to be retained. For example, the problems with gastric retention behavior described earlier, were observed in Gottingen minipigs.

Table 6 Total Transit Times in Humans and Swine

Marker	Transit time (hr)	
	Human	Swine
Food residue	15-25	17-50
Oros[a]	27 (median)	

[a]*Monolithic osmostic pump.*
Source: Data from Refs. 44 and 45.

Another problem with swine that is not directly related to the gastrointestinal physiology, but is certainly pertinent to conducting drug studies, is that the forearm veins in swine run deep and are therefore difficult to access. Therefore, most studies with repeated sampling require surgical preparation of a cannula to a deep vein such as the jugular, which adds an extra degree of complexity to the study design [R. Oberle, Ciba-Geigy, personal communication (1990)].

DOGS

Dogs have been used extensively as a model for oral drug absorption. Gastric dimensions for mongrel dogs weighing 15-25 kg are very similar to that of humans, approximately 1 L. For gastric acid, the data suggest that the basal output of humans may be higher than that of dogs. In studies at the University of Michigan using the Heidelberg capsule technique, predominantly low pH is always observed in young healthy human volunteers, whereas in dogs, the gastric pH is occasionally indistinguishable from that of the small intestine. Other groups have found higher incidences of elevated gastric pH in dogs (17/20 beagles aspirated had pH >5) [K. Sasahara, Sankyo Co., personal communication (1986)]. For testing pH-sensitive formulations, it would therefore be advisable to screen dogs for gastric pH before including them in the subject kennel. On the other hand, peak levels of acid secretion in dogs appear to be quite a bit higher than in humans. This may explain the observation that there is little elevation in gastric pH after ingestion of a meal in beagle dogs [10].

In the comparative study using 11-mm and 1-mm diameter particles rendered radiopaque by barium sulfate (see Fig. 3), Aoyagi et al. [31] found that most were emptied within 2 hr in both dog and man. Similar effects were later observed by following salicylate serum levels after administration of enteric-coated tablets. Onset of levels was observed within 1 hr in dogs and humans (see Fig. 2). These findings are in accord with the observation that the fasted-state motility cycle follows a similar pattern and periodicity in dogs and humans. Motility response to feeding is also similar in dogs and humans, with solids and nutrient liquids following zero-order emptying. The only difference of any significance in upper GI motility appears to be that the emptying of food from the stomach tends to be slower in dogs than in humans [16].

The small intestine of the dog is only about half as long as in humans. This difference in length correlates well with the observed transit times in the two species. In the fasted state, the transit time in the dog is only about half that for humans. In studies in beagles and humans, the mean residence time of a Heidelberg capsule in the small intestine was observed to be approximately 2 hr in dogs, compared with almost 4 hr in humans (Table 7) [16].

This appears to be true for dosage forms as well [46-48]. Studies by Ueda et al. [46] and Davis et al. [48] indicate that, especially for granules, intestinal

Table 7 Transit of Model Dosage Forms and Heidelberg Capsules Through the Upper GI Tract in Humans and Dogs

Species	Formulation	Transit time[a]		
		Gastric	Intestinal	Upper GI[b]
Dog	Granule (1.2 mm)	1.6	1.3	2.9
	Tablet (10 mm)	0.9	2.6	3.5
	H. capsule (7 × 14)		111 min	
Human	Granule (1 mm)	1.3	3.8	5.1
	Tablet (8 mm)	2.7	3.1	5.8
	H. capsule		238 min	

[a]Transit time is in hours, unless otherwise noted.
[b]Gastric plus intestinal.
Source: Data from Refs. 46–48.

transit times are considerably shorter in dogs than in humans. The average intestinal transit time for pellets was 1.3 hr in dogs, compared with 3.8 hr in humans, whereas for tablets, the values were a little closer, 2.6 hr for dogs and 3.1 hr for humans. For both pellets and tablets, the overall upper GI transit time was considerably shorter in dogs. This is important in terms of drug absorption, because it means that the contact time between the drug and the absorbing mucosa will be substantially lower in dogs, possibly leading to a reduction in the overall extent of absorption. This effect is likely to be exacerbated when a controlled-release dosage form is administered.

For absorption from immediate-release formulations consideration of villous morphology and lumenal diameter must be added to a comparison of intestinal lengths. The lumenal diameter in the dog is about 2.5–3.5 cm, which is very similar to that of humans, whereas the differences in intestinal length are offset, to some extent, by the morphology of the villi, which tend to be long and slender in carnivores such as dogs.

There is some suggestion in the literature that transport systems may have different efficiencies or specificities in the dog. For example, there are several compounds that are poorly absorbed in humans, such as acyclovir, methyldopa, and nadolol, but are virtually completely absorbed in the dog (see Table 5). Unfortunately, the mechanistic basis of these differences in absorption has not yet been established.

Another important point of comparison is the level of bile secretion. Table 8 shows the electrolyte composition of the bile fluid of some different species [49], and the profile looks fairly similar for dog and man, except that the total bile salt concentration is quite a bit higher in dogs. One can speculate that the higher bile salt concentrations in the dog would facilitate dissolution of poorly

Table 1 Comparison of Anatomical and Physiological Data for the Stomach of Humans, Dogs, Swine, and Rhesus Monkeys

Parameter	Human	Dog	Swine	Monkey
Volume (L)	1–1.6	1	6–8	0.1
Gastric acid secretion				
BAO: volume (mL/min)	1	0.3–1.5	1.05	Similar to humans unless stressed
rate (mEq/hr)	2–5	0.1	5.6 µg/hr	Similar to humans unless stressed
PAO: rate	18–23	39	1.25 µg/hr	
pH				
fasted	1.7 (1.4–2.1)[a]	1.5 (beagles)	2.7 3.75–4 (n = 20) 1.6–1.8 (0.8–3.0)[b]	
fed				
during meal	5.0 [4.3–5.4][a]	2.1 ± 0.1 (SD)	<2, (n = 1)	
time to return to pH 3	56 ± 41 min			

[a]Interquartile range.
[b]Range.
Source: Data from Refs. 3–24.

soluble drugs. Dogs and humans both produce cholic acid as the primary bile salt; in the dog this undergoes substantially more hydroxylation, resulting in salts with three and even four hydroxyl groups per molecule.

In the Aoyagi study [31], for example, where Gottingen minipigs demonstrated consistently longer t_{max} values than humans, the dogs had t_{max} values of less than 2 hr, irrespective of the formulation, compared with t_{max} values of 3.5-8 hr in humans.

The pancreatic juice contains both digestive enzymes and bicarbonate in dogs and appears to be secreted at a rate fairly similar to that in humans. The duodenal pH in the fasted state is 0.5-1 pH unit higher in dogs than in humans. This difference is maintained in dogs upon feeding, but is probably only of consequence for very pH-sensitive formulations, such as enteric-coated dosage forms.

Another interesting distinction between these two species is the distribution of Peyer's patches. In the dog, as in swine, they are distributed throughout the small intestine, whereas in humans they are mainly found in the ileum.

The cecums of the human and canine are quite small relative to the rest of the GI tract. In the dog this can be attributed to the carnivorous diet. The colon of the dog has a generally similar arrangement to that of humans. However, the overall length of the colon is shorter and the diameter is narrower, only about the same as in the small intestine. In contrast with humans, dogs do not have haustrae. Despite this difference, dogs exhibit mass movements in the aboral direction in a way similar to humans and also have some mixing patterns of a similar nature to haustral shuttling.

For dogs, the GI tract is most similar to that of man at the proximal end and becomes less similar as one considers more distal regions. There are only minor differences in the gastric anatomy and physiology. The occasional incidence of poor fasted-state gastric acid output should not constitute a problem for absorption studies, provided dogs are prescreened for gastric pH. The general upper GI motility patterns of dogs and humans share many commonalities. For example, in the fasted state the IMMC occurs with about the same periodicity as in humans, resulting in similar emptying patterns for liquids and solids. However, there are potentially significant differences in motility in terms of dosage form performance. These include the slower gastric-emptying times in the fed state, the short small intestinal residence time, and the shorter colonic transit. The shorter residence time in the small intestine may lead to a decrease in the extent of absorption of some compounds, especially when formulated as controlled-release dosage forms. The differences in mixing patterns in the colon and the shortness of the large bowel may also reduce the absorption of some drugs relative to humans. On the other hand, the small intestine appears to be considerably more permeable to certain drugs (see Table 5) than the small intestine of humans.

There are also some subtle points to consider in selecting a suitable breed when using dogs. For example, breeds that are traditionally housed in kennels, such

Animal Models for Oral Drug Absorption

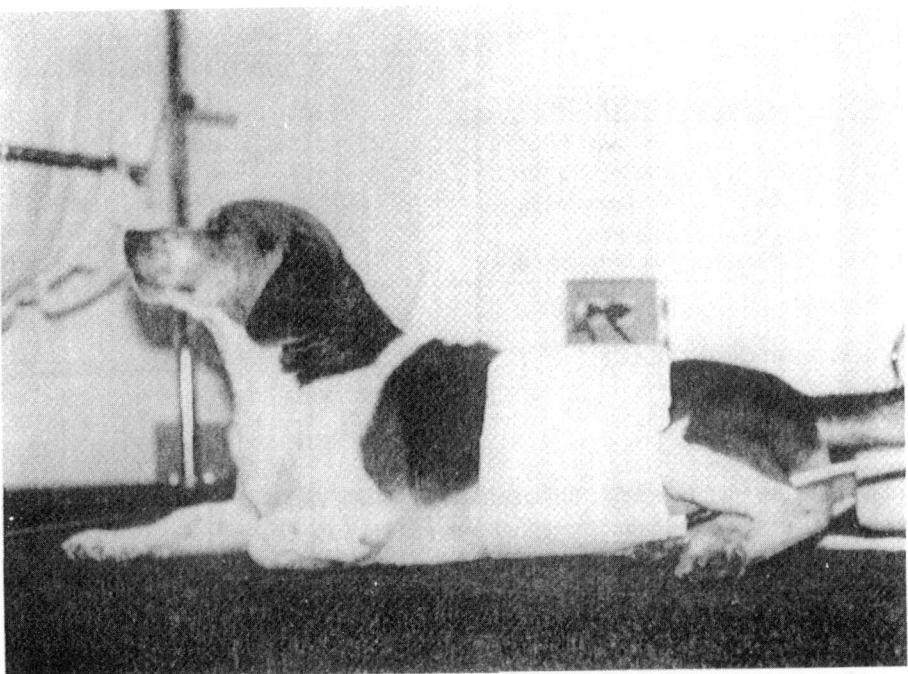

Figure 8 Beagle dog attached to Heidelberg capsule apparatus.

as hounds (Fig. 8), are thought to adapt better to the laboratory environment than those bred as house pets. Furthermore, some breeds are predisposed to certain illnesses that may affect their ability to be suitable subjects. Perhaps the best known example of this is the predisposition of German shepherds to juvenile pancreatic insufficiency [50].

The laboratory setting and handling of the animals is also of crucial importance to successful bioavailability studies. In our experience, it takes 2 or 3 weeks of acclimatization to the testing procedure for dogs to normalize in terms of GI physiology. Gastric emptying, in particular, is usually delayed for several hours when the dog is unfamiliar with the test environment.

Studies that have been conducted in dogs and humans tend to substantiate the possibility that physiological differences can lead to differences in drug absorption profiles. In work published by Ogata [51] in the Japanese literature (Table 9), correlations were established between the absorption of several drugs from conventional dosage forms in dogs and in humans. For these compounds, diazepam,

Table 9 Correlation Coefficients Between Canine and Human Pharmacokinetic Data for Five Compounds

Drug	Dosage form	N	R (correlation coefficient)		
			C_{max}	T_{max}	AUC
Diazepam	Uncoated tablet	4	0.627	0.310	0.990[b]
Griseofulvin	Uncoated tablet	4	0.388	0.711	0.306
Nalidixic acid	Uncoated tablet	5	0.895[a]	0.654	0.690
Flufenamic acid	Capsule	5	0.648	0.228	0.121
Metronidazole	Sugar-coated tablet	5	0.863	—	0.793

[a] $p < 0.05$
[b] $p < 0.01$
Source: Data from Ref. 51.

griseofulvin, nalidixic acid, flufenamic acid, and metronidazole, the correlation coefficients indicated spotty relationships between the two species.

Using the areas under the concentration–time curves (AUCs) as an example, the relationships between dog and human results ranged from excellent correlation for diazepam AUC among four formulations to essentially no correlation for five flufenamic acid capsule formulations. For griseofulvin tablets, the correlation was substantially improved when only microsize formulations were administered, since ultramicrosized formulations were much more bioavailable in dogs than in humans.

With sustained-release dosage forms, one example of poor predictability is valproic acid formulations. It is apparent from the plasma concentration–time curves shown in Figure 9 [52–54] that, although the rank order of bioavailability is retained between humans and dogs, the relative bioavailabilities of the sustained-release formulations of valproic acid are much lower in the dog. This point is more clearly illustrated using the cumulative percentage absorbed plots for the three formulations. These indicate that although availability is virtually the same among the three formulations in humans, the slowest releasing dosage form, SR-A, is incompletely available in the dog.

Similar behavior was reported for aminorex tablets (Fig. 10) by Cressman et al. [55]. In this study the sustained-release dosage form gave equivalent bioavailability in humans, but in dogs the percentage absorbed was only two-thirds that of the immediate-release formulation.

A further study [K. Yamada, unpublished data] comparing absorption from immediate- and sustained-release formulations in humans and beagle dogs involved acetaminophen formulations. Plots of plasma level of acetaminophen versus time are shown for both humans and dogs after administration of a 450 mg dose

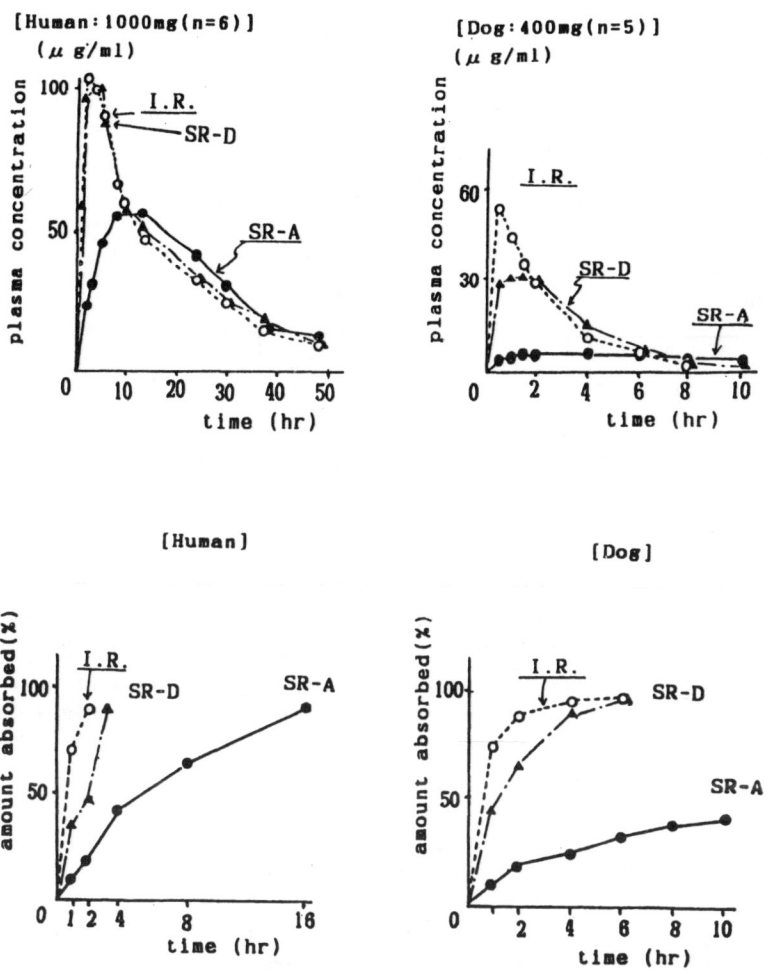

Figure 9 Valproic acid plasma levels as a function of time (top panels) and cumulative % valproic acid absorbed (lower panels) following administration of immediate (I.R.) and sustained-release (SR-A) dosage forms to humans and dogs. (Redrawn from data in Ref. 52–54.)

(Fig. 11). The sustained-release formulation had a relative bioavailability of 92% in humans, but only 57% in dogs.

One case for which the absorption behavior from sustained-release dosage forms appears to be similar in the two species is for phenylpropanolamine (Fig. 12)

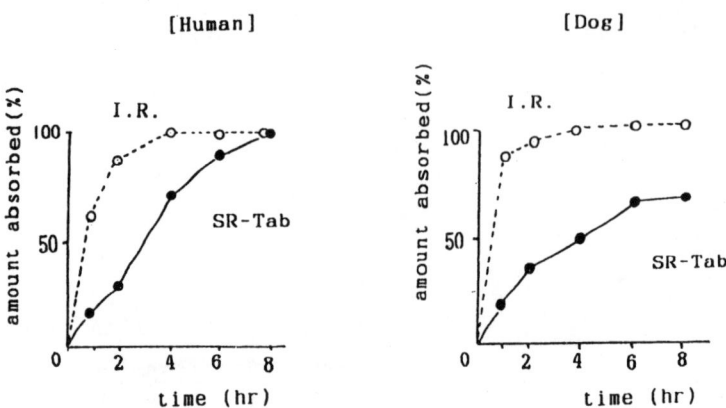

Figure 10 Cumulative percentage aminorex absorbed after administration in immediate- and sustained-release dosage forms to humans and dogs. (From Ref. 55.)

[K. Yamada, unpublished data]. One explanation for the behavior of phenylpropanolamine formulations being different from other compounds is that phenylpropanolamine is absorbed from the colon. The total residence time of the dosage forms in regions supplying absorptive sites (i.e., gastric plus small intestine plus colon) would therefore be sufficient to accommodate complete release and

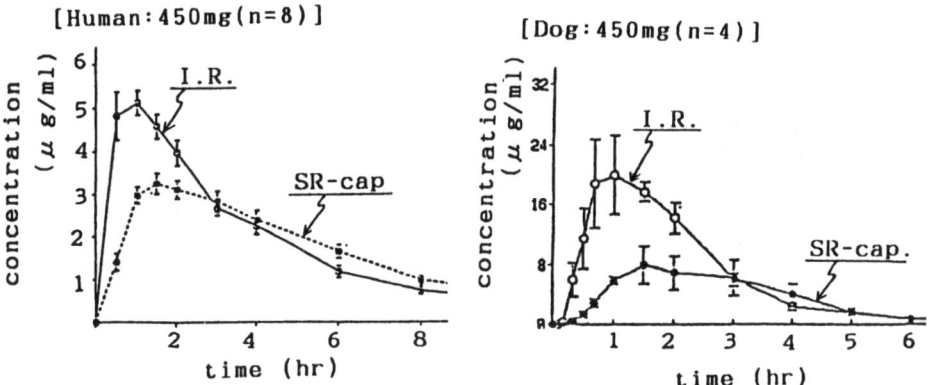

Figure 11 Acetaminophen levels after administration in immediate- and sustained-release dosage forms to humans and dogs. Bioavailability of the sustained-release capsule was 92% in humans, 57% in dogs, relative to the immediate-release formulation. (K. Yamada, unpublished data.)

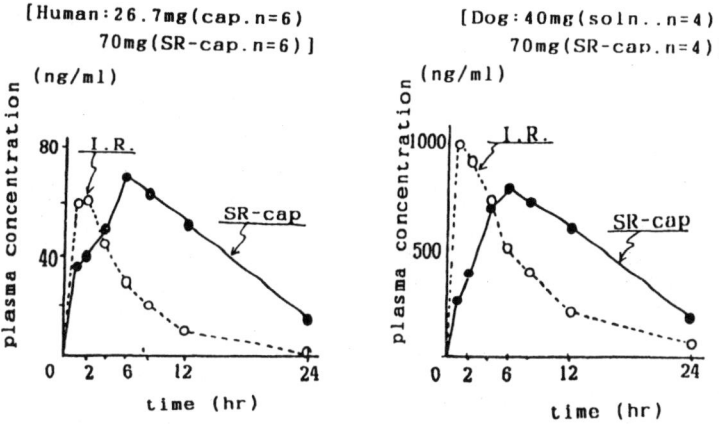

Figure 12 Phenylpropanolamine levels after administration in immediate and sustained-release dosage forms to humans and dogs. Six humans were administered 26.7 mg as an immediate-release capsule or 70 mg as a sustained-release capsule, and four dogs were administered 40 mg as a solution or 70 mg as a sustained-release capsule. (K. Yamada, unpublished data.)

absorption from a 6-hr-release formulation in the dog. For compounds not well absorbed by the colonic mucosa, this would most likely *not* be the case in the dog; therefore, one would expect incomplete availability from sustained-release dosage forms of such drugs in dogs.

Overall, if certain physiological differences, such as the short colon, slower gastric emptying rate in the fed state, and some subtle differences in GI pH, are taken into account, one can at least explain many of the discrepancies in absorption that have been observed between dogs and humans. Prediction of human results based on canine data may also be possible for sustained-release dosage forms of compounds that are absorbed to similar extents from immediate-release dosage forms in the two species.

Kimura et al. [56] have shown that absorption of phenytoin, the absorption of which is limited to the upper GI tract, can be enhanced when the subject is pretreated with propantheline bromide (Fig. 13), and similar results have been published for other compounds. It may be possible to use this kind of pharmacologic modification in dogs to enhance predictive success for sustained-release dosage forms.

Another idea to overcome the tendency of the dog to underestimate absorption from controlled-release dosage forms is to do studies in both the dog and another species that has a comparatively long GI tract, so that one is essentially

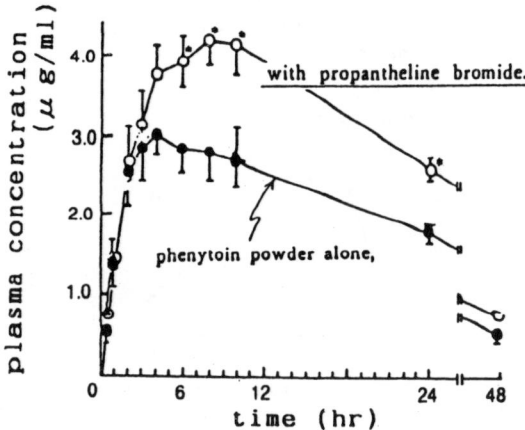

Figure 13 Plasma concentrations of phenytoin administered as a 6-mg/kg dose to humans, with and without pretreatment with propantheline. (From Ref. 56.)

bracketing the human physiology. The swine appears to be a suitable candidate for these purposes, at least from the standpoints of gastrointestinal residence time and bile concentration.

CONCLUSIONS

In conclusion then, animal testing has been shown over the years to be a crucial part of drug evaluation, including screening for oral absorption and in elucidating the sites and mechanisms of absorption of drugs. Animals with appropriate GI dimensions are also useful for pilot studies of new dosage forms. However, among the animal models currently being used, it appears that no single animal model reflects the GI physiology of the human accurately enough to enable us to predict with confidence the bioequivalence of oral formulations in humans.

REFERENCES

1. R. L. Brown, J. A. Gibson, G. E. Sladen, B. Hicks, and A. M. Dawson. *Gut* 15:999–1004 (1974).
2. J. H. Meyer. Motility of the stomach and gastroduodenal junction. In *Physiology of the Gastrointestinal Tract*, Chap. 19 (L. R. Johnson, ed.) Raven Press, New York, p. 613 (1987).
3. M. Grossman. In *Physiology of the Gastrointestinal Tract* (L. R. Johnson, ed.) Raven Press, New York, pp. 659–672 (1981).

4. H. W. Smith. *J. Pathol. Bacteriol.* 8:95 (1965).
5. W. G. Huber and R. F. Wallin. Gastric secretion and ulcer formation in the pig. In *Swine in Biomedical Research* (M. E. Tumbleson, ed.) Plenum Press, New York, p. 21 (1966).
6. P. L. Altman (Comp.). *Blood and Other Body Fluids* FASEB, Washington, D.C., 1961.
7. J. H. Maner, W. G. Pond, J. K. Loosli, R. S. Lowley. *J. Anim. Sci.* 21:49 (1962).
8. C. A. Youngberg. Radiotelemetric Determination of GI pH in Man and Dog. The University of Michigan, M. Sc. Thesis (1984).
9. J. B. Dressman, R. R. Berardi, L. C. Dermentzoglou, et al. *Pharm. Res.* 7:756–761 (1990).
10. C. A. Youngberg, J. Wlodyga, S. Schmaltz, J. B. Dressman. *Am. J. Vet. Res.* 46:1516–1521 (1985).
11. W. G. Huber and V. K. Reddy. Physiologic and anatomic features of monogastric and ruminant animals. In *Animal Health Products: Design and Evaluation*, Chap. 2 (D.C. Monkhouse, ed.) APhA/APS, Washington, D.C. (1980).
12. M J. Swenson (ed.). *Duke's Physiology of Domestic Animals*, 8th ed. Comstock Publishing, Ithaca, N.Y., p. 419 (1970).
13. J. E. Breazile (ed.). *Textbook of Veterinary Physiology*, Sect. 7. Lea & Febiger, Philadelphia, 1971.
14. R. Getty (ed.). *Sisson and Grossman's The Anatomy of Domestic Animals*, 5th ed. W. B. Saunders, Philadelphia, 1975.
15. J. W. Phillis (ed.). *Veterinary Physiology*. W. B. Saunders, Philadelphia, 1976.
16. J. B. Dressman. *Pharm. Res.* 3:123–131 (1986).
17. G. Dotevall. *Acta Med. Scand.* 170:59–69 (1969).
18. H. W. Davenport. *Physiology of the Digestive Tract*, 5th ed. Year Book Medical, Chicago, p. 54 (1982).
19. M. H. Sleisinger and J. S. Fordtran (eds.). *Gastrointestinal Disease: Pathophysiology, Diagnosis and Management*, 2nd ed. W. B. Saunders, Philadelphia (1978).
20. M. N. G. deBourne and G. H. Bourne. Histology and histochemistry. In *The Rhesus Monkey*, Chap. 6, (G. H. Bourne, ed.). Academic Press, New York, p. 178 (1975).
21. B. A. Lapin and G. M. Cherkovich. Biological normals—GI juice and motility. In *Pathology of Simian Primates*, Part I (R. N. T-W-Fiennes, ed.) S. Karger, Basel, p. 127 (1972).
22. W. G. Pond and K. A. Houpt. *Biology of the Pig*. Comstock Publishing (Cornell University Press), Ithaca, N.Y. (1978).
23. L. E. Mount and D. L. Ingram. *The Pig as a Laboratory Animal*. Academic Press, London (1971).
24. M. E. Tumbleson (ed.). *Swine in Biomedical Research*. Plenum Press, New York, p. 121 (1986).
25. W. J. Banks (ed.). *Histology and Comparative Organology: A Text Atlas*. Williams & Wilkins, Baltimore, p. 179 (1974).
26. S. S. Ozturk, B. O. Palsson, B. Donohoe, and J. B. Dressman. *Pharm. Res.* 5:550–564 (1988).
27. C. D. Clemente (ed.). *Gray's Anatomy*, 30th Am. Ed. Lea & Febiger, Philadelphia (1985).

28. J. S. Fordtran. *Am. J. Dig. Dis.* *11*:503 (1966).
29. R. A. Argenzio and M. Southworth. *Am. J. Physiol.* *228*:454 (1975).
30. E. T. Clemens, C. E. Stevens, and M. Southworth. *J. Nutr.* *105*:759 (1975).
31. N. Aoyagi. Comparative Studies of Griseofulvin Bioavailability Among Man and Animals. Kyoto University, Thesis (1986).
32. L. Okerman (R. Sundahl, trans.) *Diseases of Domestic Rabbits*. Blackwell Scientific, Oxford (1988).
33. N. Aoyagi, H. Ogata, N. Kaniwa, and A. Eima. *J. Pharm. Dyn.* *7*:630–640 (1984).
34. T. Maeda, H. Takenaka, Y. Yamahira, and T. Noguchi. *Chem. Pharm. Bull.* *27*:3066–3072 (1979).
35. B. A. Lapin. The rational use of primates in biomedical research. In *Pathology of Simian Primates*, Part I (R. N. T-W-Fiennes, ed.) S. Karger, Basel, pp. 2–10 (1972).
36. C. P. Groves. Phylogeny and classification of primates. In *The Rhesus Monkey*, vol. 1 (G. H. Bourne, ed.) Academic Press, New York, p. 23 (1975).
37. R. A. Whitney et al. (eds.). *Laboratory Primate Handbook*. Academic Press, New York (1973).
38. C. Jones. Natural diets of wild primates. In *Pathology of Simian Primates*, Part I (R. N. T-W-Fiennes, ed.) S. Karger, Basel, p. 58 (1972).
39. J. Dreyfuss, J. M. Shaw, and J. J. Ross. *Xenobiotica* *8*:503–508 (1978).
40. P. de Miranda, H. C. Krasny, D. A. Page, G. B. Elion. *J. Pharm. Exp. Ther.* *219*:309–315 (1981).
41. Merck & Co. Presented by K. C. Kwan at the PMA/FDA workshop The Use of Animals as Substitutes for Humans in Oral Bioavailability Studies, July 1989, Washington, D.C.
42. N. Aoyagi, H. Ogata, N. Kaniwa et al. *J. Pharm. Dyn.* *7*:7–14 (1984).
43. N. Aoyagi, H. Ogata, N. Kaniwa et al. *J. Pharm. Dyn.* *7*:S74 (1984).
44. V. A. John, P. A. Shotton, J. Moppert, and W. Theobold. *Br. J. Clin. Pharmacol.* *19*:203S–206S (1985).
45. K. J. Hill. Developmental and comparative aspects of digestion. In *Duke's Physiology*, 8th ed. Cornell University Press, Ithaca, N.Y., pp. 409–422 (1970).
46. Y. Ueda. In *Proceedings Second Symposium on Clinical Pharmacy* (Tokyo), pp. 12–21 (1988).
47. M. J. Mundy, C. G. Wilson, and J. G. Hardy. *Nucl. Med. Comm.* *10*:45–50 (1989).
48. S. S. Davis et al. *J. Pharm. Pharmacol.* *37*:91 (1985).
49. S. Erhlinger. Physiology of bile secretion and enterohepatic circulation. In *Physiology of the Gastrointestinal Tract*, 2nd ed. (L. R. Johnson, ed.) Raven Press, New York, p. 1557 (1987).
50. H. J. Van Kruiningen (ed.). *Comparative Gastroenterology*. Charles C. Thomas, Springfield (1982).
51. H. Ogata. *Applied Pharmacokinetics—Theory and Experimental*. Soft Science, Tokyo, p. 585 (1985).
52. M. Bialer, M. Friedman, and J. Dubrovsky. *Int. J. Pharm.* *20*:53–63 (1984).
53. M. Bialer, M. Friedman, and J. Dubrovsky. *Biopharm. Drug Dispos.* *5*:1–10 (1984).
54. M. Bialer, M. Friedman, and J. Dubrovsky. *Biopharm. Drug Dispos.* *6*:401–411 (1984).
55. W. A. Cressman et al. *J. Pharm. Sci.* *60*:132 (1971).
56. Y. Kimura et al. *Yakuzaigaku* *48*:313–317 (1988).

10
Interspecies Scaling in Pharmacokinetics

Patrick J. McNamara
University of Kentucky
Lexington, Kentucky

INTRODUCTION

Animal models are employed to examine drug safety issues. Before clinical trials, new drug candidates undergo considerable testing in animals to establish their toxicity profiles. Animal models are also employed to help establish the etiology of human disease and the impact of specific treatment regimens. The use of animal models permits examination of mechanistic phenomena without human exposure to unacceptable risk (e.g., exposure of healthy volunteers to antineoplastic drugs to estimate bioequivalence).

Interspecies scaling in pharmacokinetics may play an important role in the selection of a suitable animal model. Evolution has dictated certain species differences in anatomical structure, physiological function, and biochemical pathways, all of which can influence the time profile of drugs in the body. Nonetheless, similarities across species exist, and certain aspects of pharmacokinetic behavior can be correlated across species. Relating the specific information gained in animal testing to the human situation is an important goal in pharmacology and toxicology. An understanding of interspecies pharmacokinetic differences and similarities provides an important conceptual framework with which to interpret the clinical significance of pharmacologic and toxicological outcomes in animal models.

Pharmacokinetics was originally developed in the field of physiology [1-3], and this close interrelationship between physiology and pharmacokinetics remains. Two approaches have been utilized to extrapolate information obtained from animal studies to the human situation: physiological flow models and interspecies scaling. Both approaches rely heavily on the dependency of pharmacokinetics on fundamental physiological principles. Numerous articles and reviews [1-11] have addressed the topic of interspecies scaling of pharmacokinetics. This chapter will provide an overview of interspecies scaling of parameters and the probable physiological origins of these species similarities in pharmacokinetics.

PHYSIOLOGICAL FLOW MODELS

Physiological flow models have been in use for over 25 years with much of the pioneering work contributed by the group led by Bischoff and Dedrick [12-20]. Physiological flow models are anatomically, physiologically, and biochemically correct [1-4,13]. Flow models are composed of eliminating organs (e.g., kidney and liver) and noneliminating tissue compartments connected by the circulatory system. The number of distinct tissue compartments varies from model to model depending upon available data, the tissue sites of interest (i.e., sites of pharmacologic or toxicologic activity) and the goal of the investigation. This chapter contains only a brief discussion of physiological flow models. More complete descriptions of these models can be found elsewhere [12-20].

The physiological flow model approach appears most appropriate and is most frequently applied when the time course of drug distribution in a specific tissue is the issue of greatest concern. The major advantage of a flow model is that it provides a rational approach for extrapolating information obtained in one species to predict the time course of drug in another [1-4,13]. This is accomplished by replacing values for biochemical or physiological parameters from the test species (e.g., laboratory animal) with corresponding values for the species of interest (e.g., human).

In constructing a flow model, considerable information is required, such as organ perfusion rates and tissue volumes. In addition, estimates of tissue/blood partitioning and intrinsic clearance are required for each drug, frequently involving extensive in vitro and in vivo experimentation. A major criticism of this type of modeling is that each additional parameter introduces a constraint, thereby reducing the freedom of predicting drug concentrations in the various tissues [1]. Moreover, as the number of parameters increases, their associated error limits the quality of the prediction. A major drawback is the large amount of data required to validate the model; data that is almost impossible to obtain in humans (i.e., tissue/blood partitioning values). Nonetheless, physiological flow models remain important tools for understanding pharmacokinetic differences between species.

Methotrexate has been the most extensively studied drug with this approach, and details of its physiological model are contained in several articles [17-19]. By using a model developed in the mouse, Bischoff and co-workers were able to not only predict observed human plasma profiles [18], but also to predict the disposition of methotrexate in the stingray [19]. In the extrapolation from mice to stingrays, these investigators established the versatility of the flow model approach. Moreover, this work emphasized the importance of using intrinsic or physiological clocks for comparing pharmacokinetic events. Adjusting the x-axis from chronological time (Fig. 1, left panel) to a function of blood circulation velocity (i.e., physiological time; see Fig. 1, right panel) makes the disposition profiles for the mouse and the stingray superimposable.

The physiological flow model approach has been used to describe the time course of a number of drugs. The disposition of cytarabine hydrochloride (Ara-C) and its metabolite uracil arabinocide (Ara-U) has been successfully modeled in several species [12]. The nonlinear kinetics of ethoxybenzamide in the rabbit were accurately predicted from a physiological flow model developed in the rat [21]. Other examples of successful scale-up of physiological flow models from animals to human pharmacokinetics include cisplatin [22], diazepam [23], and digoxin [24]. Sawada et al. [25] were successful in predicting human kinetics for hexobarbital, phenytoin, phenobarbital, and quinidine, but these investigators were less successful with tolbutamide, valproate, and diazepam.

Physiological flow models offer a conceptual framework for integrating pharmacokinetics within the context of physiology. These models remain an important tool in examining species differences in pharmacokinetics. However, the experimental and mathematical complexities involved in the use of flow models have limited their widespread adaptation.

INTERSPECIES SCALING OF PHARMACOKINETIC PARAMETERS

Over the last 10 years [2,3,5-11] species comparisons have focused on interspecies extrapolation of pharmacokinetic parameters. The extrapolation between species has been based on the power function, and data from several different species are represented visually by plotting the log of the parameter of interest from a species versus the log of the species body weight. It should be noted, however, that these power functions have been criticized [26] and can be somewhat deceiving. A log-log plot visually minimizes the apparent error in the relationship. When these plots cover multiple orders of magnitude (30-g mouse to 70-kg human), a given predicted value can differ considerably from an observed value and yet visually appear to be a satisfactory prediction. Nonetheless, interspecies scaling has received considerable attention [2,3,5-11].

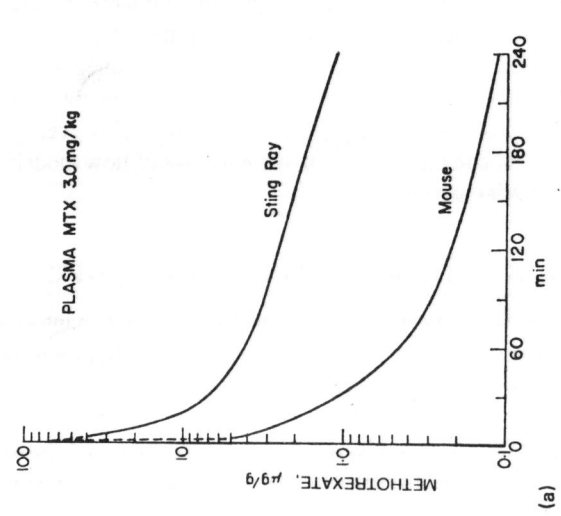

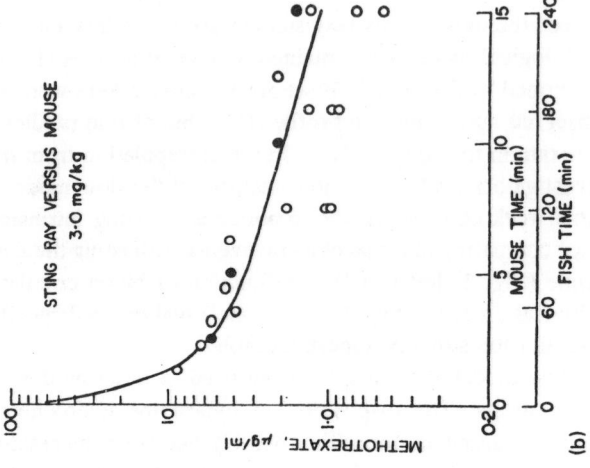

Figure 1 Comparison of plasma methotrexate concentrations in the mouse and stingray with appropriate physiological parameters used for each species (dose, 3 mg/kg IV): (a) When the time scale is an extrinsic time scale (min), the predicted plasma methotrexate concentrations appear dissimilar. (b) When the time scale is made proportional to the blood circulation velocity for each species (i.e., biological time), the plasma methotrexate concentrations in the mouse (solid circles) and stingray (open circles), are superimposable. (From Ref. 19.)

An alternative approach to the multiple-species regression analysis has been to search for correlations between the same pharmacokinetic parameters in one test species and the species of interest (i.e., humans). The pharmacokinetic data from a series of benzodiazepines in dog and humans [6], six β-lactam antibiotics in monkey and humans [27], and a number of other model drugs in rat and humans [7,28,28] have been analyzed with this approach. Reasonable correlations were obtained for several parameters, and this approach may offer some usefulness in predicting the pharmacokinetic behavior of a compound of similar structure. However, as pointed out by Wilkinson [4], ". . . it is probably unrealistic to expect this type of approach to provide precise estimates for any compound in particular." Although more time-consuming, the multiple-species comparison approach would seem to offer the more robust and stable estimates for extrapolation to the human situation. Such an approach would be less susceptible to any particular interspecies variation.

Certain parameters in pharmacokinetics (i.e., clearance and volume terms) lend themselves well to interspecies scaling. Underlying mechanisms or controlling factors dictate the numerical value of these parameters, and these physiological factors readily scale to body weight (allometry, see following discussion). It should also be noted that these values exist on a continuum and can vary over several orders of magnitude, as does body weight. Other pharmacokinetic parameters do not vary as greatly or may have a limited range of potential values. It is unlikely that parameters such as the fraction unbound, bioavailability, extraction ratio, or the fraction of the dose metabolized to a certain metabolite will scale to body weight across species.

Allometry

Mammals vary in size from a 3-g shrew to a 3000-kg elephant. Even though there is 10^6-fold variation in the weight and outward structure, most of the species have similar anatomy, physiology, biochemistry, and cellular structure. Although no animal mimics man exactly, organ weights and physiological functions of mammals have been correlated with humans on a body weight basis (allometric scaling). Huxley [30] demonstrated a linear relationship between organ weight and body weight with the following equation:

$$\log y = \beta \log BW + \log \alpha \tag{1}$$

where y is organ size, BW is body weight, log α is the value of log y for 1-kg body weight and β is the slope (shows size effects).

The antilog of this equation is termed the power function

$$y = \alpha\ BW^\beta \tag{2}$$

From the power equation, Adolph [31] compiled 33 equations relating such variables as quantitative physiological periods (time events), the output of nitrogen and sulfur, and organ weights to body weight. Stahl [32] showed a linear correlation between the log of the weight of principal organs to log body weight for several primates. Boxenbaum [5] showed that log liver weight or liver blood flow versus log body weight was linearly related in mammals (Fig. 2).

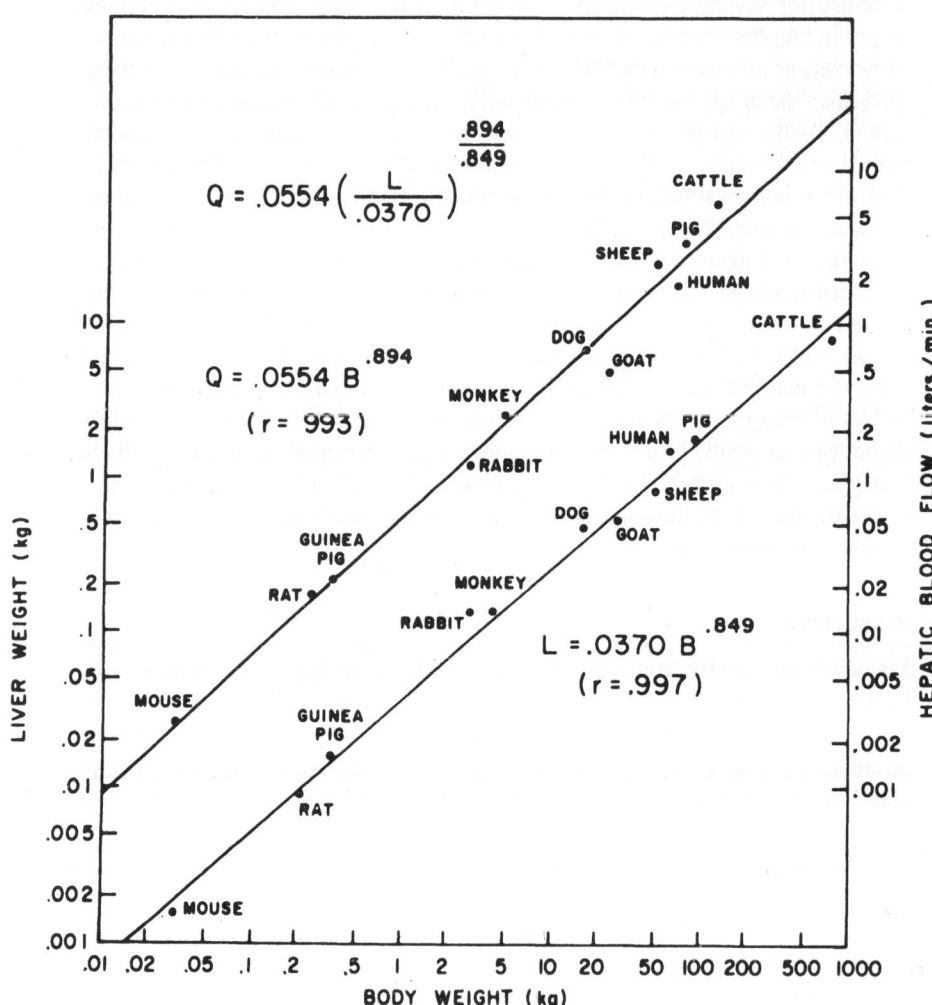

Figure 2 Liver weight and hepatic blood flow in mammals as a function of body weight: Equations were fitted using the method of least squares on unweighted, logarithmically transformed data. (From Ref. 5.)

Table 1 Hepatic and Renal Physiology Scaling Parameters[a] in Adult Animals

Parameter	Ref.	α	β	r	Predicted (70-kg human)	Observed (70-kg human)	Ref.
Liver weight (kg liver vs kg body weight)	5	0.037	0.849	0.997	1.36	1.35	36
Liver blood flow (L/min flow vs kg body weight)	5	0.0554	0.894	0.993	2.47	1.60	36
Total liver cytochrome P-450 (nmol P-450 vs kg body weight)	34	0.963	0.686	0.952	17.8	14.8	34
Kidney weight (g kidney vs g body weight)	33	0.020	0.850	0.993	263	280	37
Kidney blood flow (mL/min flow vs g body weight)	33	0.120	0.824	0.994	1179	1120	37
Glomerular filtration rate [inulin clearance] (mL/min vs kg body weight)	35	5.36	0.72		114	125	37

[a]Parameters = αBW^β; r = regression coefficient

Prothero [33] found similar relationships for kidney weight and blood flow. Allometric relationships describing physiological functions that have a significant impact on pharmacokinetics are listed in Table 1.

Clearance

Clearance is undoubtedly the most important parameter for characterizing drug removal from the body. Whether drug is removed by metabolic or excretory processes, clearance can be readily related to physiology and, thereby, can reflect species differences in pharmacokinetics.

Organ clearance (Cl) is a function of organ blood flow (Q) and the efficiency of the organ to remove the drug as blood perfuses through it (i.e., extraction ratio, E). This concept is most often viewed in the context of hepatic drug elimination; however, it can apply to all other routes of elimination as well.

$$Cl_{organ} = Q_{organ} E_{organ} \qquad (3)$$

Drug clearance through an organ is frequently described by one of two theoretical models: (1) well-stirred or venous equilibration model and (2) sinusoidal perfusion or parallel tube model [4]. Both models define *intrinsic clearance* (Cl_i) as the rate of drug elimination divided by the unbound drug concentration at the elimination site. Both models also assume distribution into the organ to be perfusion rate-limited. When the extraction ratio is small, both models predict a similar behavior in Cl_i. Different predictions emerge for the two models as the extraction ratio approaches unity [4]. For simplicity, only the well-stirred model will be considered, but the limiting cases for the parallel tube model will be identical.

Organ clearance in the well-stirred model is described by

$$Cl_{organ} = Q_{organ} \left[\frac{f_{u,b} \, Cl_{int}}{Q_{organ} + (f_{u,b} \, Cl_{int})} \right] \quad (4)$$

where $f_{u,b}$ is the fraction unbound in the blood and Cl_{int} is the maximal ability of the organ to remove a drug by all pathways in the absence of protein binding or blood flow limitations.

For drugs with high extraction ratios ($f_{u,b} \, Cl_{int} >> Q_{organ}$), the value of Cl_{organ} has a limiting value equal to

$$Cl_{organ} = Q_{organ} \quad (5)$$

As was previously described, Q_{organ} can be readily related to body weight (see Table 1). Therefore, organ clearance for high extraction ratio-type drugs should readily correlate with body size by

$$Cl_{organ} = Q_{organ} = \alpha_q \, BW^{\beta_q} \quad (6)$$

where α_q and β_q are the allometric coefficient and exponent terms relating organ blood flow to body weight (BW).

For drugs with low extraction ratios ($f_{u,b} \, Cl_{int} << Q_{organ}$), the value of Cl_{organ} has the limiting value

$$Cl_{organ} = f_{u,b} \, Cl_{int} \quad (7)$$

Plasma protein binding can be readily measured in vitro, leaving the intrinsic clearance as the parameter of interest for interspecies scaling. Although not as readily apparent as with high-extraction-ratio drugs, clearance for low-extraction-ratio drugs may also correlate with body size. In the absence of diffusional barriers into the organ of elimination, this Cl_{int} reflects the effective mass of functional units (e.g., hepatic enzymes or renal transport proteins) or the surface area available for diffusion out of the system (e.g., total glomerular surface area). This mass of functional units (or surface area) also correlates well with body weight; therefore, Cl_{int} will correlate with body weight.

Hepatic Metabolic Clearance (Animals—The Rule)

Although many drugs are metabolized by other organs in the body, the liver is the dominant metabolic organ owing to its high enzyme content compared with the other eliminating organs [4]. Table 2 documents the interspecies power function parameters for several drugs that are removed from the body principally by metabolism (e.g., antipyrine, phenytoin, cyclophosphamide, cyclosporine). Interspecies scaling of antipyrine is depicted in Figure 3. Antipyrine intrinsic clearance is well-described by a simple allometric function for all of the mammals studied, with the exception of humans (see Fig. 3a). A similar situation is observed with several other drugs in which the predicted values for humans are consistently larger than those observed (see Table 2). Nonetheless, the predictive ability of the simple allometric approach for many drugs appears quite sufficient. The predictive power of this allometric scaling in nonhuman mammals is undeniable. The exception to the rule (i.e., human metabolism) will be discussed subsequently.

Table 2 Clearance Parameters[a] (mL/min) Scaled to Body Weight (kg) in Adult Animals

Drug	Cl type[b]	Ref.	α	β	Human included?	Parameter values for a 70-kg human	
						Predicted	Observed[c]
Antipyrine	Cl_{int}	35	8.16	0.885	N	350.0	47.6
Phenytoin	Cl_{int}	35	47.1	0.915	N	2298.0	522.0
Aztreonam	T	35	4.45	0.662	Y	74.1	88.0
Ara-C	R	35	3.93	0.790	Y	113.0	91.0
Cefotetan	T	27	6.32	0.535	Y	61.3	30.2
Cefazolin	T	27	4.51	0.679	Y	80.7	53.0
Cefmetazole	T	27	12.3	0.594	Y	153.0	111.0
Methotrexate	T	35	10.9	0.690	Y	204.0	112.0
Cyclophosphamide	T	35	16.7	0.754	Y	411.0	200.0
Erythromycin	T	38	36.8	0.659	Y	605.0	492.0
Oleandomycin	T	38	30.5	0.691	Y	574.0	637.0
Cyclosporine	Cl_{int}	39	133.0	0.919	Y	6599.0	4718.0
Phencyclidine	T	40	50.0	0.640	Y	806.0	377.3
Acivicin	T	41	4.0	0.620	N	50.0	49.0
AZT	T	84	25.9	0.936	Y	1551.0	1867.0
	R	84	13.57	0.830	Y	461.0	355.0

[a]Parameter = αBW^β
[b]Cl_{int}, unbound, intrinsic clearance; T, total clearance; R, renal clearance
[c]Goodman and Gilman, 1975 or original reference

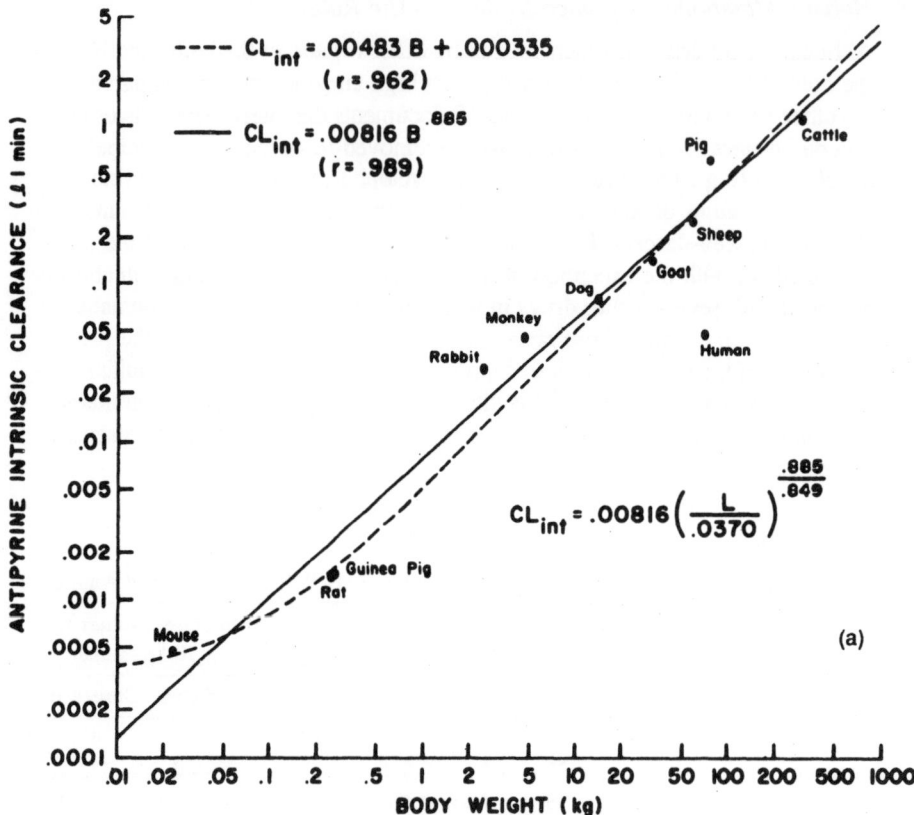

Figure 3 (a) Antipyrine intrinsic clearance in mammals as a function of body weight: Dashed line is the least-squares fit of nonlogarithmically transformed data weighted by the factor $1/y^2$. The solid line is from the equation fitted using the method of least squares on unweighted, logarithmically transformed data. (From Ref. 5.) (b) Allometric relationship between intrinsic clearance of unbound antipyrine per maximum life span potential (MLP) and body weight. (From Ref. 8.)

Hepatic intrinsic clearance, under linear conditions, is generally thought of as a reflection of hepatic enzyme content such that

$$Cl_{int} = \frac{V_{max}}{K_m} = \frac{V'_{max} P}{K_m} \quad (8)$$

where V_{max} is the maximum in vivo velocity of the metabolic reaction (expressed

Interspecies Scaling in Pharmacokinetics

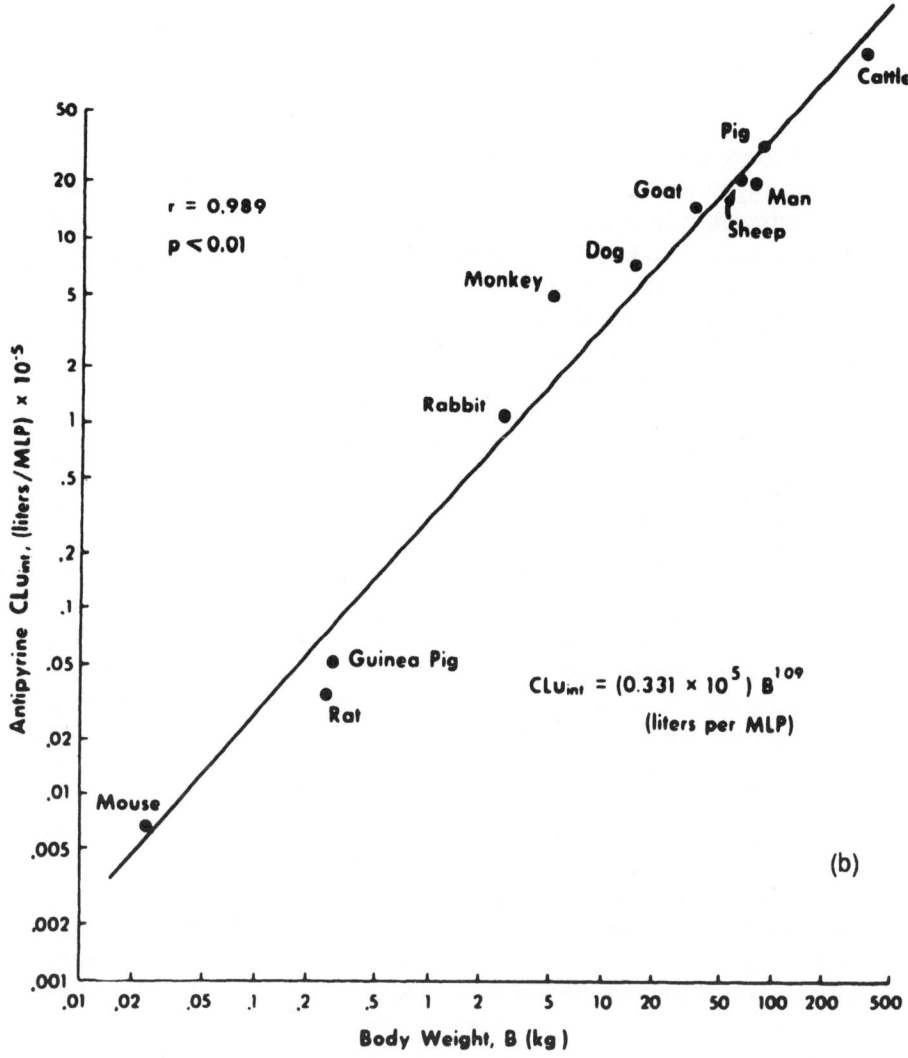

Figure 3 *(Continued)*

in terms of mass metabolized per unit time) and K_m is the corresponding in vivo Michaelis constant, V'_{max} is the maximum in vivo velocity of the metabolic reaction equivalent to in vitro V_{max} (expressed in terms of mass metabolized per unit time per enzyme basis) and P represents the total mass of cytochrome P-450.

Although not directly related, the in vivo constants have approximately the same meaning as do the more easily observed in vitro estimates; K_m reflects the affinity of drug for the enzyme site, whereas V_{max} largely reflects the amount of enzyme present. Rane et al. [42] used a similar approach to predict successfully the hepatic extraction ratio in perfused rat livers from in vitro measurements (i.e., rat liver microsomes) of V_{max} and K_m for several drugs.

Most drug-metabolizing activity of the liver is carried out by the cytochrome P-450 (mixed function oxidase) enzyme system. This enzyme is actually a family of isozymes with each isozyme varying in concentration, inducibility, and activity toward various substrates [43]. Although some homology of these isozymes exists across species, clear differences in isozyme structure, concentration, and activity have also been reported [43-47]. Interspecies differences in cytochrome P-450 isozymes is a relatively new area, and additional research will be required to address more fully the effect these multiple isozymes have on the interpretation of species differences in pharmacokinetics.

It would appear that some drugs (e.g., antipyrine, phenytoin) can be metabolized by multiple forms of hepatic cytochrome P-450, whereas over drugs are handled most efficiently by one specific isozyme (e.g., mephenytoin, debrisoquin, dextromethorphan) [43]. For drugs that are metabolized by multiple forms of hepatic cytochrome P-450, there appears to be a good correlation of intrinsic clearance with total cytochrome P-450. Total cytochrome P-450 content across species is fairly consistent when expressed on a per milligram microsomal protein or per gram of liver basis [34]. In fact, total hepatic cytochrome P-450 content also appears to correlate with body weight using the power function (Fig. 4). Although species variation in V'_{max} has been reported [34,48], the range of value is limited to one order of magnitude. Fewer reports have addressed species differences in K_m [34,48], but indications are that this term does not vary greatly across species. Given the consistency of in vitro V'_{max} and K_m across species, the dominant factor controlling Cl_{int} is total hepatic enzyme content (P). which is largely a function of liver weight, which in turn, is a function of body weight (see Table 1). As a result, Cl_{int} should readily correlate with body weight for those drugs the elimination mechanism of which is nonspecific (e.g., not dependent upon one specific isozyme or transport system). Antipyrine clearance in mammals other than humans (see Fig. 3a) clearly shows this behavior and has been widely used as an indirect, in vivo measure of hepatic mixed function oxidase activity (i.e., cytochrome P-450 content). Other examples of this nonspecific metabolic elimination include drugs such as phenytoin, diazepam, and phenobarbital.

Hepatic Metabolic Clearance (Human: The Exception)

The allometric relationship that adequately predicts the clearance of a number of drugs in animals (see Fig. 3a and Table 1) fails to predict the human situation.

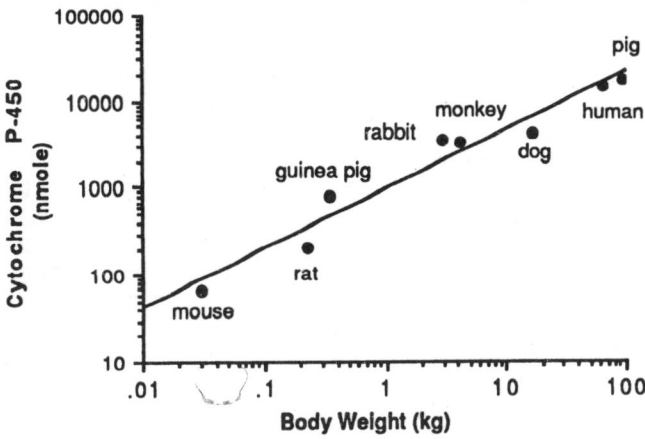

Figure 4 Total hepatic cytochrome P-450 in eight mammals as a function of body weight. (Data from Ref. 34.)

Boxenbaum has ascribed this shortcoming to a lower metabolic activity in humans relative to other mammalian species [28,35]. When the clearance data for antipyrine were replotted as unbound intrinsic clearance per maximum life span potential versus body weight on log–log coordinates (see Fig. 3b), the clearance value for humans could now be readily predicted. Table 3 contains the allometric relationship parameters for this type of plot for five compounds.

The underlying mechanism behind these observations is unknown. Boxenbaum related the diminished intrinsic clearance of these compounds to two physiological parameters that do not readily follow the allometric function: brain weight and life span [28,35]. Boxenbaum concluded that the sevenfold differences in expected and observed antipyrine clearance was attributable to an overall lower quantitative metabolic capacity in humans compared with other species. Boxenbaum [8] states that "his [man's] relatively low intrinsic clearance is paced to his longevity, i.e., activity is conserved so as to be extended over a relatively longer chronicologic MLP" (maximum lifespan potential). Yates and Kugler [50] have presented a related hypothesis neoteny, to explain why the values obtained from humans appear as outliers on simple allometric plots.

Neoteny applies particularly to humans and is thought of as a "sustained juvenilization or retarded development—an evolutionary phenomenon" [50]. Yates and Kugler [50] state that ". . . there is a similarity of body plans among mammals, but that the unfolding of that design need not be at the same relative rate for every species and that the rate of unfolding does not determine the

Table 3 Unbound, Intrinsic Clearance (Cl_{int} Normalized to Maximum Life Span Potential (L/lifetime) Scaled to Body Weight (kg) in Adult Animals[a]

Drug	Ref.	α ($\times 10^{-5}$)	β	Human included?	$Cl_{u,int}$ (mL/min) in human Predicted[b]	Observed
Antipyrine	8	0.33	1.09	N	68.0	47.6
Phenytoin	8	1.76	1.23	N	655.0	522.0
Clonazepam	8	6.73	0.92	Y	677.0	415.0
Caffeine	49	0.38	1.20	Y	122.0	153.0
Cyclosporine	39	4.25	1.47	Y	4352.0	4718.0

[a]Parameter = αBW^β
[b]Assumes a 70-kg human and a maximum life span potential of 95 years.

developmental sequence." Therefore, the lack of fit of the human values to allometric functions is attributed to the relative immaturity in their metabolic capacity. The scaling of antipyrine intrinsic clearance using maximum life span potential [28,35] brought the data for humans more closely in line with those predicted from other mammals.

Although an intriguing concept, neoteny is not intuitively satisfying when exploring mechanisms. Another, equally probable explanation of the lower drug clearance activity in humans lies in the diversity or the genetic control of the major drug metabolizing enzyme system, the cytochrome P-450 mixed function oxidases. An alternative hypothesis would hold that humans have a longer life span potential *because* their mixed function oxidase system has a diminished activity. The key to long-term survival may lie in the ability of an animal (or human) to less readily metabolize certain exogenous substances that result in harmful by-products (e.g., carcinogens, free radicals) [51].

Regardless of the underlying mechanisms, the approach of plotting the log of unbound intrinsic clearance per maximum life span potential versus log body weight seems to work well as a predictive tool. Note the good agreement between the predicted and observed (see Table 3); these predictions were superior to the previous predictions that did not adjust Cl_{int} for MLP (see Table 2). Continued efforts using this approach have considerable merit and may lead to a better understanding of the mechanism behind this phenomenon.

Hepatic Metabolic Clearance (Polymorphisms and Stereoselectivity)

Some drugs are more specifically eliminated than others. Their overall elimination appears to be dominated by one particular pathway of elimination and dependent upon one particular drug–protein interaction (e.g., drug–enzyme). Such specificity can give rise to stereospecific elimination and genetic polymorphism [43]. A good example of this phenomenon is the stereospecific metabolism of mephenytoin (Table 4). Mephenytoin is not extensively bound to plasma proteins (35% bound), and the limited binding is not stereospecific for either human or the rat [51-54]. Therefore, clearance values reported in Table 4 reflect differences in the intrinsic clearances of the two enantiomers in the rat, dog, and human. In humans, the S enantiomer of mephenytoin is rapidly metabolized to a hydroxy metabolite, whereas the R enantiomer is predominantly metabolized to a N-demethylated product [51-54]. Moreover, a marked genetic polymorphism has been noted in humans for the hydroxylation of the S enantiomer, with efficient metabolizers (95% of white population; [51,53] able to clear S-mephenytoin at a rate 150 times faster than slow metabolizers. This high degree of stereospecificity and the presence of a prominent genetic polymorphism results from a major portion of S-mephenytoin's clearance that is carried out by a particular isozyme(s) of the cytochrome P-450 system.

Given the higher clearance values for the R enantiomer in other species (on a mL/min basis, see Table 4), it appears that the rat and the dog are not suitable models for predicting mephenytoin elimination kinetics. Moreover, neither animal model could have predicted the genetic polymorphism in S-mephenytoin clearance. Similar observations have been reported for hexobarbital enantiomers in rats and humans [55,56]. In the rat, d-hexobarbital has a sevenfold greater clearance than the l isomer [55], whereas l-hexobarbital has a eightfold higher clearance than the d isomer in humans [56]. A similar phenomenon may also dominate the disposition of sparteine, debrisoquin, and dextromethorphan [43]. These observations support the concept that as the overall elimination process becomes dominated by a specific pathway or isozyme, animal predictions are less likely to be viable. In addition, this argument would suggest that *formation clearances* (i.e., clearances down particular metabolic pathways) will also be less likely to extrapolate across species. The problem of human heterogenecity for several metabolic activities and animal model extrapolation has been addressed by Calabrese [57].

Table 4 Species Differences in Mephenytoin Pharmacokinetics

Species	Ref.	Wt. (kg)	Clearance (mL/min)		Volume (L/kg)	
			R	S	R	S
Rat	52	0.27	195 ± 50	122 ± 35	1.35	1.35
Dog	53	21.5	139 ± 2.9	154 ± 5.7	1.2	1.1
Human EM	53	81	27 ± 9	4,700 ± 2,800	1.9	
PM		76	20 ± 4	29 ± 7	1.5	1.7

EM, Efficient metabolizers of mephehytoin; PM, poor metabolizers of mephehytoin.

Hepatobiliary Clearance

Species differences in this route of drug elimination have not been well studied. Smith [58] has presented a review of species variations in biliary excretion. Certain anatomical (e.g., presence or absence of a gallbladder) or physiological differences (e.g., bile flow rates) exist across species, but do not appear to cause species differences in biliary excretion per se [58]. Species variation in the efficiency of these transport systems themselves is the more probable cause. However, species differences in biliary anatomy (i.e., presence or absence of a gallbladder) can give rise to species differences in pharmacokinetics. The secondary peaks in plasma concentration versus time profiles associated with the enterohepatic recycling of certain drugs in the human and dog are due to intermittent bile release from the gallbladder. These secondary peaks are absent in time profiles in the rat, which lacks a gallbladder and secretes a constant flow of bile into the small intestines.

Most of the information on drug elimination into bile is presented in the form of percentage of the dose recovered in the bile within a given time. Pharmacokinetic information in the form of fractions cannot be correlated to body size. In addition, these fractions are frequently collected over a fixed chronologic period and may not reflect the overall disposition of the compound in the particular species.

Table 2 documents the interspecies power function parameters for clearance and body weight for several drugs in which clearance is, in part, by biliary secretion mechanisms (e.g., aztreonam, erythromycin). Although the number of examples is limited, it appears that biliary clearance correlates fairly well across species.

Renal Clearance

Renal clearance is the net result of three related processes: gomerular filtration, tubular secretion, and tubular reabsorption. Filtration and secretion pathways have been well studied across species, whereas tubular reabsorption has received less attention. As with hepatic clearance, renal clearance can be viewed as a function of blood flow and the mass of functional units. Sawada et al. [27] have used a modification of a mechanistic relationship proposed by Levy [59] describing renal clearance (Cl_r) in terms of the following:

$$Cl_r = f_{u,b} \times GFR + \left(\frac{Q_r\, f_{u,b}\, Cl_{int,r}}{Q_r + (f_{u,b}\, Cl_{int,r})} \right) \quad (9)$$

$$= \text{filtration} + \text{secretion}$$

where $f_{u,b}$ is the fraction unbound in blood, GFR is the glomerular filtration rate, Q_r is renal blood flow, and $Cl_{int,r}$ is the renal secretory intrinsic clearance of unbound drug. The modification assumes no tubular reabsorption and divides renal clearance into two components: filtration and secretion.

If the principal extretory pathway is filtration then the second term in Eq. (9) tends toward zero, and Cl_r is determined by protein binding and GFR. As mentioned earlier, $f_{u,b}$ can readily be measured in vitro, and unbound, renal clearance can be estimated. Unbound, renal clearance will readily correlate across species, since GFR has a well-recognized allometric relationship (see Table 1). The functional units of the kidney are the number of glomeruli, or more precisely, the total glomerular surface area, which also correlates with body size [33].

If the secretory pathway is very efficient at removing drug then Cl_{renal} approximates Q_r. Renal blood flow, as well as kidney weight, readily correlate with body weight (see Table 1). The removal of several substances used as markers for renal blood flow (e.g., p-aminohippurate) scale well with body size across species using an allometric function.

Drugs that are principally removed from the body by renal routes appear to follow the simple allometric relationship. Table 2 documents the interspecies power function parameters for several drugs that are removed from the body principally by renal mechanisms (e.g., cefotetan, cefazolin, cefmetazole). For renally eliminated drugs, this simple allometric approach appears to work well. Sawada et al. [27] successfully employed the approaches outlined in this review to describe and predict the disposition of several antibiotics (Fig. 5).

Total Systemic Clearance

Total systemic clearance (Cl_s) for drugs eliminated through multiple pathways is the sum of all of the clearance terms governing the individual elimination processes. For example, systemic clearance of a drug eliminated by two routes of elimination (e.g., hepatic and renal elimination) is given by

$$Cl_s = Cl_h + Cl_r \tag{10}$$

where Cl_h and Cl_r are hepatic and renal clearances, respectively.

If clearance down each elimination pathway is a function of body weight, then it follows that Cl_s will also correlate with body weight, such that

$$Cl_s = \alpha_h BW^{\beta_h} + \alpha_r BW^{\beta_r} \tag{11}$$

where α_h and α_r are the coefficients and β_h and β_r are the exponential terms for the power function relationship relating Cl_h and Cl_r, respectively, to body weight.

If one assumes that β_h and β_r are approximately the same value ($\beta = 0.75$), then Cl_s can be rewritten as

$$Cl_s = (\alpha_h + \alpha_r)BW^\beta \tag{12}$$

Hence, total systemic clearance, as well as individual pathway clearances (e.g., metabolic or renal clearance), should correlate with total body weight. Table 2 documents the interspecies power function parameters for several drugs that

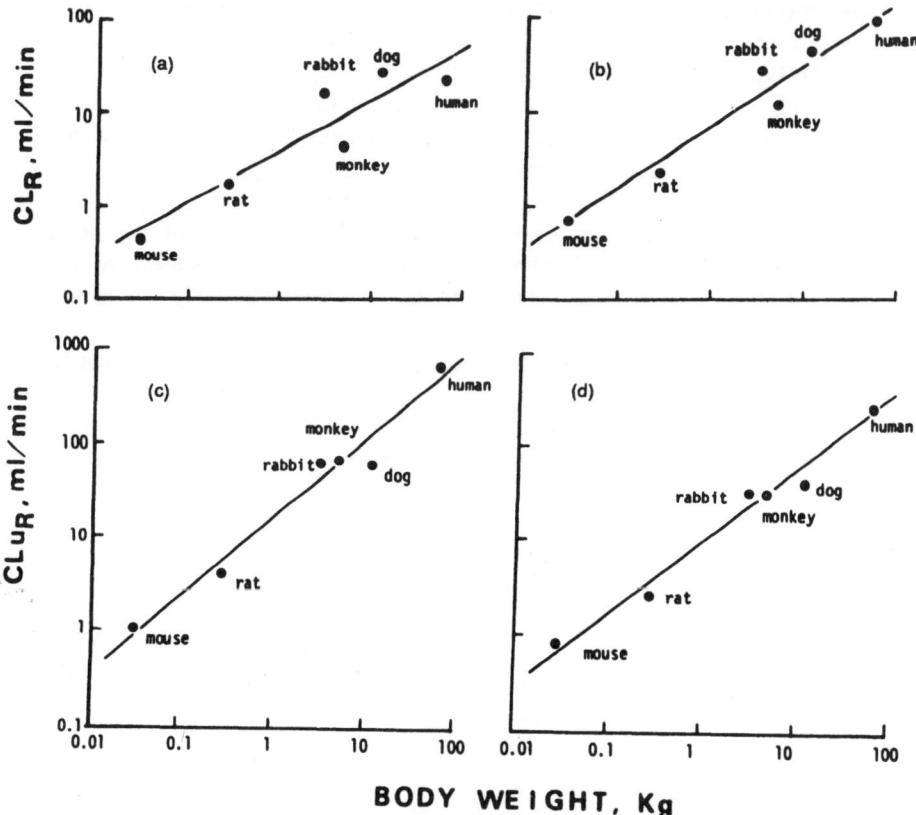

Figure 5 Renal clearance (CL_R) (a,b) and renal clearance of unbound drug (CLu_R) (c,d) in mammals as a function of body weight. (a,c) cefotetan and (b,d) cefmetazole. The solid line was calculated by the least-squares method using unweighted logarithmically transformed data. (From Ref. 27.)

are removed from the body by multiple elimination mechanism (e.g., aztreonam, methotrexate, and erythromycin). Again, the power function adequately addressed differences in clearance between species, even though the compound may be eliminated by different mechanisms in different species.

Distribution

Once a drug enters the systemic circulation, a number of physiological factors govern its distribution, including protein binding (both tissue and plasma), total body water volume, and fat content. Species variation in these physiological factors can influence the distribution aspects of pharmacokinetics.

Protein Binding

Drug binding to plasma proteins can have a marked effect on pharmacokinetics, affecting both clearance and the volume of distribution [4]. Although affinity and capacity constants may be more mechanistically useful, the free or unbound fraction (i.e., unbound/total concentration ratio; $f_{u,b}$) is more frequently reported, and $f_{u,b}$ is more useful for interpreting the influence of binding on pharmacokinetics. Among all of the pharmacokinetic parameters of interest, $f_{u,b}$ poses less of a problem for animal scaling, since $f_{u,b}$ can be readily measured in vitro.

One of the principal determinants of the extent of drug binding is the concentration of the binding proteins (e.g., albumin and α_1-acid glycoprotein). Albumin concentrations are fairly consistent across species, whereas α_1-acid glycoprotein concentrations are consistently lower in the dog and rat (Table 5). The other determinant of drug binding, binding affinity, may vary owing to known species differences in protein structure or to variations in the plasma concentration of competing endogenous ligands (e.g., free fatty acids).

Table 5 presents plasma free fraction ($f_{u,p}$) estimates for several drugs. Phenytoin, digitoxin, and diazepam are believed to bind to three separate binding sites on serum albumin [68]. To a limited extent, the species differences in the unbound fraction of these compounds can be explained on the basis of differences in their albumin concentration (see Table 5). However, the higher free fraction of diazepam in the rat compared with humans, would suggest a difference in binding affinity for the diazepam–albumin interaction as well. Sawada summarized the $f_{u,p}$ values for several antibiotics in mice, rats, rabbits, dogs, monkeys, and humans [27]. Antibiotic $f_{u,p}$ values in the monkey best correlated with human $f_{u,p}$ estimates.

Few studies have been conducted to compare the binding constants across species. Table 5 also contains results of two studies that focused on the interaction of drugs with α_1-acid glycoprotein. The lower capacity constant for propranolol, oxprenolol, and disopyramide in the rat and the dog clearly reflect the lower concentration of α_1-acid glycoprotein in their sera compared with human serum. The larger $f_{u,p}$ for propranolol, oxprenolol, and disopyramide suggests that the rabbit also has a lower α_1-acid glycoprotein concentration. There appears to be a greater similarity when comparing affinity constants across species. The free fraction estimates for propranolol, oxprenolol, and disopyramide in Table 5 also illustrate the effect of multiple binding sites/proteins on free fraction. Propranolol is also bound to albumin to a significant extent [66], hence, the impact of lower α_1-acid glycoprotein levels (e.g., rat and rabbit) is not as marked for propranolol as it is for oxprenolol and disopyramide, which do not interact with albumin to the same extent [66,67].

Table 5 Species Differences in Drug Binding to Plasma as Represented by Free Fraction Values (%)

Principal binding protein	Drug	Ref.	Species[a,b]			
			Rat	Rabbit	Dog	Human
Albumin			60 [21]	[40]	[35]	[49]
	Phenytoin	62–64	20.7	10.1	18.1	13.5
	Digitoxin	65	13.9	9.7	11.2	7.7
	Diazepam	62–64	15.9	9.3	1.6	1.4
α_1-Acid Glycoprotein		61–63	[0.19]	[nda]	[0.37]	[0.70]
	Propranolol	66	10	20	12	13
			(2.04, 1.75)	(nda)	(1.23, 6.71)	(0.58, 16.6)
	Oxprenolol	66	21	60	22	10
			(1.06, 3.18)	(nda)	(1.18, 4.37)	(1.28, 8.70)
	Disopyramide	67	96	97	68	15
			(nda)	(nda)	(0.82, 0.39)	(1.1, 6.7)

[a]Values in brackets represent normal plasma concentrations [g/L].
[b]Values in parentheses reflect affinity (μM^{-1}) and capacity (μM) constants, respectively. r_s for the high affinity binding site; nda, no data available.

Volume of Distribution

Drug distribution is frequently expressed through the use of a hypothetical space known as the apparent volume of distribution (V_d). For many drugs, V_d is constant over a wide dosage range. This hypothetical space can be as small as blood volume or can exceed total body water (owing to extensive tissue binding). The effect of species differences on the volume of distribution can be examined by considering the following theoretical relationship:

$$V_{ss} = V_p + V_t (f_{u,p} / f_{u,t}) \tag{13}$$

where V_{ss} is the present volume of distribution at steady state, V_p is the plasma volume, V_t is the physiological volume outside the plasma into which drug distributes, $f_{u,p}$ is the unbound fraction of drug in plasma, and $f_{u,t}$ is the mean weighted unbound fraction of drug outside the plasma.

Drugs extensively bound to plasma proteins (i.e., relative to tissue binding, such that $f_{u,p} << f_{u,t}$) possess small volumes of distribution, and V_{ss} approximates V_p. Blood volume (and V_p) scale to body size; hence, V_{ss} terms for drugs with limited distibution outside the vascular space will also scale across species.

Drugs that are more widely distributed would at first appear to be more problematic. For those drugs with relatively large volumes of distribution, the V_p term in equation becomes less important resulting in Eq. (13) collapsing to

$$V_{ss} = V_t (f_{u,p} / f_{u,t}) \tag{14}$$

As pointed out earlier, $f_{u,p}$ cannot readily be predicted or scaled across species; however, $f_{u,p}$ can be readily measured from in vitro experiments.

The ability of this modified volume of distribution term [see Eq. (14)] to scale across body weight for various species depends upon interspecies variation in V_t and $f_{u,t}$. It appears likely that V_t would scale to body size, since the percentage of total body water and the relative size of major organs is consistent across species [69]. Table 6 documents the interspecies power function relationship between volume of distribution and body weight for several drugs. When expressed on the body weight basis, no species difference in V_d exists for drugs that are not extensively protein bound, such as methotrexate, cyclophosphamide, and antipyrine. Figure 6 illustrates the relationship of antipyrine volume of distribution as a function of body weight. Antipyrine is bound minimally to plasma proteins and has widely been used as a marker of total body water ($V_p + V_t$), which scales well across species.

Predicting species variation in $f_{u,t}$ (a weighted mean sum of tissue unbound fractions) is difficult. One approach to this problem is a rearrangement of Eq. [(13)]:

$$V_t / f_{u,t} = (V_{ss} - V_p) / f_{u,p} \tag{15}$$

This expression represents the total amount of drug in all tissue compartments

Table 6 Volume of Distribution (L) Scaled to Body Weight (kg) in Adult Animals[a]

Drug	Ref.	α	β	Human included?	Parameter values for a 70-kg human	
					Predicted	Observed
Antipyrine	35	0.756	0.963	Y	45.2	60.8
Aztreonam	35	0.234	0.906	Y	11.0	12.1
Methotrexate	35	0.859	0.918	Y	42.4	67.2
Cyclophosphamide	35	0.883	0.989	Y	59.0	54.6
Erythromycin	38	3.71	0.729	Y	82.1	62.0
Oleandomycin	38	2.83	0.738	Y	65.1	54.0
Cyclosporine	39	5.53	0.828	Y	186.0	245.0
Phencyclidine	40	10.0	0.960	Y	647.0	477.0
Acivicin	41	0.620	0.950	N	35.1	36.5
AZT	84	1.08	1.05	Y	92.3	98.0

[a]Parameter = αBW^β

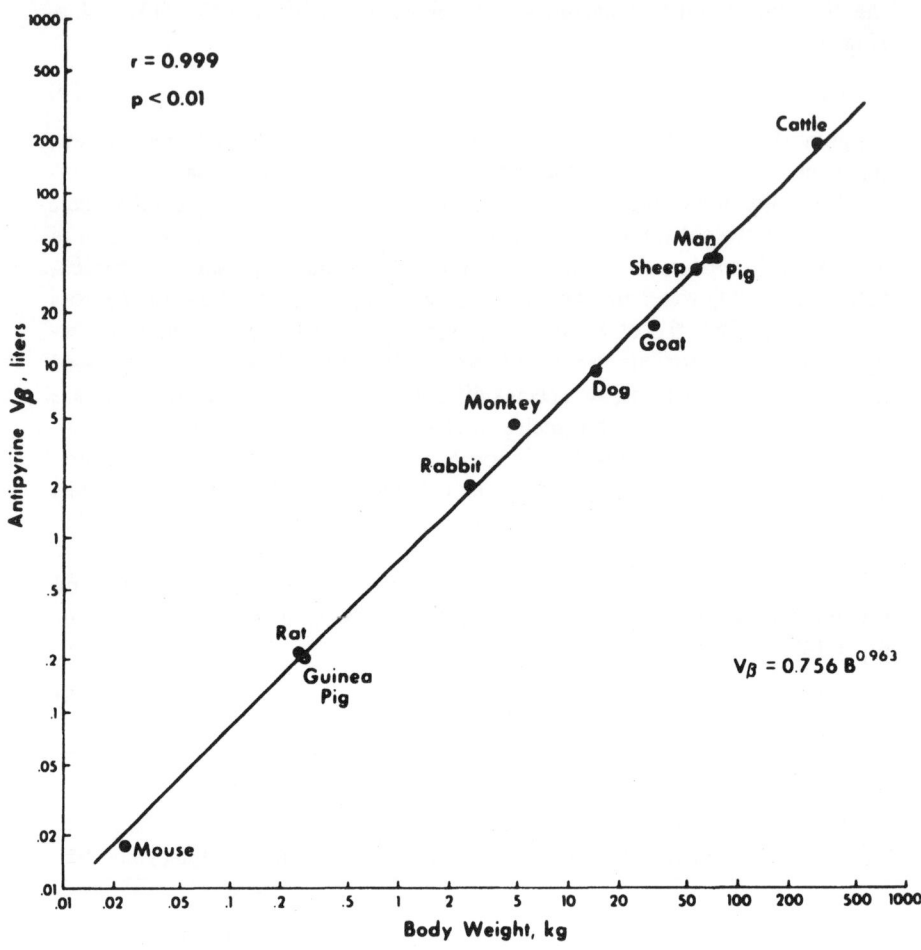

Figure 6 Allometric relationship between antipyrine volume of distribution (V_β) and body weight. (From Ref. 8.)

divided by the concentration of unbound drug in plasma and reflects the extent of extravascular distribution. Sawada et al. [27] successfully used a similar approach to correlate the distribution (i.e., $V_t/f_{u,t}$) of a variety of cationic drugs (Fig. 7). Nakashima et al. [70] examined the steady-state tissue/plasma unbound concentration ratios in rabbits and rats for the anticholinergic drug, biperiden. These investigators found a high degree of interspecies correlation across a variety

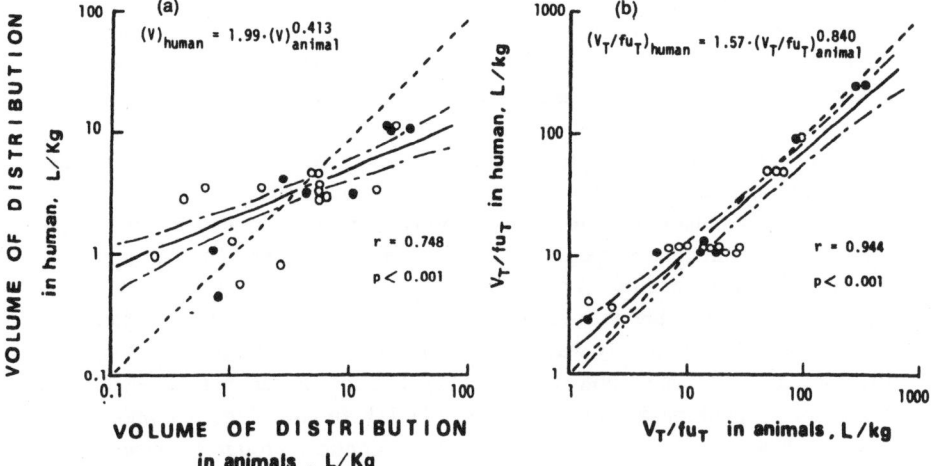

Figure 7 Correlation between the volume of distribution of ten basic drugs in animals and humans. (a) volume of distribution, V (open circles) and V_{ss} (solid circles). (b) V_T/f_T, calculated from V (open circles) and from V_{ss} (solid circles). The short-dashed line shows a positive correlation (r = 1.000), and the long-short-dashed line shows the 95% confidence limit of the estimation. (From Ref. 27.)

of tissues (e.g., lung, brain, fat, muscle, bone), suggesting that the weighted sum of biperiden $V_t / f_{u,t}$ for these two species would be similar.

Absorption

Both the rate and the extent of drug absorption are central to the evaluation of bioavailability and bioequivalence studies. The extent of drug absorption (i.e., relative or absolute bioavailability, F) is established by examining the relative area under the plasma concentration–time curve following two treatments (e.g., oral and intravenous). The absorption rate is usually reflected in the maximum plasma concentration (C_{max}) and the time of C_{max} (t_{max}). Although animal models have been used for drug absorption studies, few have critically examined the relative merit of one animal model versus another or addressed the concept of interspecies scaling. Ritschel [1] has provided an excellent review of the use of animal models for bioavailability assessment.

Animal Models

There are many reports in the literature on the absorption of drugs in animals and humans after oral administration. A number of reports have also been published on the use of animals in the area of transdermal absorption [1]. A more limited number of studies have been conducted on drug absorption in animals after intranasal, buccal, or rectal administration of drugs. Intestinal and hepatic first-pass metabolism of drugs is avoided when the drug is administered by these routes, and as a result, information on absorption from animal models may more readily extrapolate to humans. In his review, Ritschel addresses some of the issues concerning animal models for nonoral routes of administration [1].

The use of animal models for bioavailability assessment appears to work well for some drugs in certain species and to fail for other drugs. The dog appears to be a good model for lithium bioavailability, with estimates of F (75–85%) and t_{max} (1–3 hr) comparable with values obtained in humans [71,72]. The extent of oral lidocaine bioavailability was similar in human, dog, and monkey (25–31%) and less than 8% for the rabbit and the rat [1]. The dog appears to be an excellent model for propylthiouracil bioavailability [72,73]. In one of the few published bioequivalence studies using animal models, identical products appeared to generate similar values for F and t_{max} in the dog [73] and human [74].

For some drugs, there does not appear to be a suitable animal model. Orally administered ethinyl estradiol was 40% absorbed in humans, 3% in rat, 0.3% in rabbit, 9% in dog, 0.6% in monkey, and 2% in baboon [1]. The absolute bioavailability of coumarin after oral administration was only 3% in humans, whereas it was 45% in the dog and 75% in the rat [1]. Bialer et al. [75–77] reported on the bioavailability of several sustained-release formulations of valproic acid in dogs and humans. The dog model exhibited prolonged-release characteristics similar to humans for several formulations. However, the relative bioavailability estimate was 40% for one formulation in the dog [75], whereas the same formulation produced a relative bioavailability value of 96% in humans [74]. The valproic acid, ethinyl estradiol, and coumarin examples suggest that a straightforward extrapolation from animal models to humans of bioavailability assessment is not possible, especially for drugs subject to first-pass metabolism.

Recently, Amidon et al. [78] have derived a relationship for predicting the fraction of the human oral dose that is absorbed, with use of rat intestinal membrane permeability. This approach correlates as well for drugs that are carrier mediated as for those absorbed by passive processes. It is important to note that this approach estimates the fraction *absorbed*, not bioavailability, and assumes that solubility and metabolism factors are not significant [78]. Another interesting report is that by Hsu et al. [79]. These authors reported that species differences (rat, dog, and human) in the dose-dependency of the fraction absorbed versus dose expressed on a body weight basis (BW) for chlorothiazide disappeared if the dose was expressed on a body surface area (BSA) basis. The authors used an allometric approach to estimate BSA (BSA = $K \times BW^{2/3}$). It is interesting to speculate that this dose-dependent absorption actually reflects a physiological function that scales to body weight by allometry.

Although addressing bioavailability/bioequivalence problems in specific patient populations would be most clinically relevant, such studies are frequently conducted in healthy volunteers. However, ethical considerations may warrant the use of animals as models when the drugs to be studied are particularly toxic (e.g., antineoplastic agents). Because of such ethical concerns, the Food and Drug Administration (FDA) promulgated bioavailability and bioequivalence requirements for drug products that included the use of animals as models for the assessment of bioavailability [80]. Although promoted as an alternative, there are apparently no examples of a bioavailability or bioequivalence issue being resolved on the basis of animal data alone [81].

Bioavailability: Modeled

In assessing bioavailability, a parameter of particular interest is the fraction absorbed (F_{ab}). F_{ab} is the product of the "true bioavailability" of the product (i.e., drug released at the absorption site and subsequently absorbed) and that fraction of the dose escaping metabolic degradation in the gut wall or liver (i.e., the so-called first-pass effect). Factors affecting the true bioavailability were outlined earlier, as were observations on first-pass effect across species. The theoretical basis for relating the hepatic first-pass effect across species will be examined here.

If one returns to the well-stirred model and assumes no binding to serum proteins, the fraction removed by the liver (i.e., hepatic extraction ratio; E_h) can be written as

$$E_h = \frac{Cl_{i,h}}{Q_h + Cl_{i,h}} \tag{16}$$

Substituting the respective power function relationships for intrinsic hepatic clearance and blood flow ($Cl_{i,h}$ and Q_h, respectively) yields

$$E_h = \frac{\alpha_{Cli} BW^{\beta_{Cli}}}{(\alpha_{Qh} BW^{\beta_{Qh}}) + (\alpha_{Cli} BW^{\beta_{Cli}})} \tag{17}$$

where α_{Cli} and α_{Qh} are the coefficients and β_{Cli} and β_{Qh} are the exponential terms for the power function relationship relating Cl_h and Q_h, respectively to body weight.

Given the comparable values for β_{Cli} and β_{Qh}, the exponent β and, thus, body weight in the numerator and denominator cancels, resulting in the following:

$$E_h = \frac{\alpha_{Cli}}{\alpha_{Qh} + \alpha_{Cli}} \tag{18}$$

Therefore, hepatic extraction (or the first-pass effect on F) cannot be readily extrapolated across species, since the dominance of body weight in the extrapolation across species is lost. A similar argument can be made if one examines the fraction of the dose metabolized down a particular pathway or the fraction excreted in bile or urine. As a general rule, fractional parameters in pharmacokinetics do not readily extrapolate across species. If the objective of animal model development is to predict a specific pharmacokinetic parameter, such as E or F, then animal models will have to be developed and characterized on an individual basis. Unlike clearance and volume of distribution, the use of interspecies scaling to predict human bioavailability cannot be justified on a theoretical basis.

Biological Half-Life

As pointed out by Boxenbaum [35], if both V and Cl are allometrically related to body weight across species, so too will be the terminal disposition half-life ($t_{1/2}$) since

$$t_{1/2} = (0.693 \text{ V})/\text{Cl} = (0.693 \ \alpha_V BW^{\beta_V})/\alpha_{Cl} BW^{\beta_{Cl}} \tag{19}$$

where α_V and α_{Cl} are the coefficients and β_V and β_{Cl} are the exponential terms for the power function relationship relating V and Cl, respectively, to body weight.

Equation 19 can be written

$$t_{1/2} = \alpha_t BW^{\beta_t} \tag{20}$$

where α_t is the ratio of α_V and α_{Cl}, and β_t is the numerical difference between β_V and β_{Cl}.

Table 7 documents the interspecies power function relationship between the terminal disposition half-life and body weight for various drugs. It should be noted that a number of these regression analyses resulted in relatively poor correlation coefficients when compared with corresponding values for V and Cl regressions. The likely reasons for poorer correlations for $t_{1/2}$ arise because $t_{1/2}$ is a hybrid parameter (indirectly related to physiological function or mechanisms). Another shortcoming of this relationship is mathematical. The values of β_V and β_{Cl} in Tables 6 and 2 are approximately equal (β_V slightly greater); therefore, the value of β_t (i.e., $\beta_V - \beta_{Cl}$) frequently approaches zero (see Table 7). As a result, body weight raised to β_t power approaches unity. Thus, $t_{1/2}$ may not correlate well with body weight; consequently, it may be more difficult to predict across species.

Dosing Regimens

Recently, Mordenti and Chappell [3] have expanded the use of allometric extrapolation to predict therapeutic, toxic, or lethal doses across species. These authors have developed a relationship that describes the dose in one species (e.g.,

Table 7 Terminal Exponential Disposition Half-Life (min) Scaled to Body Weight (kg) in Adult Animals[a]

Drug	Ref.	α	β	Human included?	Parameter values for a 70-kg human	
					Predicted	Observed
Antipyrine	35	74.5	0.069	N	99.9	654.0
Methotrexate	35	54.6	0.228	Y	144.0	432.0
Cyclophosphamide	35	36.6	0.236	Y	99.7	450.0
Digoxin	35	983.0	0.234	Y	2660.0	2340.0
Hexobarbital	35	80.0	0.348	Y	351.0	222.0
Phenylbutazone	35	340.0	0.060	Y	439.0	3360.0
Diazepam	35	122.0	0.428	Y	752.0	2580.0
Erythromycin	38	75.5	0.141	Y	137.0	96.0
Oleandomycin	38	59.5	0.066	Y	78.8	63.0
Cyclosporine	39	411.0	0.020	Y	447.0	960.0
Phencyclidine	40	126.0	0.320	Y	505.9	960.0
Acivicin	41	108.9	0.310	N	403.1	570.0

[a] Parameter = αBW^{β}

human) required to produce equivalent steady-state plasma concentrations achieved in another species (e.g., animal) as in

$$D_{human} = D_{animal} \left[\frac{F_{animal}}{F_{human}} \right] \left[\frac{\tau_{human}}{\tau_{animal}} \right] \left[\frac{BW_{human}}{BW_{animal}} \right]^{0.7} \quad (21)$$

where D is the administered dose (in mass), F is the bioavailability factor, τ is the dosing interval, and BW is body weight for the human and animal species. If the dosing interval for the two species is constant and, assuming comparable bioavailability for the two species, Eq. (21) reduces to

$$D_{human} = D_{animal} \left[\frac{BW_{human}}{BW_{animal}} \right]^{0.7} \quad (22)$$

As pointed out by Mordenti and Chappell [3], when an allometric exponent for clearance is less than 1.0 (usually 0.7–0.8), the smaller species requires a larger dose (mg/kg) to produce an equivalent steady-state concentration. Moreover, given an allometric exponent of 1.0 for the volume of distribution, this approach will result in greater peak/trough concentration ratios for the smaller species. These authors have proposed several other dosing regimens that are based on this allometric approach.

SUPERPOSITION OF CONCENTRATION–TIME PROFILES (EQUIVALENT TIME)

In chronological time, smaller animals have higher heart and respiratory rates than larger animals. However, all mammals have the same number of heart beats and breaths in their life time [82]. It can be shown that these biological activity rates follow an allometric relationship. As pointed out by Boxenbaum [82], these body weight exponents are comparable (i.e., 0.28); hence, the ratio of these internal biological rates are relatively constant. The respiratory rate/heart rate ratio is approximately 4. Therefore, the rat and human would both have four heart beats for each breath. This species-invariant trend appears to be consistent for many biological rates, and a general trend for biological rates has been proposed (biological rate = constant $\times$ $BW^{0.25}$) [3,82].

Boxenbaum and others [3,5–11,82,83] have recognized this phenomenon and have utilized it to adjust the time scale of drugs in different species to produce curves that are superimposable. Dedrick et al. [83] first demonstrated that plasma concentration versus time profiles for a given drug (e.g., methotrexate) obtained in a variety of species could be made superimposable if corrected for dose and body weight. As can be seen in Figure 8a, the time course of methotrexate is more rapid in smaller animal species and less rapid in humans. If the concentration values are divided by dose (on a body weight basis) and the time values are divided by body weight to the 0.25 power, then the curves become superimposable (see Fig. 8b). Although the original selection of the exponent term was arbitrary, it agrees well with the physiological or biological time described earlier.

These authors appear to be the first to advocate the use of an "equivalent time" in pharmacokinetics. Boxenbaum [8] subsequently reexamined the same methotrexate data and calculated the allometric relationships for methotrexate clearance and volume of distribution. For both pharmacokinetic parameters there was a fixed relationship to species-invariant physiology (allometry). The ratio of the allometric equation for methotrexate clearance to the allometric relationship describing creatinine clearance was 1.33. A similar analysis revealed a ratio of 1.22 for methotrexate volume of distribution (relative to total body water in these species). Hence, all species appear alike in the distribution and excretion of methotrexate, if viewed in terms of their own space and time framework.

Boxenbaum [8,10,11,82] has expanded on these concepts, viewing pharmacokinetic events from the vantage point of "pharmacokinetic space-time continua." One example of the approaches advocated by Boxenbaum is depicted in Figure 9. A syndesichron plot of antipyrine is constructed in such a fashion that it accounts for species differences in dose and volume of distribution (concentration axis) and species differences in intrinsic clearance and physiological time (time axis). Clearly, the concentration–time profiles for antipyrine in species ranging from the rat to the cow (including human) appear to lie along the same line.

Interspecies Scaling in Pharmacokinetics

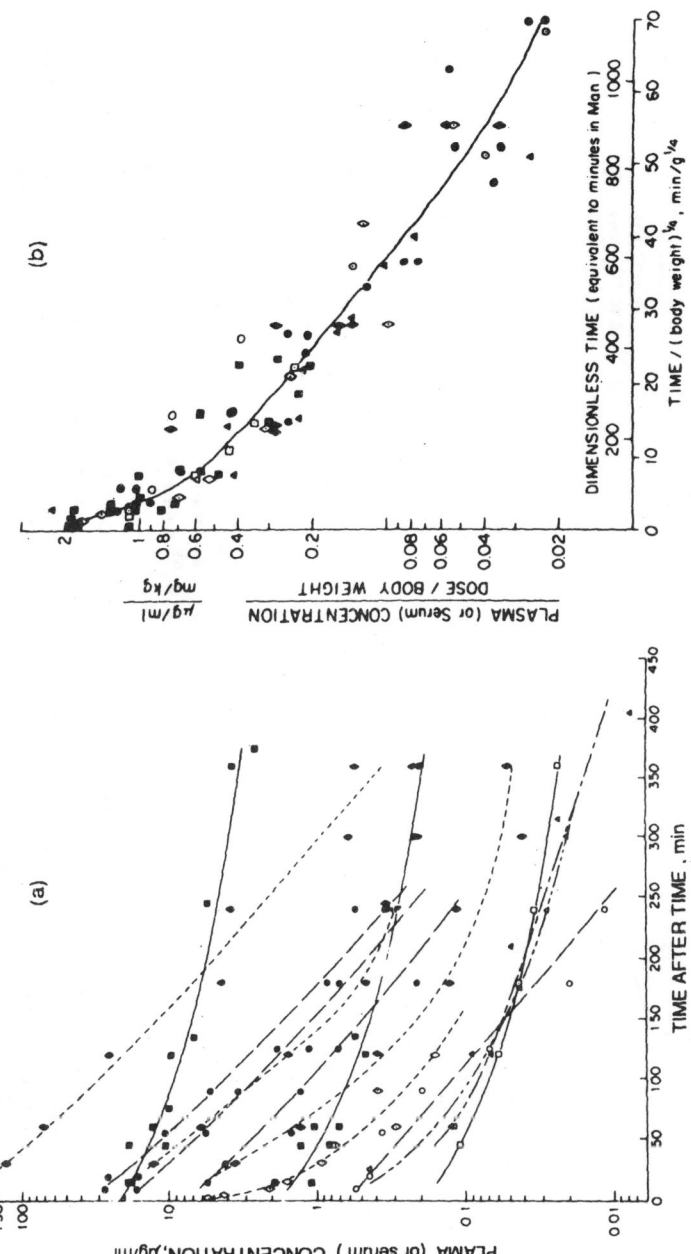

Figure 8 Plasma (or serum) concentrations of methotrexate in the mouse (-·-·-), rat (---), monkey (-- --), dog (-- -- --), and human (———) after IV or IP injection (the symbols refer to different dose levels and routes of administration): (a) semilogarithmic plots of methotrexate concentration versus time and (b) semilogarithmic plot obtained after normalization of the axes. (From Ref. 83.)

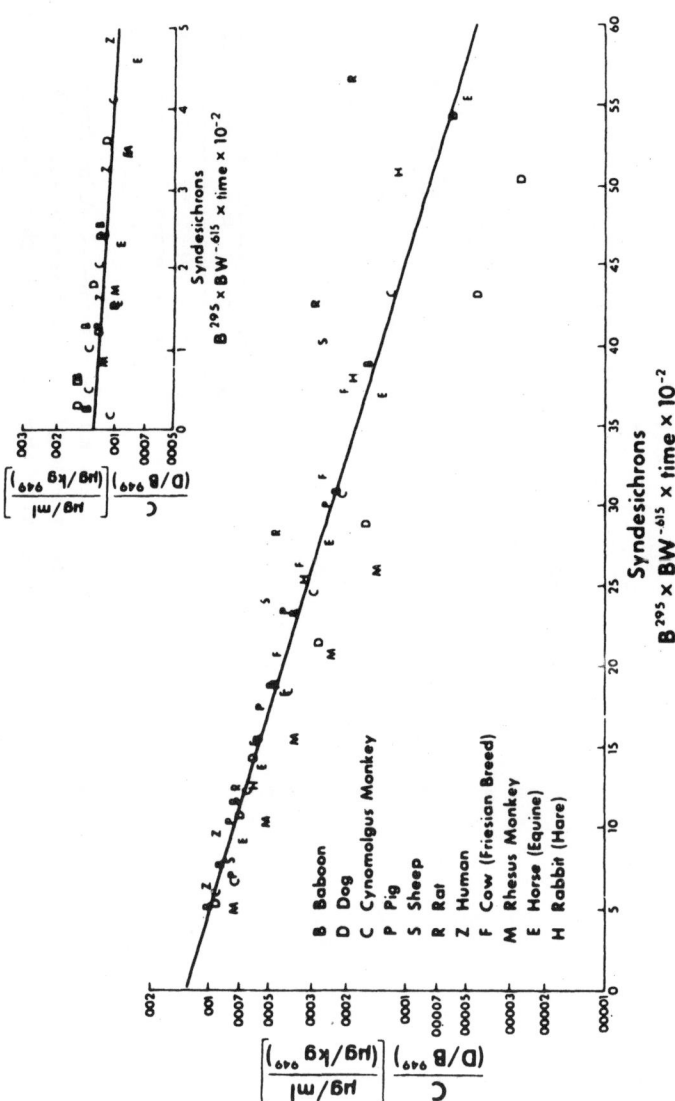

Figure 9 Semilogarithmic syndesichron plot for antipyrine disposition in 11 mammalian species (*syndesichron*: The first element of this neologism is from the word *syndes*, a transliteration of the classical Greek word meaning "a binding together." The suffix *-chron* comes from *Cronus* (*Kronos*), a word for the Greek god of time. The prefix comes from the view that space experience and temporal sequence form an integrated continuum or are inextricably bound). (From Ref. 11.)

A number of other articles address these space–time concepts in greater depth [8,10,11,82].

CONCLUSIONS

Physiology forms the basic framework for the interpretation of species differences in pharmacokinetics. Physiological flow models have been useful for scaling pharmacokinetics profiles across species, but are complex and require a considerable amount of experimental data that is frequently difficult to obtain. Interspecies scaling of pharmacokinetic parameters is considerably easier, relates well to physiological function, and addresses the relevant issues.

Numerous biological rates suggest a common species-invariant physiological clock that is not related to chronological time. This internal clock appears to play a role in controlling the time course of drugs in the body for each species. Plasma concentration–time profiles across species can be superimposed on this basis.

Physiological function and anatomical structure scale to body weight (allometry) and thus provide the basis for scaling some pharmacokinetic parameters (i.e., Cl and V). Other pharmacokinetic parameters are unrelated to body size and do not scale across species (e.g., F, $f_{u,p}$). Interspecies scaling appears to work well when scaling clearance (a function of BW), independently of the route of elimination. Metabolic clearance in humans appears to be the exception of this generalization. Human metabolic clearance can be predicted from laboratory animal profiles when the data is expressed in terms of maximum life span potential. However, interspecies scaling appears to fail if the overall fate of the drug in question becomes dependent upon a specific metabolic pathway (e.g., mephenytoin).

ACKNOWLEDGMENT

Supported in part by a grant from the National Institutes of Health GM38836.

REFERENCES

1. W. A. Ritschel. *S.T.P. Pharm.* 3:125–141 (1987).
2. J. Mordenti. *J. Pharm. Sci.* 75:1028–1040 (1986).
3. J. Mordenti and W. Chappel. In *Toxicokinetics and New Drug Development* (A. Yacobi, J. P. Skelly, and V. K. Batra, eds.) Pergamon Press, Elmsford, N.Y., p. 42 (1989).
4. G. R. Wilkinson. *Pharmacol. Rev.* 39:1–47 (1987).
5. H. Boxenbaum. *J. Pharamcokinet. Biopharm.* 8:165–176 (1980).
6. H. Boxenbaum. *J. Pharmacokinet. Biopharm.* 10:411–427 (1982).
7. Y. Sawada, M. Hanano, Y. Sugiyama, and T. Iga. *J. Pharmacokinet. Biopharm.* 13:477–492 (1985).
8. H. Boxenbaum. *J. Pharmacokinet. Biopharm.* 10:201–227 (1982).

9. H. Boxenbaum and R. D'Souza. *YIPS* pp. 49–62 (1987).
10. H. Boxenbaum and R. D'Souza. In *Pharmacokinetics* (A. Pecile and A. Rescigno, eds.) Plenum Publishing, New York, pp. 191 (1988).
11. H. Boxenbaum. *Drug Metab. Rev. 15*:1071–1121 (1984).
12. R. L. Dedrick. *J. Pharm. Sci. 75*:1047–1052 (1986).
13. K. B. Bischoff. *Bull. Math. Biol. 48*:309–322 (1986).
14. R. L. Dedrick, D. S. Zaharko, and R. J. Lutz. *J. Pharm. Sci. 62*:882–890 (1973).
15. R. L. Dedrick, D. D. Forrester, J. N. Cannon, S. M. El Dareer, and L. B. Mellett. *Biochem. Pharmacol. 22*:2405–2417 (1973).
16. R. L. Dedrick. *J. Pharmacokinet. Biopharm. 1*:435–461 (1973).
17. K. B. Bischoff, R. L. Dedrick, and D. S. Zaharko. *J. Pharm. Sci. 59*:149–154 (1970).
18. K. B. Bischoff, R. L. Dedrick, D. S. Zaharko, and J. A. Longstreth. *J. Pharm. Sci. 60*:1129–1133 (1971).
19. D. S. Zaharko, R. L. Dedrick, and V. T. Oliverio. *Comp. Biochem. Physiol. 42*:183–194 (1972).
20. R. L. Dedrick, D. D. Forrester, and D. H. W. Ho. *Biochem. Pharmacol. 21*:1–16 (1972).
21. J. H. Lin, Y. Sugiyama, S. Awazu, and M. Hanano. *J. Pharmacokinet. Biopharm. 10*:649–661 (1982).
22. F. G. King, R. L. Dedrick, and F. F. Farris. *J. Pharmacokinet. Biopharm. 14*:131–156 (1986).
23. Y. Igari, Y. Sugiyama, Y. Sawada, T. Iga, and M. Hanano. *J. Pharmacokinet. Biopharm. 11*:577–593 (1983).
24. L. I. Harrison and M. Gibaldi. *J. Pharm. Sci. 66*:1679–1683 (1977).
25. Y. Sawada, H. Harashima, M. Hanano, Y. Sugiyama, and T. Iga. *J. Pharmacobiodyn. 8*:757–766 (1985).
26. A. A. Heusner. *Annu. Rev. Physiol. 49*:121–133 (1987).
27. Y. Sawada, M. Hanano, Y. Sugiyama, and T. Iga. *J. Pharmacokinet. Biopharm. 12*:241–261 (1984).
28. H. Boxenbaum and J. B. Fertig. *Eur. J. Drug Metab. Pharmacokinet. 9*:177–183 (1984).
29. W. L. Chiou and F.-H. Hsu. *Pharm. Res. 5*:668–672 (1988).
30. J. S. Huxley. *Problems of Relative Growth*. Methuen, London, 1932.
31. E. F. Adolph. *Science 109*:579–585 (1949).
32. W. R. Stahl. *Science 150*:1039–1041 (1965).
33. J. Prothero. *Comp. Biochem. Physiol. 77A*:133–138 (1984).
34. R. Kato. Hepatic cytochrome P-450 monooxygenase system. In *International Encyclopedia Pharmacology and Therapy*, Sect. 108. Perganon Press, Oxford, p. 99 (1982).
35. H. Boxenbaum. *Drug Metab. Rev. 15*:1071–1121 (1984).
36. S. Sherlock. *Diseases of the Liver and Biliary System*, Blackwell Scientific Publications, Oxford, 1985.
37. S. G. Massy and R. J. Glassock. *Textbook of Nephrology*. Williams & Wilkins, Baltimore, 1983.
38. G. S. Duthu. *J. Pharm. Sci. 74*:943–946 (1985).

39. L. Sangalli, A. Bortolotti, L. Jiritano, and M. Bonati. *Drug Metab. Dispos.* 16:749–753 (1988).
40. S. M. Owens, W. C. Hardwick, and D. Blackall. *J. Pharmacol. Exp. Ther.* 242:96–101 (1987).
41. J. P. McGovren, M. G. Williams, and J. C. Stewart. *Drug Metab. Dispos.* 16:18–22 (1988).
42. A. Rane, G. R. Wilkinson, and D. G. Shand. *J. Pharmacol. Exp. Ther.* 199:420–424 (1977).
43. F. P. Guengerich. *Mammalian Cytochromes P-450.* CRC Press, Boca Raton, 1987.
44. H. Ohi, S. Toratani, M. Komori, T. Miura, M. Kitada, and T. Kamataki. *Biochem. Pharmacol.* 38:361–365 (1989).
45. T. Wolff and M. Strecker. *Biochem. Pharmacol.* 34:2593–2598 (1985).
46. F. P. Guengerich, M. V. Martin, P. H. Beaune, P. Kremers, T. Wolff, and D. J. Waxman. *J. Biol. Chem.* 261:5051–5060 (1986).
47. M. Komori, H. Shimada, T. Miura, and T. Kamataki. *Biochem. Pharmacol.* 38:235–240 (1989).
48. S. J. Lan, S. H. Weinstein, G. R. Keim, and B. H. Migdalof. *Xenobiotica* 13:329–335 (1983).
49. M. Bonati, R. Latini, G. Tognoni, J. F. Young, and S. Garattini. *Drug Metab. Rev.* 15:1355–1383 (1985).
50. F. E. Yates and P. N. Kugler. *J. Pharm. Sci.* 75:1019–1027 (1986).
51. E. A. Porta. *Antioxidant Defense Mechanisms*, Vol. 3 (C. K. Chow, ed.) CRC Press, New York, pp. 1–52 (1988).
52. S. H. Akrawi. Use of Chronic Porta Vein Infusion in Fats to Examine Mephenytoin Stereoselective Digestion. Ph.D. Thesis, University of Kentucky (1988).
53. A. Küpfer and J. Bircher. *J. Pharmacol. Exp. Ther.* 209:190–195 (1979).
54. P. J. Wedlund, W. S. Aslanian, E. Jacqz, C. B. McAllister, R. A. Branch, and G. R Wilkinson. *J. Pharmacol. Exp. Ther.* 234:662–669 (1985).
55. M. VanDerGraaff, N. P. E. Vermeulen, R. P. Joeves, and D. D. Brimer. *Drug Metab. Dispos.* 11:489–493 (1983).
56. M. H. H. Chandler, S. R. Scott, and R. A. Blouin. *Clin. Pharmacol. Ther.* 43:436–441 (1988).
57. E. J. Calabrese. *J. Pharm. Sci.* 75:1041–1046 (1986).
58. R. L. Smith. *The Excretory Function of Bile. The Elimination of Drugs and Toxic Substances in Bile*, Chapman & Hall, London, pp. 76–93 (1973).
59. G. Levy. *J. Pharm. Sci.* 69:482–483 (1980).
60. A. Puigdemon, A. Arboix, F. Gaspari, A. Bortolotti and M. Bonati. *Res. Commun. Chem. Pathol. Pharmacol.* 64:435–440 (1989).
61. J.-P. Lebreton, M. Hiron, D. Biou, and M. Daveau. *Inflammation* 12:413–424 (1988).
62. F. M. Belpaire, A. DeRick, C. Dello, N. Fraeyman, and M. G. Bogaert. *J. Vet. Pharmacol. Ther.* 10:43–48 (1987).
63. P. J. McNamara, R. A. Blouin, and R. K. Brazzell. *Pharm. Res.* 5:261–265 (1988).
64. J. C. Fleishaker and P. J. McNamara. *J. Pharmacol. Exp. Ther.* 244:919–924 (1988).
65. J. D. Baggot and L. E. Davis. *Res. Vet. Sci.* 15:81–87 (1973).
66. F. M. Belpaire, R. A. Braeckman, and M. G. Bogaert. *Biochem. Pharmacol.* 33:2065–2069 (1984).

67. J. J. Lima and D. B. Haughey. *Drug Metab. Dispos.* 9:582–583 (1981).
68. U. Kragh-Hansen. *Biochem. J.* 225:629–638 (1985).
69. L. E. Gerlowski and R. K. Jain. *J. Pharm. Sci.* 72:1103–1127 (1983).
70. E. Nakashima, K. Yokogawa, F. Ishimura, K. Kurata, H. Kido, N. Yamaguchi, and T. Yamana. *Chem. Pharm. Bull.* 35:718–725 (1987).
71. A. Arancibia, F. Corvalan, F. Mella, and L. Conha. *Int. J. Clin. Pharmacol. Ther. Toxicol.* 24:240–245 (1986).
72. M. Banarer and W. A. Ritschel. *Arzneim. Forsch.* 32:383–388 (1986).
73. P. Ringhanal, H. R. Maxon, W. A. Ritschel, I. W. Chen, and D. H. Bauman. *J. Clin. Pharmacol.* 20:91–97 (1980).
74. H. P. Rinyhand, W. A. Ritschel, M. C. Meyer, A. B. Straughn, and T. Hardt. *Int. J. Clin. Pharmacol.* 18:488–493 (1980).
75. M. Bialer, M. Friedman, and J. Dubrovsky. *Int. J. Pharm.* 20:53–63 (1984).
76. M. Bialer, M. Friedman, and J. Dubrovsky. *Biopharm. Drug Dispos.* 6:401–411 (1985).
77. M. Bialer, M. Friedman, and J. Dubrovsky. *Biopharm. Drug Dispos.* 5:1–10 (1984).
78. G. L. Amidon, P. J. Sinko, and D. Fleisher. *Pharm. Res.* 5:651–654 (1988).
79. F.-H. Hsu, T. Prueksaritanont, M. G. Lee, and W. L. Chiou. *J. Pharmacokinet. Biopharm.* 50:369–389 (1987).
80. Food and Drug Administration. Bioavailability and bioequivalence requirements. *Fed. Reg.* 4:1624–1653 (1977).
81. PMA/FDA Sponsored Meeting. The Use of Animals as Substitutes for Humans in Oral Bioavailability Studies. Washington, D.C. (1989).
82. H. Boxenbaum. *J. Pharm. Sci.* 75:1053–1062 (1986).
83. R. L. Dedrick, K. B. Bishoff, and D. S. Zaharko. *Cancer Chemother. Rep. 54* (Part 1): 95–01 (1970).
84. B. A. Patel, F. D. Boudinot, R. F. Schinazi, J. M. Gallo, and C. K. Chu. Personal communication (manuscript in press).

11
Pharmacodynamic Models in Bioequivalence

S. Thomas Forgue
Parke-Davis Pharmaceutical Research Division
Warner-Lambert Company
Ann Arbor, Michigan

Wayne A. Colburn
Harris Laboratories, Inc.
Scottsdale, Arizona

INTRODUCTION

The Food, Drug, and Cosmetic Act, enacted in 1938, gave the Food and Drug Administration (FDA) responsibility for ensuring that drugs marketed in the United States are safe and effective. In 1977, the FDA issued regulations that bioequivalence of a generic drug and the innovator's product must be established before marketing the generic substitute [1]. Typically, bioequivalence is established on the basis of bioavailability of the active drug moiety, as determined from pharmacokinetic data. Demonstration of therapeutic equivalence of the generic and innovator's product is not required. The association between pharmacokinetic bioequivalence and therapeutic equivalence is difficult to characterize. In 1981, Title 21 of the Food and Drug Act [2] specified criteria for identifying bioavailability differences that could lead to clinically important therapeutic or safety differences.

Conceptually, evaluation of bioequivalence in the pharmaceutical industry has come full circle. Decades ago, quality control and approval of drug products were based on pharmacological effect measurements. As bioanalytical methodology advanced, there was a trend toward chemical assay methods. Since important bioequivalence issues evolved from quality control criteria, it was natural to base assessments on chemical analyses on drug or metabolites in biological matrices. Great accuracy and precision of chemical methods elicited wide acceptance, despite that pharmacologic measures may have been more directly linked to therapeutic endpoints.

Bioequivalence can be based on pharmacokinetics, pharmacologic effect, or therapeutic (clinical) efficacy. Here, the term *efficacy* is restricted to the desired therapeutic endpoint—what the physician is trying to achieve for the patient. Efficacy of chlorpromazine, for example, may denote amelioration of signs and symptoms of psychoses. Although efficacy is the desired outcome, the time and cost of clinical efficacy trials typically preclude its use in bioequivalence testing.

Because blood and urine assays are available for nearly all drugs, and because pharmacokinetic methods are generally understood, pharmacokinetics are the current mainstay of bioequivalence assessments. The key assumption is that equivalent pharmacokinetics indicate equivalent therapeutics. Or, more precisely, that observed differences between formulations for pharmacokinetic parameters are predictive of negligible differences in clinical performance. Usually, little attempt to verify this key assumption is made [3–5]. Nonlinear pharmacokinetics or the presence of active metabolites can render the assumption unjustified, and meaningful efficacy differences can be masked. Conversely, a 20% deviation from pharmacokinetic equivalence might have negligible therapeutic consequences [6].

Measurement of effect on a (patho)physiological process as a function of time after administration of two different products can serve as the basis for bioequivalence assessment, in a manner analogous to that based on concentration data. In this context, a pharmacodynamic assessment denotes determination of effect as a function of time, in a manner analogous to a pharmacokinetic assessment of drug concentration with time. Effect parameters do not necessarily avoid problems inherent in use of concentration parameters for assessment of bioavailability. Effect data, although perceived as closely allied to efficacy, may actually be less relevant than drug concentration data. Effect measurements may be so imprecise that statistical criteria can be met only with an unreasonably large number of subjects. However, the effects of many drug classes are amenable to accurate, precise, and reproducible quantification (e.g., the miotic response of the pupil elicited by chlorpromazine) [7]. Pharmacodynamic methods for bioavailability evaluation are evolving rapidly, and their potential appears great.

Pharmacodynamics (PD) can be an alternative to pharmacokinetics (PK) in bioavailability assessment, or an adjunct to substantiate the relevance of pharmacokinetic measures. Understanding the concentration and effect relationship (CER) is important to predict the limitations of either pharmacokinetic or pharmacodynamic assessments. Thus, pharmacokinetics and pharmacodynamics are complementary approaches. Furthermore, integrated PK/PD methods can provide a comprehensive description of the relationships among dose, concentration, effect, and time. As with bioequivalence tests that are solely based on pharmacokinetics, assumptions are needed [e.g., that single-dose assessment is predictive of multiple-dose treatment (steady state), and that studies with healthy subjects are predictive of therapeutic response in patients].

The usefulness of pharmacodynamics in bioequivalence assessment is explored in this chapter. Assessment of pharmacologic effect as a function of time, pharmacodynamic models for characterization of CERs, and combined PK/PD models are reviewed. Examples of insight into fundamental bioequivalence issues that can be gained with pharmacodynamic concepts are provided by means of a novel simulation.

FUNDAMENTALS OF PHARMACODYNAMIC MODELS

Terminology

For purposes of this discussion terms need qualification. *Pharmacokinetics* denotes characterization of drug concentration, C, in a biological matrix as a function of time. Concentration in the sampled matrix, typically plasma, is denoted $C_p(t)$, emphasizing time dependence of the parameter. Concentration at the site of drug action (effector/receptor), C_e, is a hypothetical concentration estimable by mathematical modeling. *Pharmacologic effects*, E, can be categorized as either continuous variables (e.g., heart rate) or as fixed (all-or-none; quantal) effects (e.g., occurrence of somnolence or a seizure). Only continuous responses are considered in this discussion.

Although use of the term in the literature includes characterization of E as a function of C, especially in the context of *pharmacodynamic models*, in this chapter *pharmacodynamics* denotes characterization of drug effect as a function of time, E(t). To minimize confusion, E as a function of C will be designated a *concentration–effect relationship*, CER.

A *pharmacokinetic–pharmacodynamic* (PK/PD) model denotes a set of integrated equations that specifies relationships among C_p, C_e, E, and time. That is, the PK/PD model describes the pharmacokinetics, the CER, and the pharmacodynamics. Sometimes, the PK/PD model may be adequate without an explicit equation linking $C_p(t)$ with $C_e(t)$.

Pharamcodynamic Objectives and Study Design Considerations

A voluminous literature has been developed over the last 25 years on investigation of bioequivalence of different dosage forms and therapeutic regimens. The bulk of this literature has focused on pharmacokinetic, statistical, and regulatory dimensions. Bioequivalence tests that are based on pharmacokinetic parameters are largely standardized. Corresponding statistical evaluation methods are sophisticated, and acceptance criteria are well defined. Bioequivalence testing based solely on measurement of effect over time is less well established.

Current FDA guidelines for metaproterenol and albuterol aerosols for inhalation are based on pulmonary function tests (e.g., forced expiratory volume in 1 sec; FEV_1). These measurements are considered more representative of bioavailability at the site of action than are C_p data. Statistical evaluation (analysis of variance; ANOVA and confidence intervals) of area under the effect curve (AUEC), maximal effect (E_{max}), and corresponding time (tE_{max}) can be performed in a manner analogous to that for pharmacokinetic data. The pharmacodynamic assessment is dependent on pulmonary function test precision, but typically 60–90 patients with asthma, rather than 24 normal volunteers, are likely to be needed for reliable study results. In this example of β-adrenergic agonists, effect measures are the same as used to assess efficacy in relief of bronchospasm, and pharmacodynamic bioequivalence testing is conceptually indistinguishable from a clinical efficacy trial in which the control treatment is the reference drug product. Thus, pharmacodynamic bioequivalence testing—direct comparison of E(t) profiles for two products—can be a complex, expensive alternative to the pharmacokinetic bioequivalence trial. Furthermore, it can prove a less discriminating approach to product comparison.

But evaluation of $C_p(t)$ data has no intrinsic value; it is meaningful if, and only if, there is a vital relationship between $C_p(t)$ and E(t), and between E(t) and clinical effectiveness. As noted by Levy [8] in 1972: "Bioavailability problems are, in essence, problems concerning clinical effectiveness." Pharmacodynamic modeling or, more specifically, PK/PD modeling, serves to bridge the gap between basic pharmacokinetic bioequivalency testing and clinical efficacy trials by complementing blood and urine data with therapeutically relevant effect data. The fundamental question is: What information of value in resolving bioequivalence issues will accrue with additional cost and subject risk associated with complementing pharmacokinetics with pharmacodynamic modeling? The answer is not now known.

It is known that PK/PD modeling can provide a quantitative description of the CER and the potential for accurate prediction of consequences of altered bioavailability on intensity and duration of effect. Predictions can facilitate establishment of rational bioequivalence criteria tailored to drug substance, delivery system, formulation, and treatment regimen. Meaningful comparison of conventional and controlled-release products, and other evaluations that are difficult with standard pharmacokinetic bioequivalence testing, can be addressed.

The PK/PD assessment is built on the precept of a causal relationship between a (patho)physiological assessment and amount of drug somewhere in the body. In the last decade, there has been a remarkable growth in the number of applications of PK/PD models for a variety of drugs, along with appreciation of limitations of older approaches to CERs. Much growth is attributable to development by Sheiner, and others [9-14; reviewed in 15-22] of effect compartment modeling that has provided a pragmatic and intuitively reasonable approach. Commercial availability of sophisticated nonlinear regression programs, such as PCNONLIN [23] and the NLIN procedure of SAS [24], for fitting pharmacokinetic and pharmacodynamic data, has undoubtedly helped.

Considerations in design of a PK/PD study aimed at complementation of conventional bioequivalence data (Table 1) are as discussed previously in other contexts [25]. In contrast with current bioequivalence test guidelines, PK/PD study designs are currently the purview of the individual investigator. In contrast with standardized routines for calculation of pharmacokinetic parameters and statistical evaluation thereof, PK/PD analyses are invariably novel. The PK/PD evaluations produce large amounts of data, and compartmental analyses and curve-fitting procedures are notoriously time-consuming. Pooling of data within or between subjects may be a practical necessity, as well as a means of minimizing variability in parameter estimates. Yet, as with pharmacokinetic data analysis, evaluation of data for each individual subject is the preferred approach. A strategy for establishing an effect baseline is a basic design element, and may necessitate a separate placebo treatment period. The experimental period must be long enough for measurement of both $C_p(t)$ and $E(t)$, preferably to the lower limit of quantification. Blood sampling may conflict with or perturb effect measurements [e.g., psychomotor test values or electrocardiograph (ECK) tracings]. Fortunately, concomitant blood sampling and effect measurement is not necessary, because with compartmental data analysis, interpolation of drug concentration data is readily accomplished.

Pharmacodynamic (Concentration-Effect) Models

CER relationships are mathematical models that relate a pharmacologic effect to a measured or calculated concentration—in plasma, in a matrix anatomically close to the site of action such as cerebrospinal fluid, or at the effect site. The models can be derived from receptor theory, but are typically handled empirically in conjunction with data-fitting routines. Complex pharmacodynamic models, corresponding to multiple agonists, antagonists, or receptors, have been developed to address complications such as active metabolites, endogenous agonists, and drug interactions [17,25-29]. The basic equations discussed in the following have been reviewed extensively [15 22,30 32].

Linear Relationships

Observed pharmacologic effect may be directly proportional to concentration, in which case, the relationship may be described as:

$$E = P \cdot C + E_0 \tag{1}$$

Table 1 Some Considerations in Design and Conduct of a PK/PD Study to Complement Pharmacokinetic Bioequivalence Testing

Objective
    Use PK/PD modeling to characterize CER and to predict consequences of altered rate and extent of absorption.

Study Design
    Normal subjects vs patients
    Number of subjects/patients
    Inclusion and exclusion criteria; exclusion of nonresponders
    Crossover vs parallel vs dose-escalation design
    Single-dose vs steady-state assessment
    Determination of baseline effect; placebo control period

Pharmacokinetic Assessment
    Sampling schedule relative to effect measurement
    Effect of nonlinearity in pharmacokinetic behavior
    Analyses of free vs total drug concentration
    Selection of pharmacokinetic model and evaluation methods

Pharmacodynamic Assessment
    Relevance of measurable effect to therapy
    Precision and reproducibility of effect measurements
    Subjective vs objective measurements; (patho)physiological, psychomotor vs behavioral endpoints
    Timing and duration of effect monitoring relative to pharmacokinetic assessment
    Dispersion of data over entire effect range
    Compensation for tolerance, sensitization, learning, fatigue physiological reflexes, and homeostatis

PK/PD modeling
    Baseline compensation model
    Data reduction; pooling within and between subjects and treatments
    Nonlinear regression program availability
    Simultaneous fitting vs initial optimization of pharmacokinetic parameters

Statistical evaluation
    Criteria for selection among alternative models

Model validation
    Accurate description of collected data
    Uniqueness of PK/PD model; verification of model predictions

Conclusion/model application
    Prediction of consequences of alteration in bioavailability with respect to onset duration and intensity or response. Establishment of criteria for bioequivalence of the drug substance.

where the proportionality constant, P, can be obtained as the slope term corresponding to linear regression of E on C. The baseline effect, E_0, is intensity or rate of the (patho)physiological process in the absence of drug, which can be subtracted from all E measurements after dosing. Alternatively, E_0 can be obtained as the intercept of the effect axis; a negative intercept value is suggestive of an effect threshold. A linear function may be useful to describe available data, and statistical criteria may not justify higher parameterization of the model. However, the simplicity of the linear function inevitably belies a more complex CER.

Holford et al. [13] found a linear function adequate to describe the CER for quinidine's alteration of ECK intervals. Observed E values were corrected by subtracting E_0 measured during a placebo treatment phase. The slope estimate corresponding to oral administration was greater than that for IV administration, which was taken as evidence for active quinidine metabolites. Active metabolites may contribute to the finding that the pharmacodynamic bioavailability of oral quinidine was nearly 100% of that for IV dosing, whereas pharmacokinetic (absolute) bioavailability, based on AUC for intact quinidine, was only 70%. Myerburg and co-workers [33] described reduction in preventricular contraction (PVC) rate by procainamide with a linear model based on pooled data.

In a series of studies on α-adrenergic antagonists, Meredith, Donnelly, Elliott, Kelman, and their colleagues [35–38] have noted that a linear function can be more suitable than the E_{max} model for describing antihypertensive response, especially when data are restricted to low ranges of the CER. With the linear equation, patient responsiveness can be conveniently quantified by the P parameter, expressed as unit decrease in blood pressure per unit drug concentration.

If the CER does not conform to a simple linear function, a logarithmic transformation of the data

$$E = P \cdot \log(C) + I \tag{2}$$

may prove useful, where I is an empirically determined constant of no conceptual relevance. Equation (2) is analogous to linearization of a log dose–response curve. Intuitively, extrapolation beyond available data is problematic; for example, there is no upper bound on E as C increases, and a negative E is predicted as C approaches zero. Linear and log-linear CERs are commonly characterized by linear regression, with a high coefficient of determination (r^2) taken as the criterion of a meaningful relationship. However, this statistic neither validates nor indicates predictive ability of the CER.

Application of the logarithmic function was more prevalent in earlier literature than in the last decade. Many investigators used it to describe anticoagulant effects of warfarin, as reviewed by Holford [20]. A recent variation of the logarithmic transformation was reported by Sandberg et al. [39], based on pooled data from 12 patients who received the β-blocker, metoprolol as both conventional and controlled-release tablets. Time-averaged decrease in exercise-induced tachycardia was expressed as a linear function of logarithm of time-averaged steady-state C_p. Blycert et al. [40] found that reduction in supine diastolic blood pressure was closely approximated by a log-linear function.

E_{max} Models

The E_{max} models are a family of functions describing nonlinear CERs. The minimal model capable of accounting for constraints on drug action over the entire dose range is a hyperbolic function:

$$E = \frac{E_{max} \cdot C}{C_{50} + C} \tag{3}$$

where E_{max} is the maximal effect that can be elicited by the drug, and C_{50} is the value of C when response is half maximal ($E_{max}/2$). Equation (3) is a model of a saturable process; as C becomes large, E approaches E_{max} asymptotically, and no further increase in effect is possible (Fig. 1). Absence of effect is predicted in the absence of drug. These constraints on the model are intuitively reasonable.

The essential form of the equation has been applied in diverse areas of biology, chemistry, and physics, and disparate terminology has been applied. In enzyme kinetics it is known as the Michaelis–Menton equation, and linearization techniques, such as Lineweaver–Burk plots can be applied to Eq. (3), as noted years ago by Wagner [41–43]. Langmuir derived similar equations to describe the volume of gas bound to a solid surface at equilibrium; hence, references to "Langmuir adsorption isotherms" in the pharmacodynamic literature. Hill [44] used a function analogous to the sigmoidal E_{max} model [Eq. (4)] to describe binding of oxygen to hemoglobin, hence, references to the "Hill equation." The hyperbolic function has also been invaluable for description of nonlinear pharmacokinetic processes.

When $C << C_{50}$, Eq. (3) reduces to $E = (E_{max}/C_{50}) \cdot C$, and a linear relationship is described. In the range of 20–80% E_{max}, the E_{max} model is well approximated by Eq. (2), but if E_{max} cannot be estimated, then the range represented by the data is indeterminate. Linear and logarithmic functions are best considered approximations of, rather than alternatives to the essential E_{max} model.

Addition of a power term (σ) to form the sigmoidal E_{max} model allows one to describe more diverse data sets:

$$E = \frac{E_{max} \cdot C^\sigma}{C_{50}^\sigma + C^\sigma} \tag{4}$$

where the σ exponent is termed the sigmoidicity or slope factor, because it markedly affects curve slope without alteration in E_{max} or C_{50} (Fig. 2). When $\sigma = 1$, the function is the basic E_{max} model. When $\sigma > 1$, the slope of the curve in the

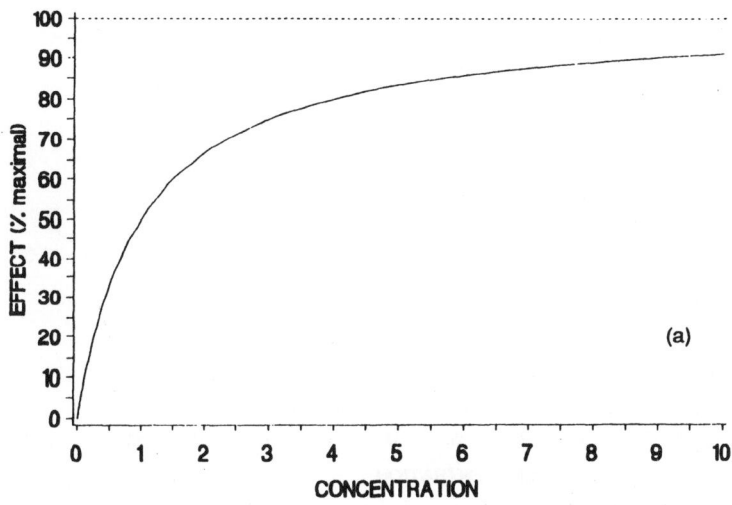

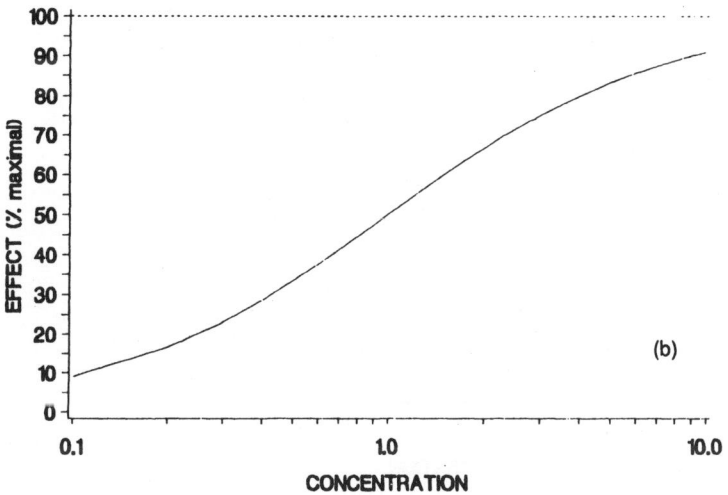

Figure 1 CER simulations based on E_{max} model [Eq. (3); $E_{max} = 100$, $C_{50} = 1$]. (a) The CER can be approximated as a linear function when $C << C_{50}$. (b) Approximation of the CER as a linear function of log C is feasible when $20 < E < 80$.

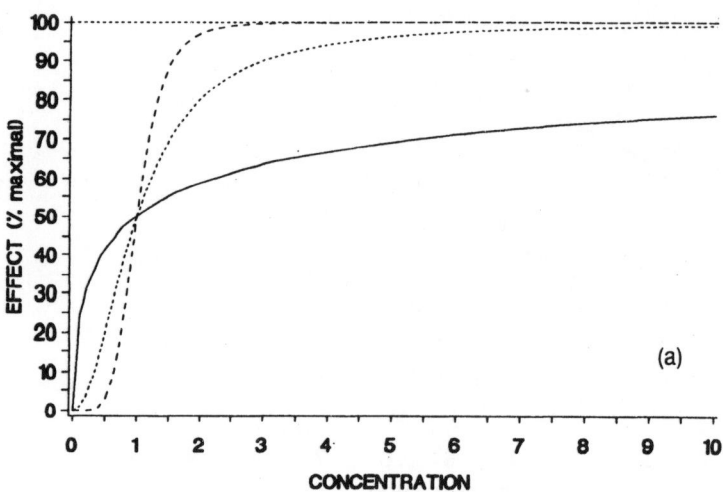

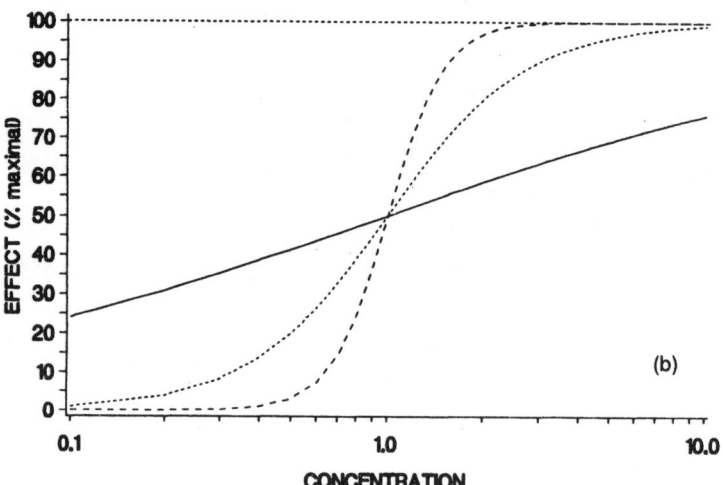

Figure 2 CER simulations based on sigmoidal E_{max} model [Eq. (4); $E_{max} = 100$, $C_{50} = 1$]. Different values for the σ power term correspond to CERs with various sensitivities (slopes) to an increase in concentration. Note that C_{50} is invariant relative to σ. (———, $\sigma = 0.2$; - - - -, $\sigma = 2$; — — —, $\sigma = 5$)

region of E_{50} (i.e., the sensitivity of response to a change in amount of drug) is increased.

Once initial estimates of the values of σ, E_{max}, and C_{50} are determined, best estimates of the model parameters are readily obtained by fitting corresponding $C(t)$ and $E(t)$ data points by means of an iterative least-squares nonlinear regression program. The ability to fit data to the sigmoidal E_{max} equation, does not necessarily mean that it is the correct model. Equations with many variables are flexible. Complex models may not be justified by the quantity and variability of the data, which will be apparent in the curve-fitting statistics (e.g., a high correlation between ostensibly independent variables).

Inhibitory E_{max} Models

The drug may cause a diminution in rate or intensity of a (patho)physiological process (e.g., decrease in arrhythmia rate or airway resistance), in which case, an inhibitory E_{max} model is useful:

$$E = E_0 - \left(\frac{E_{max} \cdot C}{C_{50} + C}\right) \tag{5}$$

where C_{50} denotes the concentration that produces 50% of maximal inhibition attainable. If the drug is capable of abolishing the effect, then $E_{max} = E_0$ and Eq. (5) reduces to

$$E = E_0 \left[1 - \left(\frac{C}{C_{50} + C}\right)\right] = E_0 \left(\frac{C_{50}}{C_{50} + C}\right) \tag{6}$$

This equation is known as the "fractional E_{max} model," since it describes intensity or rate in the presence of drug as a fraction of that in the untreated individual.

Baseline Compensation

Although complex equations may be needed, the CER model is usually based on the simple difference between rate or intensity of a (patho)physiological process in the presence and absence of drug. Accurate measurement of, and compensation for, the baseline effect, E_0, is crucial because assumptions about E_0 affect CER model predictions.

The E_0 parameter can be estimated as a variable or assigned a constant value, depending on the certainty with which the baseline is known and assumptions about its error structure. The baseline can be established in a crossover study during a placebo treatment phase in which all experimental variables are the same as during the drug treatment phase. Nevertheless, intrasubject variability may be large and interfere with measurement of the drug effect. If E_0 is known accurately and is subject only to random error, then it can be simply incorporated into the model as a constant, which tends to decrease the variance in estimates of other variables in the model. Other things being equal, the fewer variables in the model used for least-squares data fitting, the more precise the estimates of any given parameter. E_0 may be confounded by sources of variation caused by food, circadian rhythms, learning, fatigue, or drug tolerance. If E_0 error arises from such systematic variation, then $E_0(t)$ should be determined during the placebo phase, and entered as a variable into the model to compensate the corresponding $E(t)$ observed during drug treatment.

The simplest approach is to treat observed effect as the sum of endogenous rate/intensity and drug response:

$$E = E_0 + \frac{E_{max} \cdot C}{C_{50} + C} \tag{7}$$

or

$$[E - E_0] = \frac{E_{max} \cdot C}{C_{50} + C} \tag{8}$$

Implicit in use of this "baseline subtraction" model is the assumption that the drug response can simply be superimposed on the endogenous biological process. As noted by Colburn [25,29], a baseline "inclusion" model such as

$$E = \frac{E_{max} (C + C_0)}{C_{50} + (C + C_0)} \tag{9}$$

may be more correct, where C_0 can be thought of as concentration of drug equivalents needed to account for the baseline effect in the absence of exogenous drug. This model is theoretically appealing for a narcotic competing with endorphins, or a corticosteroid competing with endogenous steroid for receptor occupancy. Comparison of the CERs that would be derived from the same hypothetical uncorrected effect data using either Eq. (8) or (9) are shown in Figure 3.

Threshold Effects

If sensitivity and precision in measurement of C_p exceeds that for E, estimation of model parameters may be improved by inclusion of a threshold concentration, C_{th}, below which negligible effect occurs. A recent publication by Koopmans and coworkers [45] provides an informative example. They quantified neurophysiologic effects of the benzodiazepine, midazolam, and modeled results with both a sigmoidal E_{max} model and the following threshold effect model:

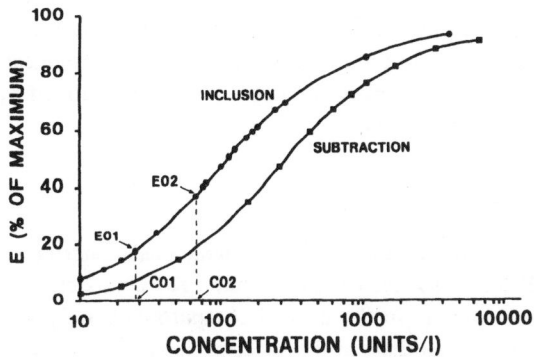

Figure 3 Comparison of predicted CERs corresponding to baseline subtraction model [Eq. (8); $E_0 = 20$] and baseline inclusion model [Eq. (9); $C_0 = 25$], when $E_{max} = 100$ and $C_{50} = 100$. An E_0 value of 20 corresponds to a concentration of 25 in the basic E_{max} model. (From Ref. 25).

$$E = E_0 + \frac{(E_{max} - E_0)(C_e - C_{th})}{(C_{50} - C_{th}) + (C_e - C_{th})} \qquad (10)$$

The percentage decrease in α-band activity in the EEG was quantified, and E_{max} was fixed at 0%, because it was known that midazolam could abolish this activity. Inclusion of the C_{th} parameter was as effective as was a sigmoidal E_{max} model. Equation (10) was linked to a two-compartment pharmacokinetic model for oral absorption by use of an effect compartment model to achieve a comprehensive description of C_p, C_e, and α-band activity with time. The combined PK/PD model could subsequently be used for theoretically sound projections of consequences of altered midazolam bioavailability.

FUNDAMENTALS OF INTEGRATED PHARMACOKINETIC–PHARMACODYNAMIC MODELS

Objectives

An integrated PK/PD model completely describes the time course of drug in the body, the CER, and the time course of pharmacologic effect—all we need to know about C, E, and time. Quantitative prediction of effect onset, intensity, and duration, associated with alterations in bioavailability can be reduced to a mathematical exercise. Straightforward PK/PD relationships were described by Levy [46–48] over 25 years ago. For a drug conforming to a one-compartmental pharmacokinetic model with a log-linear CER, the effect will decline linearly (zero order) with time. Given a minimal effective concentration, calculation of pharmacologic response duration is a simple task. The work of Levy, as well as their own pioneering efforts in defining CERs and the kinetics of drug response, are compiled by Wagner [43] and Gibaldi [49] in their texts.

Effects Related Directly to Sampled Matrix

For some drugs, E(t) can be related directly to $C_p(t)$, in which case pharmacokinetics combined with a CER model suffice to describe the PK/PD model. This does not mean the putative receptor is in the central compartment, only that equilibrium between drug in blood and drug at the receptor is rapid relative to bulk transfer of drug in the body.

The effect site may have an obvious relationship to C_p. Lees and Reid [50] used a sigmoidal E_{max} model to describe inhibition of plasma angiotensin-converting enzyme (ACE) by a metabolite of the antihypertensive perindopril. Since they knew that complete ACE inhibition was possible with the compound, they entered 100% as a constant for E_{max} during data fitting. A C_p of 1.8 ng/mL, produced 50% ACE inhibition. There was low intersubject variability in the σ parameter, which ranged from 0.53 to 0.98.

Lalonde et al. [51] fitted propranolol effect data expressed as percentage reduction in exercise-induced tachycardia to a sigmoidal E_{max} model. Absence of hysteresis in C_p versus E plots obviated the need to compensate for time course differences (equilibration delays). A CER was constructed for each individual patient with data pooled across two treatments that entailed both conventional and controlled-release formulations. Free, as well as total plasma propranolol concentration data were evaluated. Interestingly, model fits for free drug, the pharmacologically active form, were not much better than for total drug. Such information would be evidence that bioequivalence data that are based on total serum drug are meaningful. Their PK/PD equations allowed them to predict the time course of the tachycardia effect and, thereby, the duration of β-blockade by propranolol for both dosage forms.

A concise and informative application of PK/PD methods relevant to bioequivalence issues was provided by Thibonnier et al. [52], who used both free and total disopyramide concentrations along with QT interval duration data for PK/PD modeling. Pharmacokinetics, based on total concentration of this important antiarrhythmic agent are nonlinear, because of saturable protein binding. Unbound drug displays linear pharmacokinetic behavior. An innovator's capsule formulation (Norpace), two different generic capsules, as well as a solution dosage form were administered to 12 subjects according to a four-way Latin-square design. Data for each subject were evaluated individually. The pharmacokinetics for unbound disopyramide were adequately described by a one-compartment model with zero-order absorption after a brief lag time. Prolongation in QT interval was described as a linear function of C_p. Pharmacokinetic and pharmacodynamic parameters were estimated simultaneously by least-squares nonlinear iteration; unbound C_p data gave better fits than did total drug data. Interestingly, earlier modeling by Whiting and colleagues [10] had required compensation for a time (phase) lag between effect and total disopyramide concentration.

There was no significant pharmacokinetic difference between the three capsule formulations, albeit the discriminating power of the statistical tests and confidence intervals were not calculated. Pharmacodynamic parameter values for the three capsule products were indistinguishable from one another. Thus, pharmacokinetic bioequivalence was verifiable in terms of a simple, yet rigorous PK/PD model that, together with their variance model, would enable these workers to predict consequences of altered bioavailability from the capsules.

A common observation is that CER plots are not mathematical functions, owing to lack of a 1:1 correspondence between E and C_p data. Effect magnitude depends on time after dosing as well as on C_p, and hysteresis in CER plots is apparent. That is, the time sequence of points in the plot describes a counterclockwise loop (Fig. 4) with effect tending to be greater at later sampling times. *Hysteresis*, a term familiar to engineers, denotes a time lag between force and response; $C_p(t)$ and $E(t)$ are out of phase. This finding has been misinterpreted as "clear" evidence for lack of a CER. There are several approaches to compensating for hysteresis. One is to sample from a matrix in apparent equilibrium with the effector site. Galezzi and associates [54] noted counterclockwise hysteresis in a plot of change in QT interval versus C_p after IV infusion of procainamide. Hystersis was not apparent when this effect was plotted against procainamide concentration in saliva, and a linear CER was achieved. The role of procainamide's active metabolite (*N*-acetylprocainamide; NAPA) was dismissed as negligible.

Relating effect to amount of drug in a peripheral pharmacokinetic compartment is a reasonable approach, but has not often been useful in practice. The time course of the minute fraction of the dose in the proximity of the receptor (an effect compartment) need not parallel bulk transfer of drug between pharmacokinetically identifiable compartments. A classic example of a CER entailing a peripheral pharmacokinetic compartment has been described in detail by Wagner [43,55] for decrease in arithmetic test performance after IV administration of lysergic acid diethylamide (LSD).

Inotropic response to digoxin was studied by Kramer et al. [56] by measurement of electromechanical systole (QS_2 interval) after IV bolus dosing of healthy subjects. Baseline correction was based on data from a separate group of untreated volunteers. Response kinetics bore little resemblance to the drugs pharmacokinetics. Amounts of digoxin in two peripheral compartments of a three-compartment model were calculated from C_p data by conventional pharmacokinetic methods. It was then possible to apply an E_{max} model to relate change

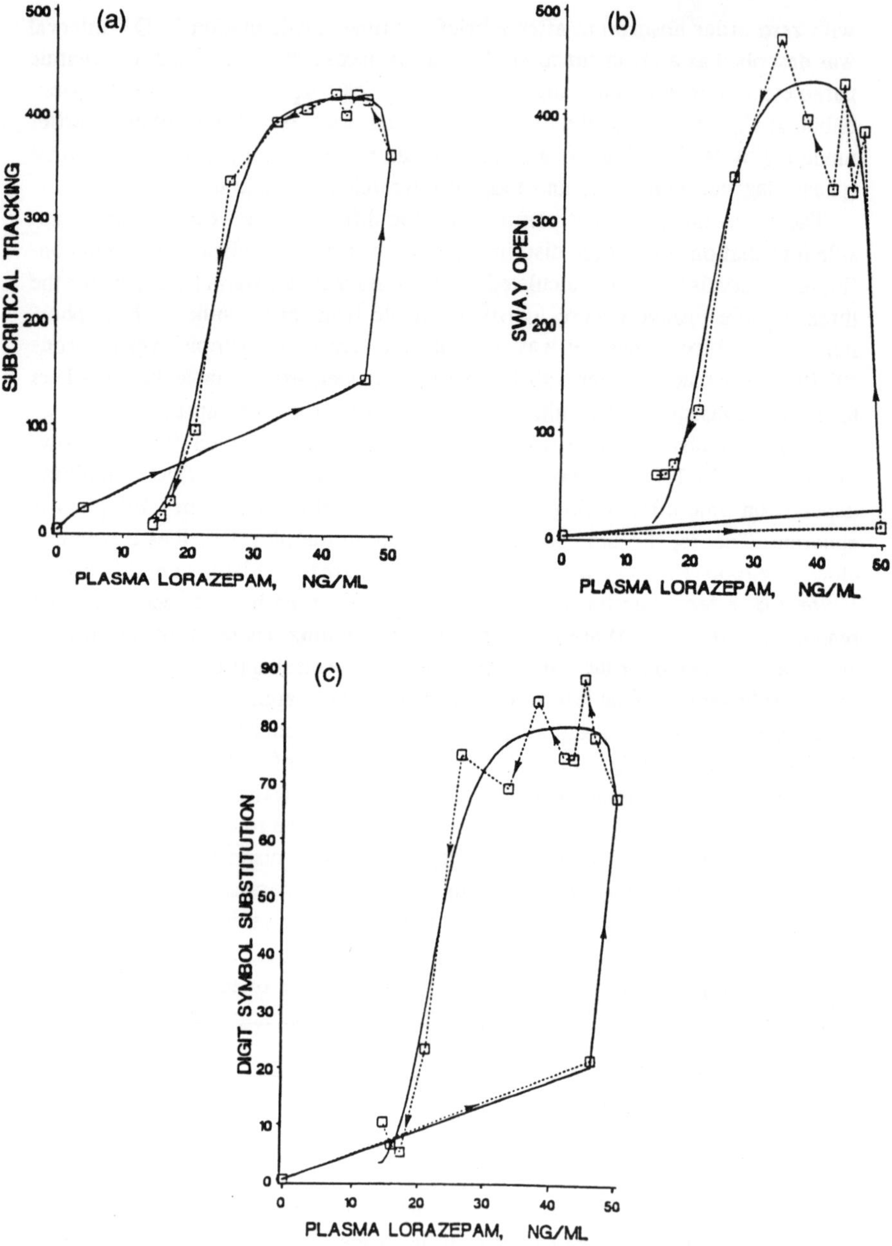

Figure 4 Hystersis loops for three psychomotor effect parameters after oral administration of the benzodiazepine, lorazepam. The temporal sequence of data points (squares) is indicated by the arrows. Solid lines are based on the PK/PD model developed by Gupta et al. (From Ref. 53.)

in QS_2 interval to amount of digoxin in the deep compartment. Data were averaged across all subjects; hence, it is not possible to tell if the relationship was representative of any individual.

Steady-State Measurements

A second approach to compensating for equilibration delays is to evaluate the CER at pharmacokinetic steady state, such as during constant IV infusion. At steady state, free drug is in equilibrium, and C_p and C_e are proportional to one another. An exceptionally rigorous and informative study that serves to contrast single-dose and steady-state PK/PD evaluations was published recently by Schwartz and colleagues [57]. Unfortunately, steady-state assessments are technically difficult, requiring protracted patient experimental time. It is subject to systematic error (e.g., from tolerance or fatigue), and verification of equilibrium may be a problem. For each steady state, only one (C, E) datapoint is obtained; accrual of data across the CER range may prove impracticable. A compelling alternative to steady-state assessment is effect compartment modeling.

Effect Compartment Models

Effect kinetics need not be congruous with the time course of drug in any pharmacokinetically identifiable compartment for a causal CER to exist. What is needed is compensation for delay in equilibration between sampling site and site of drug action. An intuitively reasonable concept is to use E(t) data itself to define the time lag. Inherent in the $C_p(t)$, E(t) data is the information necessary to define the rate of drug transfer between compartments. This does not mean that equilibration of drug concentrations is the only step leading to drug effect. The hypothetical effect compartment is a mathematical expediency. Invariably, complex physiological and biochemical processes intervene between the time the drug compound leaves the circulation and the time response is manifested.

In 1968 Segre [58] applied the effect compartment concept to describe a CER for norepinephrine. Subsequently Forrester et al. [59] defined response equilibration times for various cardiac glycosides. In 1978, Hull et al. [60] derived a first-order rate constant to describe the phase lag between C_p and C_e and, thereby, predict time of peak effect.

In 1979, formal development of an "effect compartment model" (Fig. 5) linked to a central compartment by a first-order rate constant, k_{eo}, was presented in a classic paper by Sheiner et al. [9] to describe an integrated PK/PD model for d-tubocurarine. The neuromuscular blocking agents such as this curare derivative have been extensively studied as prototypal drugs for PK/PD modeling, because reduction in muscle twitch can be accurately and precisely measured in patients undergoing surgery. Intravenous administration simplifies the PK/PD description and the phase lag beteen $C_p(t)$ and E(t), as exemplified by the data of

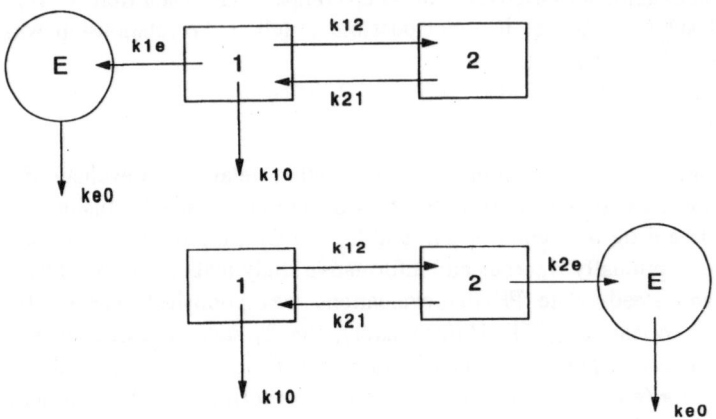

Figure 5 Schematic of effect compartment models with a link to either the central (upper) or peripheral (lower) compartment of a two-compartmental pharmacokinetic model. First-order rate constants for drug transfer between compartments are indicated. Note exclusion of a rate constant for return of drug to the driving compartment.

Evans et al. [61] for pancuronium, is shorter than for most drug classes (Fig. 6). Soon after application to neuromuscular blockers, effect compartment modeling was extended to disopyramide [10], theophylline [12], and quinidine [13]. Fundamental concepts, assumptions, and equations to support the models have been extensively reviewed by Holford and Sheiner [15–17].

The hypothetical effect compartment is not needed in pharmacokinetic characterization of the drug; it is irrelevant to description of mass transfer within the body. Its relevance is in describing the temporal relationship between of C_p and C_e, where C_e can be operationally defined as the concentration that, when used in the PK/PD model equation, describes a CER without hysteresis.

The two concentrations are related to one another by a "link" model, which, for the simplest case, is defined by the differential equation:

$$dA_e/dt = (k_{1e} \cdot A_1) - (k_{eo} \cdot A_e) \tag{11}$$

where A_e and A_1 are amounts of drug in the effect and central compartments and k_{1e} and k_{eo} are first-order rate constants for transfer into and out of the effect compartment, respectively. With a few reasonable assumptions, K_{1e} cancels out

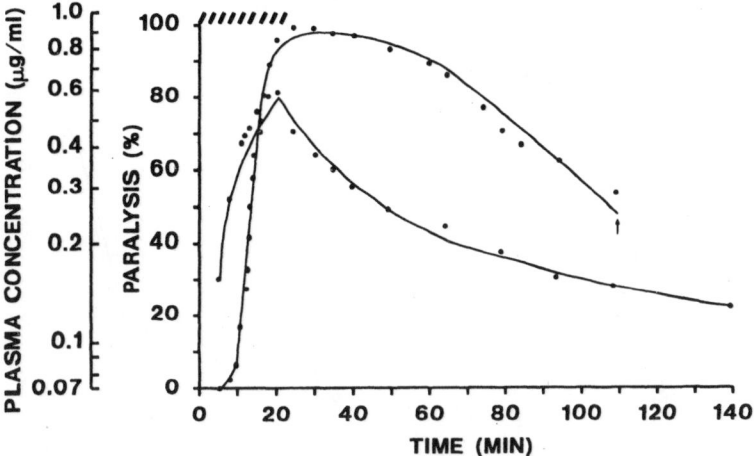

Figure 6 Contrast in time course of C_p and of neuromuscular blockade (upper curve) by pancuronium as assessed by mechanical twitch response in an individual patient under anesthesia. Striped bar indicates duration of IV infusion; the arrow shows time at which reversal agents were administered. Average (10 patients) half-time for effect compartment equilibration (ln $2/k_{eo}$) was 1.43 min. (From Ref. 61.)

in the expression for C_e, which for a drug conforming to a one-compartment pharmacokinetic model is

$$C_e = \frac{F \cdot D \cdot k_{eo}}{V(k_{eo} - k_e)} (e^{-k_e t} - e^{-k_{eo} t}) \tag{12}$$

where F is bioavailability, V is distribution volume, D is dose and k_e is elimination rate constant based on $C_p(t)$ data. The remarkable feature of Eq. (12) is that the only unknown parameter is k_{eo}, which is estimable by simultaneous fitting of (C_p, t) and (E, t) datapoints. If modeling is successful, then E can be plotted as a function of C_e, with no hysteresis present (Fig. 7). Since $C_p(t)$ is known and the equilibration delay between $C_p(t)$ and $C_e(t)$ is given by k_{eo}, and since the CER is a function of C_e, an integrated PK/PD mathematical model relating the three quantifiable variables $C_p(t)$, $E(t)$, and time is achieved. The value of this PK/PD model in assessment of bioequivalence is embodied in prediction of consequences of altered bioavailability on onset, intensity and duration of the (patho)pharmacological response.

The effect compartment model was tested by Colburn [14] with simulations over a wide range of pharmacokinetic and pharmacodynamic parameter values and was found versatile for a variety of pharmacokinetic behaviors. He extended

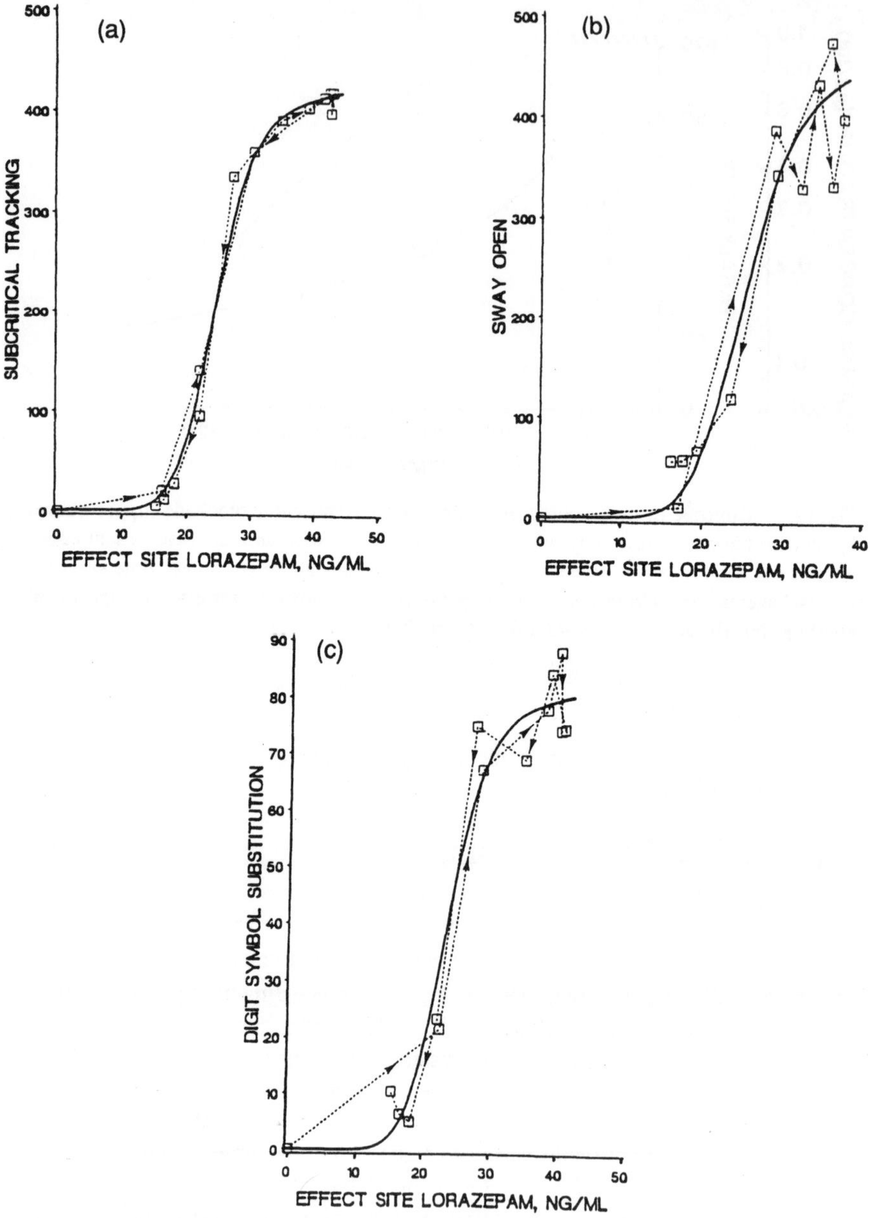

Figure 7 Relationship between three psychomotor effect parameters and calculated C_e after oral administration of the benzodiazepine, lorazepam. Symbols are actual data and solid lines indicate the CER defined by the PK/PD model. Comparison with Figure 4 indicates collapse of the hysteresis loop. (From Ref. 53.)

the concept to an effect compartment model linked to a peripheral, rather than central, compartment (see Fig. 5) and derived the necessary PK/PD equations for this model.

Complexities in Pharmacokinetic–Pharmacodynamic Assessment

An awareness of factors that alter the PK/PD relationship is necessary to conceptualize difficulties in application of any model in assessment of bioavailability. Examples of complications of practical importance are compiled in Table 2. Each of these is represented in the pharmacodynamic literature. A recent consideration of problematic factors in PK/PD investigations is given by Abernathy [62].

Formation of agonistic or antagonistic metabolites are a real concern in PK/PD modeling. A well-studied example is the antiarrhythmic procainamide and its active metabolite N-acetylprocainamide (NAPA). The contribution of active metabolites to observed benzodiazepine psychomotor activity is well known. Application of PK/PD modeling to assess pharmacodynamic consequences of altered

Table 2 Complicating Factors in Pharmacokinetic–Pharmacodynamic Assessments

Heterogeneous subject/patient population (between-subject variability)
Within-subject variability, especially in establishing baseline effect
Alteration of PK/PD relationships by disease state, circadian rhythms, meals, and demographic factors
Artifacts caused by data pooling, and rejection of "nonresponders"
Drug interactions—either pharmacokinetic or pharmacodynamic
Formation of active (agonist or antagonist) metabolites
Compensation within model for protein binding
Multiple receptors mediating opposing effects
Stereoisomers with distinct PK/PD properties
Nonlinear pharmacokinetic behavior
Insufficient concentration–effect data across response range
Indistinct, insensitive, or nonspecific pharmacologic endpoint
Errors in effect measures caused by learning and fatigue
Confounding physiological reflexes or homeostatic mechanisms
Development of tolerance or sensitization to drug
Nonequilibrium between sampled site and effect site (e.g., $k_{1e} \ll k_{12}$)
Extrapolation beyond model
Overparametrization of model; imprecise or highly correlated parameter estimates
Inappropriate model assumptions; nonunique model; failure to valdiate model (e.g., by predicting steady state from single-dose data)

oral bioavailability when active metabolites are formed is a complex matter addressed by Rowland [28]. Enantiomers of racemic drugs may have distinct pharmacokinetic and pharmacodynamic properties and present complications somewhat analogous to those for metabolites [34].

The first application of PK/PD effect compartment modeling to account for an active metabolite was published in 1983 by Meredith et al. [35]. They noted that after bolus IV injection the hypotensive effect time course for the α_1-adrenergic antagonist, trimazosin, was complex, having multiple maxima. They derived a PK/PD model that entailed production of hydroxytrimazosin by a first-order process, and an effect compartment linked to the central compartment. An optional model involved an additional metabolite effect compartment characterized with its own k_{eo} term. Total effect could be described as a linear combination of parent C_e and metabolite C_e. Alternative PK/PD models were compared by application of an F test, Akaike's information criterion [63], and evaluation of residuals, and thereby additional parameters of the more complex model were justified.

These investigators subsequently [37] described a trimazosin PK/PD model based on simultaneous fitting of C,E data derived from both oral and IV data. In this manner, the same valid model could be used to describe the complicated effect time course, irrespective of administration route (Fig. 8). The best of alternative models indicated that the sustained hypotensive action of trimazosin was primarily owing to the metabolite. A bioequivalence assessment of this chronically administered drug based solely on evaluation of single-dose pharmacokinetics for the parent compound would appear an oversimplification.

Few reports specifically address use of unbound, as opposed to total, drug concentrations, despite ubiquitous literature notes that only unbound drug is pharmacologically active. As noted earlier for propranolol's reduction of exercise-induced tachycardia [51], the PK/PD model fits for unbound propranolol were not much better than for total drug, as might be expected for a drug displaying linear binding behavior. In contrast are the findings of Thibonnier et al. [52], noted before for disopyramide, which displays nonlinear binding to plasma proteins.

Development of tolerance in drug response is common. Acute tolerance (tachyphylaxis) manifests itself as a clockwise hysteresis in CER plots. An informative example of clockwise hysteresis, attributed to tolerance development, is given by Ellinwood et al. [64] in a PK/PD study of the benzodiazepines, lorazepam, alprazolam, and diazepam. Distinct hysteretic behavior was exhibited by the different congeners, a finding with intriguing implications for interaction of the three congeners at the receptor site. Differentiating between tolerance and other possible causes of clockwise hysteresis (e.g., formation of an antagonistic metabolite or onset of fatigue) may not be easy. The possibility also exists that clockwise and counterclockwise hysteresis, arising from equilibration delay or

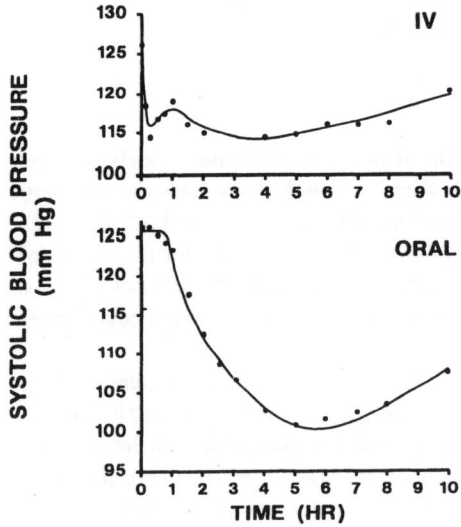

Figure 8 Description of a complex effect time course in an individual subject by means of a PK/PD model. Observed systolic blood pressure points and model predictions (solid lines) based on simultaneous fitting of C,E data for both trimazosin and its hydroxylated metabolite are shown. (From Ref. 36.)

from formation of an active metabolite, could offset one another. A direct relationship between C_p and E could be observed; however, the predictive value of the resultant PK/PD model would be suspect.

Undoubtedly, the most serious difficulty is validation of the PK/PD model that is to be used to predict the consequences of altered bioavailability. The ability to fit data to a set of equations does not necessarily mean they are the correct, unique set. A high coefficient of determination from a regression program does not validate the model or indicate the accuracy of predictions. Validation of PK/PD models is a complex task, addressed previously [14,25]. Overcoming problems of model validation may be the greatest impediment to acceptance of PK/PD methods in bioequivalence assessment.

POTENTIAL OF PHARMACOKINETIC–PHARMACODYNAMIC MODELS IN BIOEQUIVALENCE STUDIES

Pharmacodynamic Literature Relevant to Bioavailability Assessment

Recent literature illustrating application of pharmacodynamic models to assess bioavailability is reviewed in the following. In some cases, pharmacodynamic results based on effect parameters, such as CE_{max}, tE_{max}, and AUEC, were treated independent of corresponding pharmacokinetic results for the tested formulations. Occasionally, PK/PD modeling was pursued. We are not aware of any published study in which PK/PD modeling was directed toward development of bioequivalence criteria.

In a pioneering study, Smolen et al. [7] showed that rate and extent of chlorpromazine absorption could be precisely assessed by measuring pupil diameter as a function of time and, thereby, demonstrated bioavailability differences between dosage forms. Interestingly, pupilometry was a specific assay for chlorpromazine, whereas a concomitant effect, intraocular pressure, was nonspecific (i.e., dependent on chlorpromazine metabolites as well as unchanged drug). Subsequently, Smolen elaborated theoretical considerations based on systems analyses of bioavailability, [65,66]. Perhaps, because of mathematical complexity, this approach has not enjoyed widespread application.

Galeazzi [31] observed that absolute bioavailability of an oral dose of isosorbide dinitrate was only 25%. Comparison of AUEC based on peripheral vascular flow measurements for oral and IV dosing indicated pharmacodynamic bioavailability approached 90%. Galeazzi attributed this large difference between pharmacokinetic and pharmacodynamic bioavailability to the nature of the nonlinear log dose–response relationship that plateaus at high concentrations. Concentrations achieved after IV administration contributed much to AUC and little to AUEC.

Miller et al. [67] determined bioavailability of two tablet formulations of the diuretic metolazone on both pharmacokinetic and pharmacodynamic bases. Effect modeling was not reported. An enhancement in rate of absorption, apparent from plasma concentration data, corresponded to more rapid urinary excretion of salt. A large difference in pharmacokinetic bioavailability corresponded to a much smaller difference in bioavailability, based on diuresis.

Two allopurinol tablets were identified as pharmacokinetically bioequivalent by Nissen and Pedersen [68], who confirmed the finding by showing negligible differences between products in reducing plasma urate concentrations.

Molz and co-workers [69] subjected two glyburide (glibenclamide) formulations to bioequivalence testing using conventional pharmacokinetic methods. No statistically significant differences between mean pharmacokinetic parameters were observed. The plasma glucose time courses for the two hypoglycemic drug preparations were virtually identical. Thus, pharmacokinetic and pharmacodynamic equivalence was demonstrated for these specific conditions. A contrasting study on glyburide was performed by Ayanoglu et al. [70], who assessed test capsules relative to a marketed tablet (Euglucon). Rate and extent of glyburide absorption were much lower for the test formulation. Even though significant differences in blood glucose levels were identified, the pharmacodynamic differences were much smaller than the pharmacokinetic ones. Although the pharmacokinetic evaluation appeared the more discriminating test here, the therapeutic relevance of the pharmacokinetic data for this drug is questionable.

Olson et al. [71] found that pharmacodynamic measures that were based on serum glucose showed much smaller differences than could be demonstrated with serum tolbutamide concentrations when they studied the effects of food and tablet age on two tablet formulations. The two tablets were inequivalent from both a pharmacokinetic and pharmacodynamics perspective.

Propranolol pharmacokinetics and pharmacodynamics in healthy male subjects after administration of 80-mg and 160-mg doses of controlled-release propranolol capsules were studied by Flouvat et al. [72]. Doubling the dose approximately doubled systemically available drug; nevertheless, the magnitude and time course of reduction in exercise-induced tachycardia were similar for the two dose strengths. Thus, for these controlled-release products, it was easier to discriminate between the two strengths on a pharmacokinetic basis than on a pharmacodynamic one.

Pharmacokinetic and pharmacodynamic properties of a controlled-release tablet of the β_1-adrenergic antagonist metoprolol were compared with those of a conventional formulation in a study by Sanburg et al. [39]. Release of metoprolol from the controlled-release formulation was approximately zero-order over a 24-hr interval. The plasma concentration profile for dosing of the controlled-release tablet every 6 hr was distinct from that for twice-daily administration of the conventional tablet when determined at steady state (fifth day of dosing). Bioavailability of the controlled-release formulation was only a third of that for the conventional tablet. Nevertheless, the time courses for reduction in exercise-induced tachycardia for the two dosage forms were similar. Thus, metoprolol was more efficiently utilized after administration of the controlled-release product. Essentially similar results for comparison of controlled-release and conventional metoprolol formulations were reported recently by Lee and coworkers [73]. Oosteruis et al. [74] compared two controlled-release formulations of metoprolol on the basis of both pharmacokinetic and pharmacodynamic parameters. Mean (90% confidence interval) C_{max} for metoprolol CR/ZOK was 57% (46-69%) of that for the reference tablet. In contrast, mean CE_{max} was 95% (88-104%) of the reference mean. Thus, in all three studies of this β-blocker, pharmacokinetic comparisons were more discriminating than pharmacodynamic ones.

Krol et al. [75] studied bioavailability of nitrendipine tablets relative to a suspension dosage form of the antihypertensive. The C_{max} values coincided with maximal decrease in systolic blood pressure. Differences between tablet and suspension formulations were more apparent from nitrendipine C_p data than from pharmacodynamic data. These investigators noted a hysteresis loop for the relationship between C_p and blood pressure lowering, but did not pursue pharmacodynamic modeling.

The dromotropic effect of verapamil was investigated by Reiter et al. [76], who observed quite different CERs after administration of verapamil by three different administration routes. Higher C_p values relative to those for IV administration were necessary after oral administration to achieve the same degree of PR interval prolongation. They concluded that the drug was less potent when given orally and suggested route-dependent metabolism or physiological delay as possible mechanisms. That differences in rate of absorption of verapamil could affect the different CERs was put on sound theoretical footing by Colburn and co-workers [77]. With use of a PK/PD model based on two-compartmental pharmacokinetics, a central effect compartment, and a sigmoidal E_{max} function, they explained how absorption rate could influence effect compartment kinetics, resulting in divergent CERs (Fig. 9). More specifically, this theory indicated that a first-order input rate could significantly affect onset and duration of pharmacologic effect.

Holazo and associates [78] performed PK/PD modeling of the antiarrhythmic cibenzoline during multiple oral dose administration in a dose-escalation study. They also studied the impact on model parameter estimates of pooling the data. The premature ventricular contration (PVC) rate data were obtained from continuous ECK leads (Holter monitors) from four patients. The effect data were fitted to an inhibitory E_{max} model; baseline frequency data (E_0) were averaged over 6-hr intervals during a placebo treatment phase. A modeling assumption was that PVC rate could be abolished at high cibenzoline concentrations. Their PK/PD model based on pooled data was capable of characterizing antiarrhythmic activity at steady state.

Comparison of a soft gelatin capsule and an uncoated tablet of temazepam (hydroxydiazepam) was performed by Toumainen [79] with use of both pharmacokinetic and pharmacodynamic measures. Psychomotor performance (digit symbol substitution, letter cancellation, and Maddox wing test) and subjective measures (visual analog scales) were employed. Attempts to construct a CER were unsuccessful.

Triazolam is a 1,4-benzodiazepine, the major metabolites of which do not contribute to pharmacologic effects and, hence, do not complicate PK/PD modeling. In a recent study [80], Gupta and his co-workers modeled three psychomotor parameters by use of a sigmoidal E_{max} model, with a baseline determined during the placebo treatment of a two-way crossover study. The influence of learning

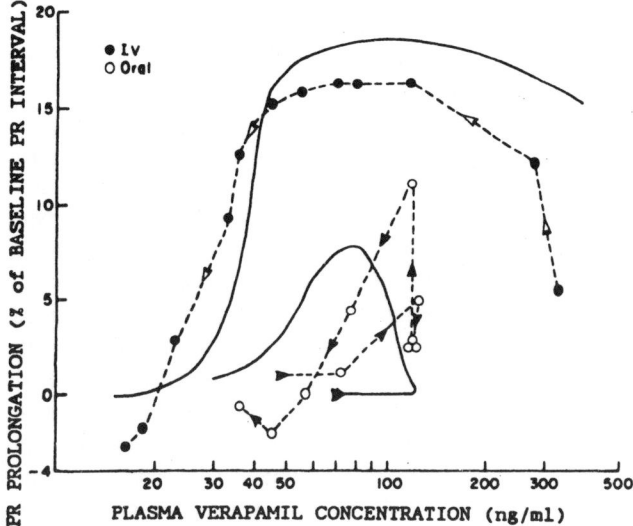

Figure 9 Explanation of administration route differences in CER for verapamil. Mean C_p and PR interval prolongation data originally reported by Reiter et al. [76] are indicated with circles with the temporal sequence denoted by arrows. Predictions of a PK/PD model derived by simultaneous fitting of (C_p E) oral and IV data are indicated by solid lines. (From Ref. 77.)

was minimized by prior training of subjects to a standardized level of performance in each test. Triazolam pharmacokinetics for individual subjects conformed to one- or two-compartment models, and fitted parameters were used for subsequent effect data fitting with an effect compartment model. Satisfactory fits to the data were obtained, although data extended only to two-thirds of E_{max}, suggesting that parameter estimates could be suspect. Mean parameter estimates for the various effects were similar to one another, and consistent with the assumptions of the model. The half-life for equilibration between the central and effect compartments was approximately 10 min.

The integrated PK/PD model for triazolam and the analogous PK/PD evaluation of lorazepam, published recently by Gupta and co-workers [53], are invaluable for prediction of how variations in benzodiazepine bioavailability from different formulations would affect pharmacodynamics of these anxiolytic agents. Comparison of discriminating ability of pharmacokinetic parameters relative to pharmacodynamic measures would be informative. It would be interesting to extend PK/PD modeling of lorazepam or triazolam to computer-analyzed EEG pharmacodynamic evaluations as applied by Itil and Itil [81]. By using this sophisticated brain-scanning method, these investigators could discern differences between diazepam (Valium) and a generic diazepam formulation deemed bioequivalent, according to FDA pharmacokinetic criteria. It is possible that higher discrimating ability of certain pharmacodynamic parameters is predictable.

Pharmacokinetics and pharmacodynamics of the β-adrenergic agonist terbutaline were modeled by Oosterhuis et al. [82] after subcutaneous administration of this bronchodilator. They noted little hysteresis in $C_p(t)$, $E(t)$ plots and suggested that the receptors were in closer proximity to the central compartment than to the peripheral one of a two-compartment model. Inclusion of an equilibrium delay (k_{eo}) improved the fit only slightly as evaluated by Akaike's statistical criterion for least-squares fitting. An average k_{eo} value of 5.5 hr^{-1} was observed for the FEV_1 respiratory parameter, corresponding to a mean equilibration half-life of approximately 10 min. The k_{eo} values for the various effect parameters were similar, as would be expected for effects mediated by the same receptor(s). Their PK/PD model provided a comprehensive description of the interrelationships between drug in the body, drug in the effect compartment, bronchodilatation, and time. However, it should be noted that first-order input can be rate-limiting and obscure relationships between pharmacokinetics and pharmacodynamics that might be discernible with bolus IV input [29].

The work by Cook et al. [83] represents an interesting variation on the PK/PD modeling theme. They modeled the natriuretic action of the loop diuretic bumetanide relative to drug excretion rate, not C_p data. Absolute bioavailability of an oral dose was only 81%; however, cumulative pharmacodynamic response was essentially the same for both administration routes. Thus, efficiency of the oral dose was greater than for IV administration. The sodium excretion rate was well described by a sigmoidal E_{max} model. The value of their study was enhanced by inclusion of patients with congestive heart failure, as well as normal subjects. Significantly lower E_{max} values were found for patients. No significant difference between the two groups was reported for C_{50}. Thus, it was possible to evaluate alterations in rate and extent of absorption, and differences in clinical status on pharmacodynamic parameters.

Use of Pharmacokinetic–Pharmacodynamic Models to Predict Consequences of Altered Bioavailability

Two drug products are deemed bioequivalent if they have the same bioavailability. From a pharmacokinetic perspective this means that the same amount of drug reaches the systemic circulation in any given time interval, regardless of drug product. From a pharmacodynamic perspective, this means the effect magnitude at any point in time, $E(t)$, is the same, regardless of drug product. Presumably, an equivalent $C_p(t)$ time course produces an equivalent concentration time course for the therapeutic substance(s) at the site of action, which yields an equivalent

E(t) time course. But, in the absence of a quantitative model linking $C_p(t)$, $C_e(t)$, and E(t) the validity of this assumption is difficult to verify.

Irrespective of the complexity of the PK/PD relationship, the presence of active metabolites, intra- and intersubject variability, tolerance, and so forth, if the two treatments have *identical* pharmacokinetics, it is difficult to argue that they really differ in effect parameters. The problem is prediction of the effect a 10 or 20% difference in bioavailability parameter estimates on onset, intensity, and duration of a therapeutic or adverse response. Another problem is comparison of dosage forms with different release characteristics. What criteria based solely on pharmacokinetics are meaningful for comparison of an controlled release capsule with a conventional one?

The PK/PD modeling can serve to test the validity of pharmacokinetic-based bioavailability—to affirm or negate the relevance of $C_p(t)$ data. Without such an evaluation, one has to rely on arbitrary criteria. The mathematical model enables comparison of relative rates of pharmacokinetic and pharmacodynamic processes and, thereby, identification of the parameters that will be most discriminating between products. Benefits beyond the bioequivalence issue considered in this chapter are projections of optimal dose and dose frequency for a particular drug and delivery system and enhancement of therapeutic drug monitoring.

Equations defining the kinetics of pharmacologic effects corresponding to classic compartmental pharmacokinetics and effect models were delineated through pioneering works of Levy, Gibaldi, Wagner, and others [41–43,46–49]. The time course of pharmacologic effect can be described for effect-compartment models in an analogous manner. With specification of a minimal effective concentration or an effect threshold, onset and duration of drug response can be predicted with a reasonable degree of confidence.

Application of PK/PD models to bioequivalence problems is illustrated by the work of Olson et al. [84]. They expanded upon principles noted by Levy [8] concerning consequences on pharmacologic effect of a 50% decrease in extent of absorption. Given a hyperbolic CER (Fig. 10), there is little consequence when $C >> C_{50}$. The influence on effect increases with decreasing dose or concentration. From simulations of an E_{max} model for a drug conforming to a one-compartment pharmacokinetic model, Olson and his co-workers found that differences in effect duration caused by bioavailability differences allowed under bioequivalence guidelines, were likely to be minor when compared with those caused by natural variability (Fig. 11). Their conclusion is consistent with the aforementioned literature, suggesting that it is often easier to detect differences in pharmacokinetics than in effect parameters, even when biological variation in response is eliminated.

The complementation of conventional bioequivalence assessment with pharmacodynamics facilitates comparison of dosage forms that are different by design. Comparison of a controlled-release tablet with an immediate-release capsule on

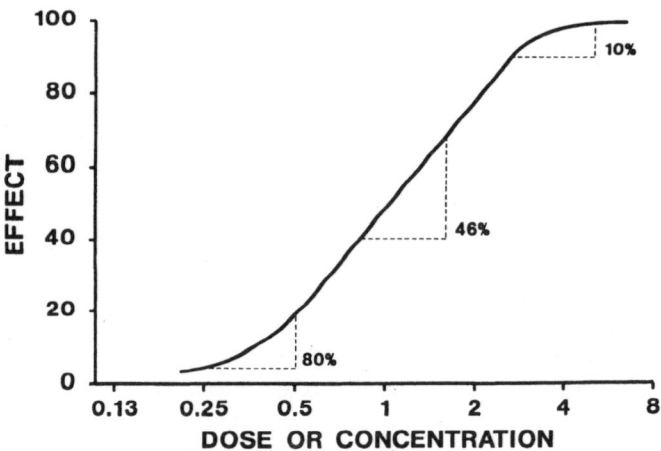

Figure 10 Consequence of 50% decrease in bioavailability on pharmacologic effect. (From Ref. 8.)

the basis of C_p data lone is discordant. The extent of absorption from the controlled-release product may be relatively low; however, if drug concentrations do not exceed the log-linear region of the E_{max} curve, whereas concentrations for the immediate-release product saturate the effect, the two dosage forms may be have equivalent effectiveness. In the range in which E is proportional to log C_p, fluctuation in response tends to be attenuated relative to fluctuations in C_p. Examples are noted in the preceding section.

An informative assessment of the impact of altered bioavailability during repeated dosing was published by Grével et al. [85,86], who used suppression of plasma prolactin by an experimental dopamine antagonist as the prototype. By assuming two-compartmental pharmacokinetics and a sigmoidal E_{max} equation, they predicted the influence on steady-state effect measurements of a sudden drop in bioavailability, such as would occur with substitution of an inferior product (Fig. 12). Simulations indicated that the impact would depend on dose regimen, as well as the PK/PD model characteristics for the individual patient. Their model was derived from fitting (C_p, E) data after a single oral dose, and it may not provide a unique mathematical solution; a different model would yield different multiple-dose projections. Undoubtedly, validation of PK/PD modeling projections is the preeminent problem that must be addressed in future studies.

Pharmacodynamic Models in Bioequivalence

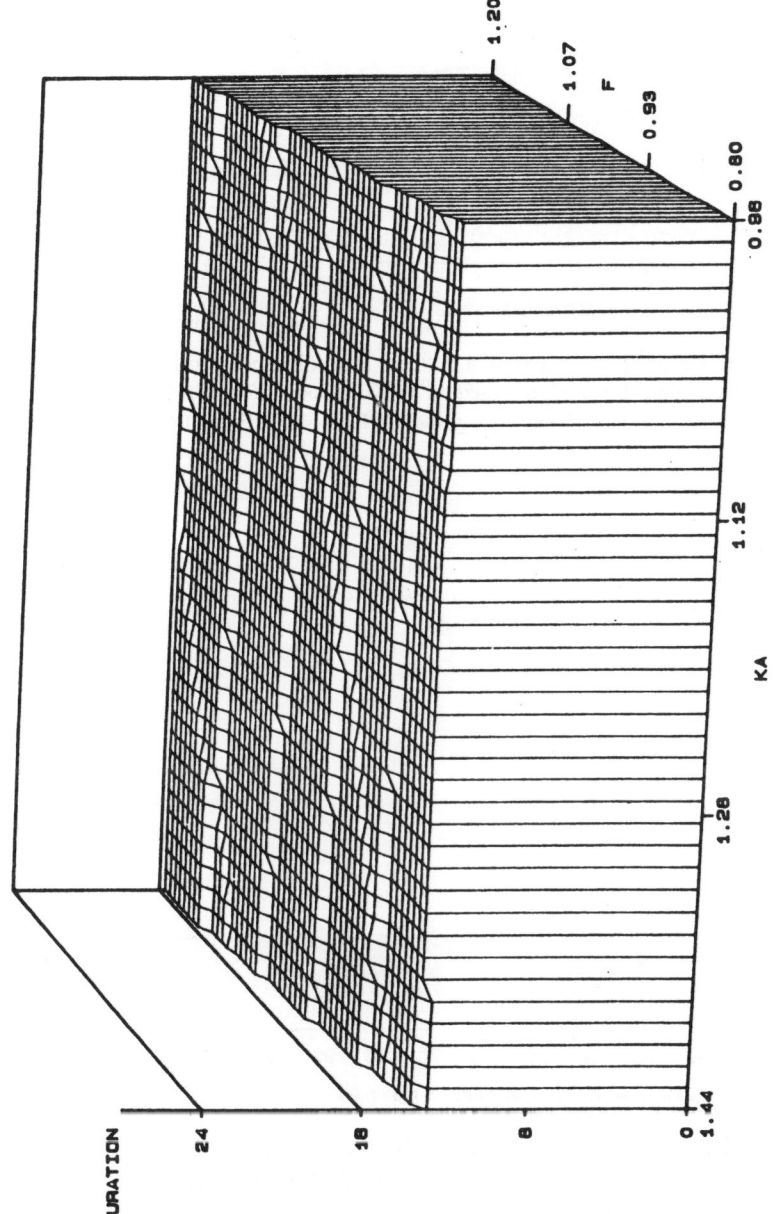

Figure 11 Impact of a 20% variation in absorption rate constant, k_a, and extent of absorption, F, after a single oral dose of a hypothetical drug with a 3-hr half-life. The simulation was based on a PK/PD model entailing monoexponential pharmacokinetics, an effect compartment ($k_{eo} = 0.25$ hr^{-1}) and an E_{max} model. (From Ref. 84.)

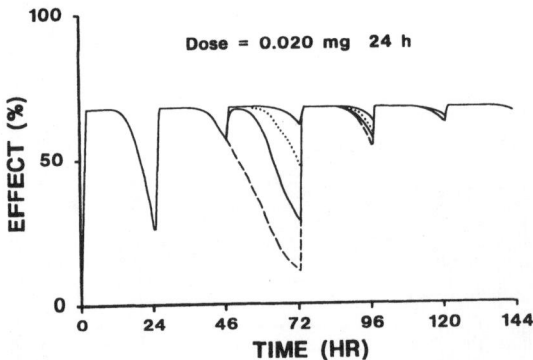

Figure 12 Pharmacodynamic impact of a decrease in absolute bioavailability, F, occurring with the third dose. Simulations based on a PK/PD model for an individual subject after oral administration of a dopamine agonist CQP201-403. (From Ref. 86.)

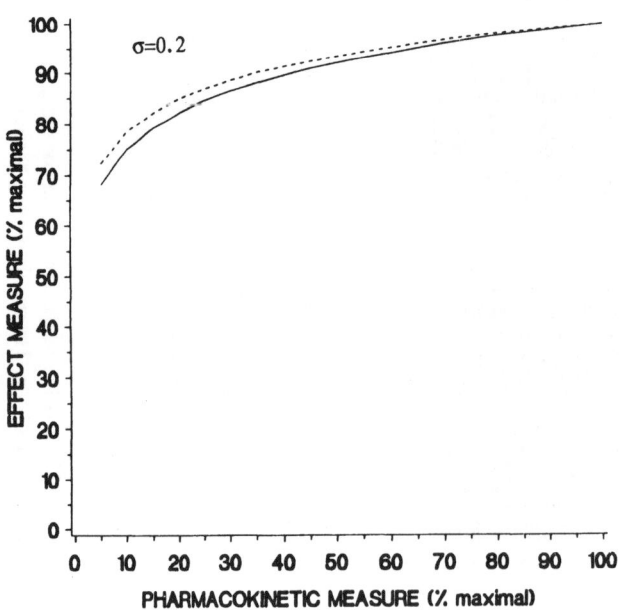

Figure 13 Relationship between pharmacokinetic parameters and pharmacodynamic parameters as F decreases from 100% [the point (100,100)] to 5% (point nearest origin). Simulations for a hypothetical PK/PD model based on monoexponential IV pharmacokinetics, a sigmoidal E_{max} CER, and an effect compartment described by a first-order rate constant, k_{eo}. For each of the three panels, corresponding to σ values of 0.2, 1, and 10, the two curves are C_0 vs E_{att}/E_{max} (------) and AUC vs AUEC (———).

Pharmacodynamic Models in Bioequivalence

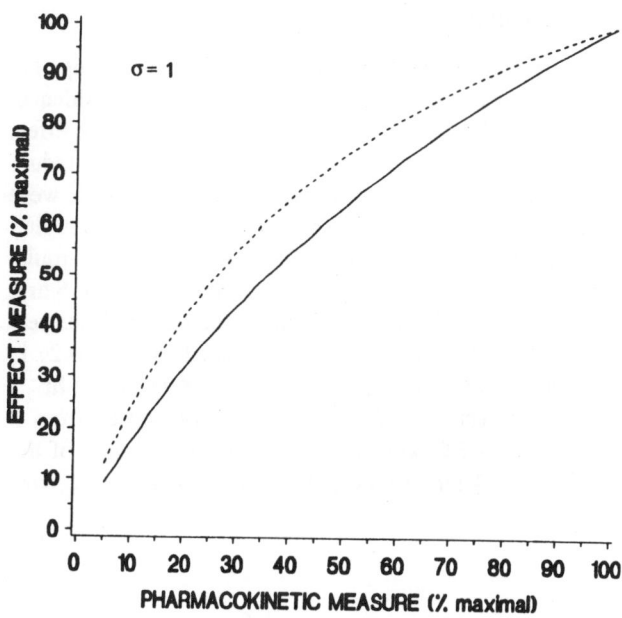

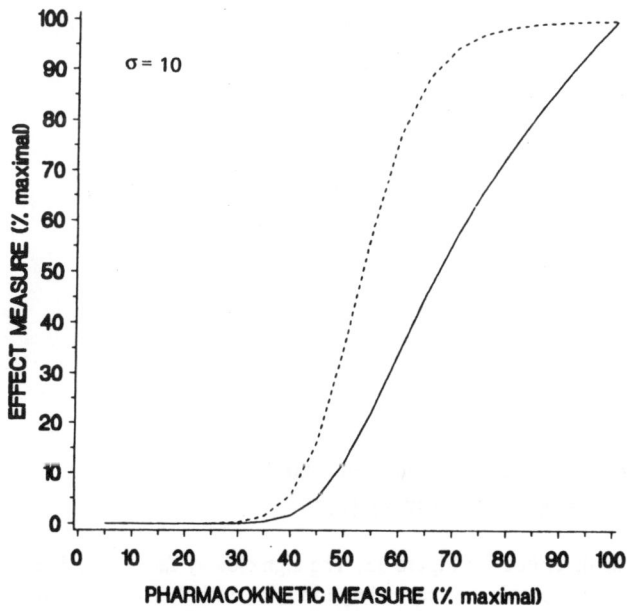

Figure 13 *(Continued)*

Pharmacokinetic–Pharmacodynamic Model Simulations

To illustrate application of PK/PD modeling for evaluation of relationships between pharmacokinetic and pharmacodynamic parameters of bioequivalence, simulations based on a sigmoidal E_{max} CER [see Eq. (4)] and the simple effect compartment model [see Eq. (12)] were performed. Consequences of a reduction in extent of absorption, F, on pharmacokinetic variables C_0 and AUC were compared with the effects on pharmacodynamic parameters E'_{max} and AUEC. Here E'_{max} was maximal attainable effect for F < 100%. Constants for simulation were C_0 = FD/V = 100 µg/mL, k_e = 0.116 (elimination half-life of 6 hr), E_{max} = 100, and C_{50} = 40 µg/mL. Five pharmacodynamic parameter value sets were used. With k_{eo} = 1.0 hr^{-1}, effect curves were simulated for σ = 0.2, 1, and 10. With σ = 1, effect curves were simulated for k_{eo} = 0.0693 and 25 hr^{-1}, as well as for k_{eo} = 1 hr^{-1}. For each of the five cases, F was varied from 5 to 100% of the dose. E'_{max} and AUEC were expressed as a percentage of the parameter value when F = 100%. Time of maximal attainable effect, tE_{max}, was also calculated.

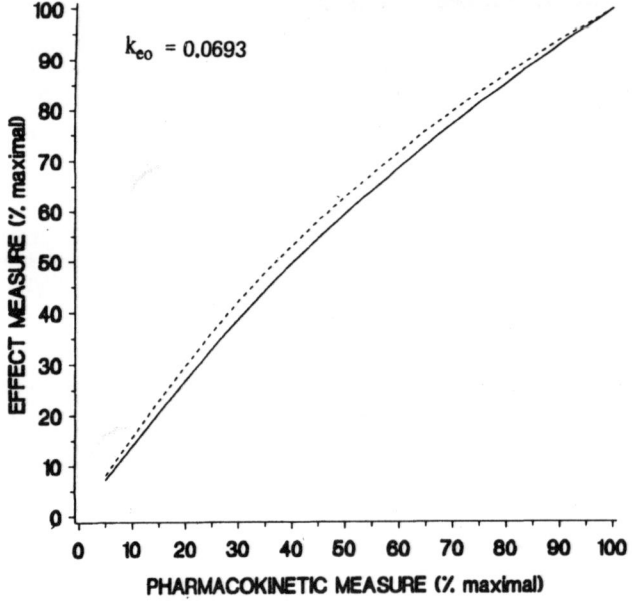

Figure 14 Simulations as described for Figure 13. The sigmoidicity factor was fixed at σ = 1. For each of the three panels, corresponding to k_{eo} = 0.0693, 1.0, or 25, the two curves are C_0 vs E_{att}/E_{max} (----) and AUC vs AUEC (———). The case of σ = 1 and k_{eo} = 1 is repeated from Figure 13.

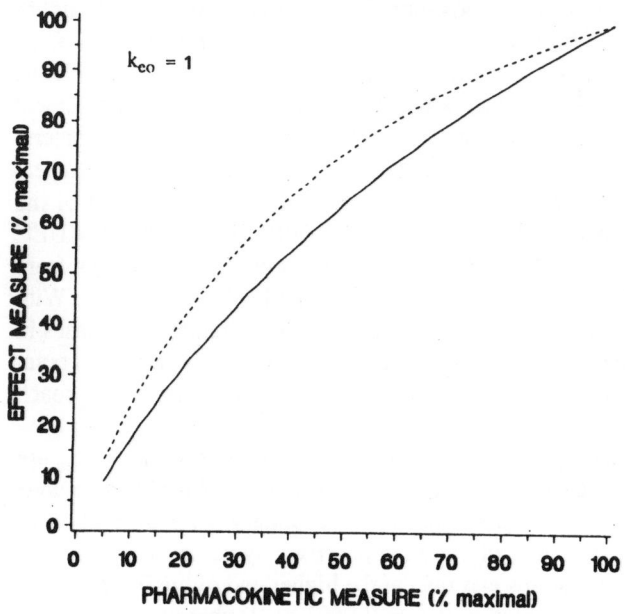

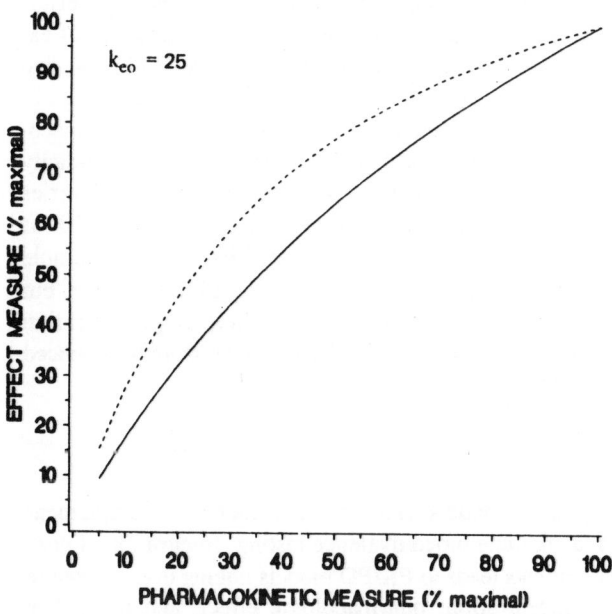

Figure 14 *(Continued)*

Simulations for $k_{eo} = 1$ hr^{-1}, corresponding to an half-life of 0.693 hr for effect compartment equilibration, are shown in Fig. 13. For a shallow CER ($\sigma = 0.2$), decreases in effect parameters with decreasing F are small relative to decreases in C_{max} and AUC. Only when F falls below 10% is the decrement in E'_{max} and AUEC proportionally greater than for pharmacokinetic parameters. For a moderate CER slope ($\sigma = 1$), decreases in pharmacodynamic parameters are proportional to decreases in pharmacokinetic parameters over most of the range. For example, when AUC declines from 50 to 40% (20% decline), AUEC declines from 64 to 55% (15% decline). Similarly, when AUC declines from 10 to 8% (20% decline), AUEC declines from 17 to 14% (19% decline). With a steep CER ($\sigma = 10$), small decreases in F can result in dramatic decreases in AUEC, with little change in E'_{max} until C_{max} declines below 70%, at which point E'_{max} declines precipitously. For F < 30%, AUEC and E'_{max} values approach zero.

Simulations for a fixed sigmoidicity value ($\sigma = 1$) and three values of k_{eo} are shown in Fig. 14, with the $k_{eo} = 1$ hr^{-1} hr case repeated from the previous figure. For $k_{eo} = 25$ hr^{-1}, representing nearly instantaneous equilibration of plasma and effect compartments, alteration in pharmacodynamic parameters are proportionately greater at the low end than at the higher end of the F range. For slow-effect compartment equilibration ($k_{eo} = 0.0693$ hr^{-1}) pharmacokinetic and pharmacodynamic parameters generally change in proportion to one another.

The tE_{max} parameter is a function of k_{eo}, but not σ or F. That is, peak effect time depends on the rate of effect compartment equilibration, irrespective of extent of absorption. With k_{eo} values of 25, 1, and 0.0693, tE_{max} is 0.22, 2.4, and 11 hr, respectively.

Comparison of Figs. 13 and 14 reveals that the relationship between pharmacodynamic and pharmacokinetic parameters depends more on the sigmoidicity parameter than on k_{eo}. When $\sigma = 1$, similar curves are obtained as k_{eo} varies from 0.0693 to 25 hr^{-1}. Curves corresponding to σ values of 0.2, 1, and 10 for a fixed k_{eo} of 1 are markedly different from one another. That is, in this simple model, the relationship is relatively insensitive to in vivo equilibration time, but sensitive to CER curve slope in the region of C_{50}. For a steep slope, alteration in pharmacologic response with decreased bioavailability can be more pronounced than alteration in C_{max} and AUC.

CONCLUSION

In this chapter pharmacodynamic models have been considered as complementary to conventional pharmacokinetic bioequivalence testing. Integration of concentration and effect measurements leads to PK/PD models linking dose, systemic concentration, effect site concentration, pharmacologic effect, and time. The PK/PD modeling based on a hypothetical effect compartment provides a practical,

Table 3 Potential Applications of Pharmacodynamic Models in Bioequivalence Assessment

---
Determination of pharmacokinetic parameters that are most relevant to therapeutic equivalence

Evaluation of alternative dosage forms and administration routes

Identification of active drug moieties

Prediction of impact of altered bioavailability on onset, intensity, and duration of pharmacologic or adverse response

Extrapolation of single-dose data to multiple-dose regimens

Establishment of bioequivalence criteria tailored to special patient populations

---

reasonable approach to understanding concentration–effect relationships for many drug classes. The PK/PD models are useful for predicting consequences of an alteration in rate or extent of absorption.

In this sense, PK/PD modeling is the logical step beyond pharmacokinetics toward verification of therapeutic equivalence (Table 3). It serves to verify the relevance of pharmacokinetic measures by quantitative description of how alterations in drug concentrations affect onset, intensity and duration of pharmacologic response. The relative discriminating power of pharmacokinetic and pharmacodynamic measures under specific conditions can be described quantitatively. If the measured drug effect is an efficacy surrogate, then pharmacokinetic bioequivalence can be linked to therapeutic equivalence. In this manner, pitfalls inherent in exclusive use of either pharmacokinetic or pharmacodynamic parameters to assess performance of a drug substance and formulation can be mimimized.

Application of pharmacodynamic models to bioequivalence assessment represents a union of two complex fields of study. In comparison with conventional pharmacokinetic testing and statistical criteria, use of PK/PD methods in pursuit of the most rational bioequivalence criteria is at a rudimentary stage. The potential of PK/PD modeling to provide practical solutions to bioequivalence issues will be understood only as specific drug products are subjected to rigorous PK/PD analysis. If survey of recent literature is any indication, then realization of this potential is assured.

REFERENCES

1. Bioequivalence requirements and in vivo bioavailability procedure. *Fed. Reg.* 42:1624–1653 (1977).
2. Code of Federal Regulations (revised) Title 21: Food and Drugs, Part 320. Bioavailability and bioequivalence requirements (April 1, 1981).

3. J. C. Somberg. Bioequivalence or therapeutic equivalence. *J. Clin. Pharmacol.* 26:1 (1986).
4. H. R. Dettelbach. A time to speak out on bioequivalence and therapeutic equivalence. *J. Clin. Pharmacol.* 26:307–308 (1986).
5. P. P. Lamy. Generic equivalents: Issues and concerns. *J. Clin. Pharmacol.* 26:309–316 (1986).
6. L. K. Paalzow. Integrated pharmacokinetic–dynamic modeling of drugs acting on the CNS. *Drug Metab. Rev.* 15:383–400 (1984).
7. V. F. Smolen, E. J. Williams, and P. B. Kuehn. Bioavailability and pharmacokinetic analysis of chlorpromazine in humans and animals using pharmacological data. *Can. J. Pharm. Sci.* 10:95–106 (1975).
8. G. Levy. Bioavailability, clinical effectiveness, and the public interest. *Pharmacology* 8:33–43 (1972).
9. L. B. Sheiner, D. R. Stanski, S. Vozeh, R. D. Miller, and J. Ham. Simultaneous modeling of pharmacokinetics and pharmacodynamics: Application to *d*-tubocurarine. *Clin. Pharmacol. Ther.* 25:358–371 (1979).
10. B. Whiting, N. H. G. Holford, and L. B. Sheiner. Quantitative analysis of the disopyramide concentration–effect relationship. *Br. J. Clin. Pharmacol.* 9:67–75 (1980).
11. A. W. Kelman and B. Whiting. Modeling of drug response in individual subjects. *J. Pharmacokinet. Biopharm.* 8:115–130 (1980).
12. B. Whiting, A. W. Kelman, J. Barclay, G. J. Addis. Modelling theophylline response in individual patients with chronic bronchitis. *Br. J. Clin. Pharmacol.* 12:481–487 (1981).
13. N. H. G. Holford, P. E. Coates. T. W. Guentert, S. Riegelman, and L. B. Sheiner. The effect of quinidine and its metabolites on the electrocardiogram and systolic time intervals: Concentration–effect relationships. *Br. J. Clin. Pharmacol.* 11:187–195 (1981).
14. W. A. Colburn. Simultaneous pharmacokinetic and pharmacodynamic modeling. *J. Pharmacokinet. Biopharm.* 9:367–388 (1981).
15. N. H. G. Holford and L. B. Sheiner. Pharmacokinetic and pharmacodynamic modeling in vivo. *CRC Crit. Rev. Bioeng.* 5:273–322 (1981).
16. N. H. G. Holford and L. B. Sheiner. Understanding the dose–effect relationship: Clinical application of pharmacokinetic–pharmacodynamic models. *Clin. Pharmacokinet.* 6:429–453 (1981).
17. N. H. G. Holford and L. B. Sheiner. Kinetics of pharmacologic response. *Pharmacol. Ther.* 16:143–166 (1982).
18. W. A. Ritschel and A. Hussain. Review on correlation between pharmacologic response and drug disposition. *Methods Find. Exp. Clin. Pharmacol.* 6:627–640 (1984).
19. W. A. Colburn and R. K. Brazzell. Pharmacokinetics as an aid to understanding drug effects. In *Advances in Pain Research and Therapy*, Vol. 8 (K. M. Foley and C. E. Inturrisi, eds.) Raven Press, New York, pp. 427–440 (1986).
20. N. H. G. Holford. Clinical pharmacokinetics and pharmacodynamics of warfarin. Understanding the dose–effect relationship. *Clin. Pharmacokinet.* 11:483–504 (1986).

21. B. Oosterhuis and C. J. van Boxtel. Kinetics of drug effects in man. *Ther. Drug Monit.* *10*:121–132 (1988).
22. J. Dingemanse, M. Danhof, and D. D. Breimer. Pharmacokinetic-pharmacodynamic modeling of CNS drug effects: An overview. *Pharm. Ther.* *38*:1–52 (1988).
23. PCNONLIN, Statistical Consultants, Inc., 300 East Main St., Suite 400, Lexington, Kentucky 40507-1539.
24. SAS Institute Inc., Box 8000, Cary, North Carolina, 27511-8000.
25. W. A. Colburn. Pharmacokinetic/pharmacodynamic modeling: Study design considerations. In *Pharmacokinetics and Pharmacodynamics: Research Design and Analysis* (R. B. Smith, P. D. Kroboth, and R. P. Juhl, eds.) Harvey Whitney Books, Cincinnati, pp. 65–84 (1986).
26. L. K. Paalzow and P. O. Edlund. Multiple receptor responses: A new concept to describe the relationship between pharmacological effects and pharmacokinetics of a drug: Studies on clonidine in the rat and the cat. *J. Pharmacokinet. Biopharm.* *7*:495–510 (1979).
27. A. Wellstein, D. Palm, H. F. Pitchner, and G. G. Belz. Receptor binding of propranolol is the missing link between plasma concentration kinetics and the effect-time course in man. *Eur. J. Clin. Pharmacol.* *29*:131–147 (1985).
28. M. Rowland. Bioavailability assessment and pharmacologic response: Impact of first-pass loss when drug and metabolites are active. *J. Pharmacokinet. Biopharm.* *16*:573–593 (1988).
29. W. A. Colburn and D. M. Gibson. Endogenous agonists and pharmacokinetic/pharmacodynamic modeling of baseline effects. In *Pharmacokinetics and Pharmacodynamics, Vol. 2, Current Problems and Potential Solutions* (P. D. Kroboth, R. B. Smith, and R. P. Juhl, eds.) Harvey Whitney Books, Cincinnati, pp. 168–184 (1988).
30. W. A. Colburn. Pharmacokinetics/pharmacodynamics: Measures, models and manipulations. In *Simulation at the Frontiers of Science* (J. Young, V. W. Ingalls, and R. Hawkins, eds.) Society for Computer Simulation, San Diego, pp. 7–11 (1986).
31. R. L. Galeazzi. Simultaneous modeling of pharmacodynamics and pharmacokinetics. *J. Pharmacol. (Paris)* *17*(Suppl. 1):63–70 (1986).
32. T. L. Swinghammer and P. D. Kroboth. Basic concepts in pharmacodynamic modeling. *J. Clin. Pharmacol.* *28*:388–394 (1988).
33. R. J. Myerburg, K. M. Kessler, I. Kiem, K. C. Pekfaros, C. A. Conde, D. Cooper, and A. Castellanos. Relationship between plasma levels of procainamide, suppression of ventricular complexes and prevention of recurrent ventricular tachycardia. *Circulation* *64*:280–290 (1981).
34. J. B. Schuttler, D. Stanksi, P. F. White, A. J. Trevor, Y. Horai, D. Verotta, and L. B. Sheiner. Pharmacodynamic modeling of the EEG effects of ketamine and its enantiomers in man. *J. Pharmacokinet. Biopharm.* *15*:241–253 (1987).
35. P. A. Meredith, A. W. Kelman, H. L. Elliot, and J. L. Reid. Pharmacokinetic and pharmacodynamic modeling of trimazosin and it major metabolite. *J. Pharmacokinet. Biopharm.* *11*:323–330 (1983).
36. A. W. Kelman, P. A. Meredith, H. L. Elliot, and J. L. Reid. Modeling the pharmacokinetics and pharmacodynamics of trimazosin. *Biopharm. Drug Dispos.* *7*:373–388 (1986).

37. H. L. Elliot, R. Donnelly, P. A. Meredith, and J. L. Reid. Predictability of antihypertensive responsiveness and α-antagonism during prazosin treatment. *Clin. Pharmacol. Ther.* 46:576–583 (1989).
38. R. Donnelly, P. A. Meredith, and H. L. Elliot. Pharmacokinetic–pharmacodynamic relationships of α-adrenoceptor antagonists. *Clin. Pharmacokinet.* 17:264–274 (1989).
39. A. Sandberg, I. Blomqvist, U. E. Jonsson, and P. Lundborg. Pharmacokinetic and pharmacodynamic properties of a new controlled-release formulation of metoprolol: A comparison with conventional tablets. *Eur. J. Clin. Pharmacol.* 33 (Suppl): S9–S14 (1988).
40. E. Blychert, T. Hedner, C. Dahlof, and D. Elmfeldt. Plasma concentration–effect relationships of intravenous and extended-release oral felodipine in hypertensive patients. *J. Cardiovasc. Pharmacol.* 15:428–435 (1990).
41. J. G. Wagner. Kinetics of pharmacologic response. I. Proposed relationships between response and drug concentrations in the intact animal and man. *J. Theor. Biol.* 20:173–201 (1968).
42. J. G. Wagner. Relations between drug concentrations and response. *J. Mond. Pharm.* 4:14–31 (1971).
43. J. G. Wagner. *Fundamentals of Clinical Pharmacokinetics*. Drug Intelligence Publications, Hamilton, Ill., pp. 307–335 (1975).
44. A. V. Hill. The possible effects of the aggregation of the molecules of haemoglobin on its dissociation curves, *J. Physiol. (Lond.)* 40:IV–VII, (1910).
45. R. Koopmans, J. Dingemanse, M. Danhof, G. P. M. Horsten, and C. J. van Boxtel. Pharmacokinetic–pharmacodynamic modeling of midazolam effects on the human central nervous system. *Clin. Pharmacol. ther.* 44:14–22 (1988).
46. G. Levy and E. Nelson. Theoretical relationship between dose, elimination rate and duration of pharmacologic effect of drugs. *J. Pharm. Sci.* 54:812 (1965).
47. G. Levy. Kinetics of pharmacologic effects. *Clin. Pharmacol. Ther.* 7:362–372 (1966).
48. G. Levy, M. Gibaldi, and W. Jusko. Multicompartment pharmacokinetic models and pharmacologic effects. *J. Pharm. Sci.* 58:422–424 (1969).
49. M. Gibaldi and D. Perrier. *Pharmacokinetics*, 2nd ed. Marcel Dekker, New York, pp. 221–269 (1982).
50. K. R. Lees and J. L. Reid. Effects of intravenous S-9780, an angiotensin-converting enzyme inhibitor, in normotensive subjects *J. Cardiovasc. Pharmacol.* 10:129–135 (1987).
51. R. L. Lalonde, R. J. Straka, J. A. Pieper, M. B. Bottorff, and D. M. Mirvis. Propranolol pharmacodynamic modeling using unbound and total concentrations in healthy volunteers, *J. Pharmacokinet. Biopharm.* 15:569–582 (1987).
52. M. Thibonnier, N. H. G. Holford, R. A. Upton, C. D. Blume, and R. L. Williams. Pharmacokinetic–pharmacodynamic analysis of unbound disopyramide directly measured in serial plasma samples in man. *J. Pharmacokinet. Biopharm.* 12:559–573 (1984).
53. S. K. Gupta, E. H. Ellinwood, A. M. Nikaido, and D. G. Heatherly. Simultaneous modeling of the pharmacokinetic and pharmacodynamic properties of benzodiazepines. I. Lorazepam. *J. Pharmacokinet. Biopharm.* 18:89–102 (1990).
54. R. L. Galeazzi, L. Z. Benet, and L. B. Sheiner. Relationship between the

pharmacokinetics and pharmacodynamics of procainamide. *Clin. Pharmacol. Ther.* 20:278-289 (1976).
55. J. G. Wagner, G. K. Agahajanian, and O. H. Bing. Correlation of performance test scores with "tissue concentrations" of LSD in human subjects. *Clin. Pharmacol. Ther.* 9:635-638 (1968).
56. W. G. Kramer, A. J. Kolibash, R. P. Lewis, M. S. Bathala, J. A. Visconti, and R. H. Reuning. Pharmacokinetics of digoxin: Relationship between intensity and predicted compartmental drug levels in man. *J. Pharmacokinet. Biopharm.* 7:47-61 (1979).
57. J. B. Schwartz, D. Verotta, and L. B. Sheiner. Pharmacodynamic modeling of verapamil effects under steady-state and nonsteady-state conditions. *J. Pharmacol. Exp. Ther.* 251:1032-1038 (1989).
58. G. Segre. Kinetics of interaction between drugs and biological systems. *Il Farm.* 23:907-918 (1968).
59. W. Forrester, R. P. Lewis, A. M. Weissler, and T. A. Wilke. The onset and magnitude of the contractile response to commonly used digitalis glycosides in normal subjects. *Circulation* 49:517-521 (1974).
60. C. J. Hull, H. B. H. van Beem, K. McLeod, A. Sibbald, and M. J. Watson. A pharmacodynamic model for pancuronium. *Br. J. Anesth.* 50:1113-1123 (1978).
61. M. A. Evans, C. A. Shanks, K. F. Brown, and E. J. Triggs. Pharmacokinetic and pharmacodynamic modeling with pancuronium. *Eur. J. Clin. Pharmacol.* 26:243-250 (1984).
62. D. R. Abernethy. Problematic factors in pharmacodynamic studies. In *Pharmacodynamic and Pharmacodynamics*, Vol. 2, *Current Problems and Potential Solutions* (P. D. Kroboth, R. B. Smith, and R. P. Juhl, eds.) Harvey Whitney Books, Cincinnati, pp. 60-74 (1988).
63. K. Yamaoka, T. Nakgawa, and T. Uno. Application of Akaike's information criterion (AIC) in the evaluation of linear pharmacokinetic equations. *J. Pharmacokinet. Biopharm.* 6:165-175 (1978).
64. E. H. Ellinwood, D. G. Heatherly, A. M. Kikaido, T. D. Bjornsson, and C. Kilts. Comparative pharmacokinetics and pharmacodynamics of lorazepam, alprazolam and diazepam. *Psychopharmacology* 86:392-399 (1985).
65. V. F. Smolen. Theoretical and computational basis for drug bioavailability determinations using pharmacological data. I. General considerations and procedures. *J. Pharmacokinet. Biopharm.* 4:337-353 (1976).
66. V. F. Smolen. Bioavailability and pharmacokinetic analysis of drug responding systems. *Annu. Rev. Pharmacol. Toxicol.* 18:493-522 (1978).
67. R. P. Miller, J. R. Woodworth, D. A. Graves, C. S. Locke, B. W. Steiger, and K. S. Rotenberg. Comparison of three formulations of metolazone: Bioavailability and pharmacologic effects. *Curr. Ther. Res.* 43:1133-1142 (1988).
68. P. Nissen and L. Pedersen. Allopurinol: A comparative study of the bioavailability and effect on plasma uric acid of two products in tablet form. *Biopharm. Drug Dispos.* 6:441-446 (1985).
69. K. H. Molz, R. Klimmek, C. Dilger, G. Pabst, W. Weber, M. Müller, and H. Jaeger.

Bioequivalence and pharmacodynamics of a modified glibenclamide formulation in healthy volunteers, *Arzneim. Forsch.* 39:1280–1282 (1989).
70. G. Ayanoglu, P. U. Witte, and M. Badian. Bioavailability and pharmacodynamics of a sustained-release glibenclamide product (Deroctyl) in comparison to a standard tablet formulation (Euglucon, Daonil). *Int. J. Clin. Pharmacol. ther. Toxicol.* 9:479–482 (1983).
71. S. C. Olson, J. W. Ayres, E. J. Antal, and K. S. Albert. Effect of food and tablet age on relative bioavailability and pharmacodynamics of two tolbutamide products. *J. Pharm. Sci.* 74:735–740 (1985).
72. B. Flouvat, I. Berlin, A. Cournot, D. Robinet, J. Duchier, H. Sarmini, and A. Rossi. Pharmacokinetic and pharmacodynamic comparison of two doses of long acting propranolol (80 and 160 mg) in healthy subjects. *Br. J. Clin. Pharmacol.* 27:539–545 (1989).
73. Y.-T. Lee, C.-S. Lian, E. C. K. Wong, W.-J. Chen, M.-F. Chen, and C.-C. Chen. Pharmacokinetic and pharmacodynamic comparison of conventional and controlled release formulations of metroprolol in healthy Chinese subjects. *Cardiovasc. Drugs Ther.* 3:529–533 (1989).
74. B. Oosterhuis, J. Jonkman, P. Zuiderwijk, and F. Sollie. A pharmacokinetic and pharmacodynamic comparison of metoprolol CR/ZOK with a conventional slow release preparation. *J. Clin. Pharmacol.* 30:S33–S38 (1990).
75. G. J. Krol, J. T. Lettieri, A. L. Mazzu, D. E. Burkholder, J. P. Birkett, R. J. Taylor, and C. Bon. Bioequivalence of different nitrendipine tablet dosage formulations. *J. Cardiovasc. Pharmacol.* 9(Suppl. 4):S129–S135 (1987).
76. M. J. Reiter, D. G. Shand, and E. L. C. Pritchett. Comparison of intravenous and oral verapamil dosing. *Clin. Pharmacol. Ther.* 32:711–720 (1982).
77. W. A. Colburn, R. K. Brazzell, and A. A. Holazo. Verapamil pharmacodynamics following IV and oral administration: Theoretical considerations. *J. Clin. Pharmacol.* 26:71–73 (1986).
78. A. A. Holazo, R. K. Brazzell, and W. A. Colburn. Pharmacokinetic and pharmacodynamic modeling of cibenzoline plasma concentrations and antiarrhythmic effect. *J. Clin. Pharmacol.* 26:336–345 (1986).
79. P. Tuomainen. A methodological comparison of two formulations of temazepam in pharmacokinetic and pharmacodynamic aspects. *Pharmacol. Toxicol.* 64:28–32 (1989).
80. S. K. Gupta, E. H. Ellinwood, A. M. Nikaido, and D. G. Heatherly. Simultaneous modeling of the pharmacokinetic and pharmacodynamic properties of benzodiazepines. II. Triazolam. *Pharm. Res.* 7:570–576 (1990).
81. T. M. Itil and K. Z. Itil. The significance of pharmacodynamic measurements in the assessment of bioavailability and bioequivalence of psychotropic drugs using CEEG and dynamic brain mapping. *J. Clin. Psychiatry* 47:20–27 (1986).
82. B. Oosterhuis, M. C. P. Braat, C. M. Roos, J. Wemer, and C. J. van Boxtel. Pharmacokinetic–pharmacodynamic modeling of terbutaline bronchodilation in asthma. *Clin. Pharmacol. Ther.* 40:469–475 (1986).
83. J. A. Cook, D. E. Smith, L. A. Cornish, R. M. Tankanow, J. M. Nicklas, and M. L. Hyneck. Kinetics, dynamics, and bioavailability of bumetanide in healthy

subjects and patients with congestive heart failure. *Clin. Pharmacol. Ther.* 44:487–500 (1988).
84. S. C. Olson, M. A. Eldon, R. D. Toothaker, J. J. Ferry, and W. A. Colburn. Controversy II: Bioequivalence as an indicator of therapeutic equivalence: Modeling the theoretic influence of bioinequivalence on single-dose drug effect. *J. Clin. Pharmacol.* 27:342–435 (1987).
85. J. Grevel. Description of the time course of the prolactin suppressant effect of the dopamine agonist CQP201-403 by an integrated pharmacokinetic–pharmacodynamic model. *Br. J. Clin. Pharmacol.* 22:1–13 (1986).
86. J. Grevel. Kinetic-effect models and their applications. *Pharm. Res.* 4:86–91 (1987).
87. D. B. Campbell. The use of kinetic–dynamic interactions in the evaluation of drugs. *Psychopharmacology* 100:433–450 (1990).

Part Three
Perspectives of Regulatory Agencies, Worldwide, on Bioequivalence Testing

12
Bioequivalence: A United States Regulatory Perspective

Shrikant V. Dighe and Wallace P. Adams
Center for Drug Evaluation and Research
Food and Drug Administration
Rockville, Maryland

INTRODUCTION

Bioavailability and bioequivalence of drug products have emerged as important national and international issues during the last two decades. The phenomenal growth of the generic pharmaceutical industry in the United States, Canada, the European Common Market countries, and developing countries, such as India, has added a new dimension to the issue of quality of drug products, namely, bioequivalence. To be interchangeable with the pioneer (innovator or brand name) drug product, a generic drug product must be not only pharmaceutically equivalent, but also bioequivalent. (*Pharmaceutic equivalents* are drug products that contain the same active ingredient(s) and are identical in strength or concentration, dosage form, and route of administration. They are formulated to meet the same or compendial or other applicable standards of strength, quality, purity, and identity, but they may differ in certain aspects, including shape, scoring configuration, packaging, excipients (including colors, flavors, preservatives), expiration time, and, within certain limits, labeling [1].) For a generic product to be considered *bioequivalent* to a pioneer drug product, it must be shown to have the same rate and extent of absorption as the pioneer drug product when administered at the same molar dose of the active therapeutic moiety under similar experimental conditions. Bioequivalence thus plays a pivotal role in assuring the therapeutic quality of multisource drug products in the marketplace.

The literature is replete with examples of how composition and manufacture of the finished dosage form can alter the effectiveness of the drug [2]. Product efficacy can depend on how much of the drug is ultimately absorbed from its formulation and how rapidly the drug is absorbed. Thus, the two considerations—the extent of absorption of the drug from its formulation and the rate at which it is absorbed—form the basis of bioavailability and bioequivalence testing. Bioequivalence studies are essentially investigations designed to compare the bioavailability of two or more drug products. *Bioequivalence testing* is based on the assumption that the therapeutic effect of a drug product is a function of the concentration of the active ingredient or active moiety in the systemic circulation and, hence, is related to its bioavailability. Thus, if two preparations containing equivalent amounts of the same drug produce similar concentrations of the drug entity in blood, they are bioequivalent and, therefore, assumed to be therapeutically equivalent.

BIOEQUIVALENCE IN THE UNITED STATES: A HISTORICAL PERSPECTIVE

The pioneering work on vitamins by Melnick et al. in 1945 [3], its application to multisource vitamin drug products by Morrison et al. in 1959 and 1960 [4,5] and Middleton et al. in 1964 [6], and Gerhard Levy's work on aspirin tablets [7] and tolbutamide tablets [8] in the early 1960s gave the first intimations of bioequivalence problems with multisource drug products. Until about 1965, our understanding of the contributions of the dosage form to the clinical activity of the drug was rather poor. There were many contributing factors. The sciences of pharmacokinetics and biopharmaceutics were in their infancy and pharmaceutical scientists had not yet gained sufficient insight into the processes of absorption of a drug in the body, the biotransformation pathways of a drug, and its disappearance from the body. Available analytical techniques permitted quantification of drugs administered only in relatively high doses. Mathematical interpretation of blood drug concentration–time profiles (i.e., the distinction between rate and extent of drug absorption) was not well recognized [9].

Introduction in the late 1960s and early 1970s of sophisticated methods of measurement of analytes in biological fluids, such as gas–liquid chromatography, high-pressure liquid chromatography, and mass spectrometry, represented a major improvement in the analytical methodology available to pharmaceutical scientists. The new analytical techniques made possible measurement of drugs and their metabolites in biological fluids in concentrations as low as a few nanograms per milliliter. The disposition of low doses of drugs in the human body could now be investigated pharmacokinetically. The analytical capability to quantify extremely low concentrations of drugs in the body enabled scientists to study the rate processes of absorption, distribution, metabolism, and excretion (ADME) of the administered drug and their relationship with pharmacologic effects. From these data, the process of absorption could be quantified and correlated with dosage formulation factors and pharmacodynamic effects. The seminal work of John Wagner, Eino Nelson, Gerhard Levy, Sidney Riegelman, Edward Garrett, Milo Gibaldi, and others, in the 1960s and 1970s contributed significantly toward the advancement of pharmacokinetics and biopharmaceutics. The scientific basis was now in place to study and compare the performance of dosage forms in terms of their bioavailability.

As these advances in analytical technology were applied to investigations involving bioavailability of marketed drug products, some interesting circumstances were uncovered. Some generic formulations were superior [10,11] in bioavailability to the innovator products, whereas others were inferior [12]. Neither circumstance was desirable, since the products were not equivalent. By 1974, reports of bioinequivalence included drugs such as digoxin, aminosalicylate, phenytoin, chloramphenicol, chlorpropamide, nitrofurantoin, oxytetracycline, tetracycline, and phenylbutazone [13,14].

The *Drug Amendments Act of 1962* (Kefauver-Harris Amendments) amended the new drug definition to incorporate the requirement of general recognition of effectiveness, as well as safety [15,16]. A firm submitting a New Drug Application (NDA) was required to present "substantial evidence" in the form of "adequate and well controlled" studies to demonstrate the effectiveness of the drug under the conditions of use described in its labeling. The new drug effectiveness provision of the law applied retrospectively to all drugs that were approved between 1938 and 1962 on the basis of safety only. The Food and Drug Administration (FDA) contracted with the National Academy of Sciences/National Research Council (NAS/NRC) to conduct a review of this group of drugs for effectiveness. The NAS/NRC appointed 30 panels of experts and initiated a study of approximately 3400 drug formulations. This study was known as the Drug Efficacy Study of the NAS/NRC. On the basis of the available data, the formulations were classified by the NAS/NRC panels as effective or less than effective. The FDA reviewed the reports of the panels, as well as the evidence the panels relied upon, and any additional data in FDA files, and published its own conclusions in the *Federal Register* as *Drug Efficacy Study Implementation* (DESI) notices. Many of these notices included, as a requirement for approval of the drug application, presentation of evidence to demonstrate that the "biologic availability" of the test product was similar to that of the reference (usually the innovator) product.

In determining the mechanism by which DESI drugs would be approved for marketing, the FDA believed that a simpler and shorter drug application could be adequate, as drug products that would be reviewed under this new procedure would be identical, similar, or related to drugs previously approved as safe and effective. The FDA decided that it would not be necessary for drug firms seeking approval of DESI drug products to establish the safety and efficacy of each new product identical in active ingredient and dosage form with the previously approved drug product that had already been determined to be safe and effective. The Abbreviated New Drug Application (ANDA) mechanism for approval of DESI drugs was established in 1970 [17] as an outgrowth of the DESI review program. In 1974, the FDA established a new division—the Division of Biopharmaceutics—within the Bureau of Drugs (now the Center for Drug Evaluation and Research) to tackle the problems and issues of bioavailability, bioequivalence, and pharmacokinetics.

About the same time the U.S. Congress created a special Office of Technology Assessment (OTA), which was to provide to the Congress timely and thorough assessment and advice on scientific issues. The second task undertaken by the OTA was the bioequivalence of drug products. The Drug Bioequivalence Study Panel, assembled on 12 April 1974 under the chairmanship of Dr. Robert Berliner, consisted of seven physicians, two pharmaceutical scientists (Drs. Sidney Riegelman and James Doluisio) and a statistician. The panel was asked "to determine whether or not the technological capability is now available to assure that drug products with the same physical and chemical composition will produce comparable therapeutic effects." The panel studied the issues intensively for about 3 months and met with representatives of the FDA, pharmaceutical industry, consumers, health economists, and professional and trade organizations.

On 15 July 1974, the study panel submitted its report, entitled *Drug Bioequivalence* [18,19] to the U.S. Congress. Some of the conclusions of the report were

1. Current standards and regulatory practices do not assure bioequivalence among drug products.
2. Variations in the bioavailability of drug products have been recognized as responsible for a few therapeutic failures, and other failures of a similar origin have probably escaped recognition.
3. Most of the analytical methodology and experimental procedures for the conduct of bioavailability studies in human subjects are available.
4. It is neither feasible nor desirable that bioavailability studies be conducted for all drugs or drug products. Certain classes of drugs for which evidence of bioequivalence is critical should be identified on the basis of clinical importance, therapeutic/toxic concentration ratios in blood, and certain pharmaceutical characteristics.

The panel report recommended that

1. New compendial standards for active ingredients, excipients, and finished

drug products should be developed and revised on a continuing basis to reflect the best available technology to assure quality and uniform bioavailability. Appropriate statistical procedures should be specified to make certain that the purposes of the standards are objectively satisfied. The guidelines for Current Good Manufacturing Practices (CGMPs) should be expanded to include specific descriptions of all significant aspects of manufacturing processes from the raw materials to the final product.
2. Additional research aimed at improving the assessment and prediction of bioequivalence is needed. This research should include efforts to develop in vitro tests or animal models that will be valid predictors of bioavailability in humans.
3. A system should be organized as rapidly as possible to generate an official list of interchangeable drug products. In the development of this list, distinctions should be made between two classes of drugs and drug products:
   a. Those for which evidence of bioequivalence is not considered essential. These could be added to the list as soon as standards of pharmaceutical equivalence have been established.
   b. Those for which evidence of bioequivalence is critical. Such products should be listed only after they have been shown to be bioequivalent or have satisfied standards of pharmaceutical equivalence that have been shown to assure bioequivalence.

Thus, by the end of 1974, four important developments converged to focus the attention of the FDA on bioequivalence and bioavailability problems and issues:

1. The availability of analytical technology capable of measuring nanogram levels of drugs in blood resulted in a greatly increased understanding of biotransformation pathways and pharmacokinetics.
2. The growing awareness within the scientific and regulatory communities of bioavailability problems with marketed drug products.
3. The establishment of the Division of Biopharmaceutics within the FDA's Bureau of Drugs.
4. The publication of the Office of Technology Assessment report on bioequivalence problems with drug products.

In response, on 20 June 1975, the FDA proposed its *Bioavailability and Bioequivalence Regulations* [15] and invited comments from interested persons. After due consideration of all comments submitted to the FDA, the proposed regulations were modified and the modified version was finalized on 7 January 1977 [20,21].

The ANDA process and the demonstration of bioequivalence to an approved drug product in lieu of clinical studies were applicable only to DESI drugs (i.e., those drugs originally approved between 1938 and 1962 that had been evaluated for safety, but not effectiveness) that were determined to be effective through a

DESI review. The ANDA process could not be used to obtain approval to manufacture and market generic versions of drugs first approved on or after 10 October 1962 (post-1962 drugs). Firms seeking to market generic copies of post-1962 drugs were required either to submit a full NDA, including animal safety data and clinical trial data in patients for safety and efficacy, or to file a "Paper NDA," which involved submitting, as part of the NDA, published literature of adequate and well-controlled studies documenting safety and efficacy. For most drugs, the Paper NDA route of approval was not workable, the main reason being the unavailability of published clinical data on safety and efficacy.

In September 1984, the U.S. Congress passed the *Drug Price Competition and Patent Term Restoration Act of 1984* (the Waxman-Hatch Amendments of 1984), which provided for the submission of ANDAs for generic versions of drug products first approved on or after 10 October 1962 [22].

BIOAVAILABILITY AND BIOEQUIVALENCE REGULATIONS OF 1977

The bioavailability and bioequivalence regulations [20,21] put into effect on 7 January 1977 were a distinct landmark in the drug regulation history of the United States. The regulations greatly aided the rational development of dosage forms of both new chemical entities and generic drugs, as well as the subsequent evaluation of their performance. The regulations were purposely divided into two sets: subpart B—*Procedures for Determining the Bioavailability of Drug Products*, and subpart C—*Bioequivalence Requirements*. Subpart B deals mainly with issues of bioavailability and pharmacokinetics to characterize new drug products and to support drug labeling, whereas subpart C addresses the majority of elements dealing with bioequivalence issues. However, portions of each subpart apply to the other and, therefore, the two sets of regulations should not be viewed as totally independent.

The key provisions of the bioavailability regulations (subpart B) are summarized in Table 1; the key provisions of the bioequivalence regulations (subpart C) are summarized in Table 2 [23].

Table 1 Key Provisions of the Bioavailability Regulations

1. Defines bioavailability in terms of both the rate and extent of drug absorption
2. Describes procedures for determining the bioavailability of drug products
3. Sets forth requirements for submission of in vivo bioavailability data
4. Sets forth criteria for waiver of in vivo bioavailability studies
5. Provides general guidelines for the conduct of in vivo bioavailability studies
6. Sets forth requirements for filing a *Notice of Claimed Investigational Exemption for a New Drug*

Table 2 Key Provisions of the Bioequivalence Regulations

1. Describes procedures for establishing a bioequivalence requirement
2. Sets forth criteria to establish a bioequivalence requirement
3. Describes types of bioequivalence requirements
4. Sets forth requirements for in vivo bioequivalence testing
5. Sets forth requirements for in vitro batch testing and certification
6. Describes requirements for marketing a drug product subject to a bioequivalence requirement
7. Sets forth requirements for in vivo testing of a drug product not meeting an in vitro bioequivalence standard

The 1977 bioequivalence regulations set forth the following criteria and evidence for consideration of which pharmaceutical equivalents would ordinarily be required to demonstrate bioequivalence [24]:

1. Evidence from well-controlled clinical trials or controlled observations in patients that such drug products do not give comparable therapeutic effects.
2. Evidence from well-controlled bioequivalence studies that such products are not bioequivalent drug products.
3. Evidence that the drug products exhibit a narrow therapeutic ratio [e.g., there is less than a twofold difference in median lethal dose (LD_{50}) and median effective dose (ED_{50}) values, or there is less than a twofold difference in the minimum toxic concentrations and minimum effective concentrations in the blood], and safe and effective use of the drug products requires careful dosage titration and patient monitoring.
4. Competent medical determination that a lack of bioequivalence would have a serious adverse effect in the treatment or prevention of a serious disease or condition.
5. Physicochemical evidence that:
    a. The drug has low aqueous solubility.
    b. The dissolution rate of the drug from the drug product is slow.
    c. The particle size and/or surface area of the active drug ingredient is critical to its bioavailability.
    d. Polymorphs, solvates, complexes, and such, exist that could contribute to poor dissolution and may affect absorption.
    e. There is a high excipient/active drug ratio present in the drug product.
    f. The presence of inactive ingredients could promote or interfere with absorption.
6. Pharmacokinetic evidence that:
    a. The drug undergoes site-specific absorption from the gastrointestinal tract.
    b. Drug absorption, even from solution, is poor.

c. The drug undergoes first-pass metabolism.
d. The drug is rapidly metabolized or excreted, requiring rapid dissolution and absorption for effectiveness.
e. Chemical instability of the drug in the gastrointestinal tract exists, requiring special coatings or formulations.
f. The drug follows nonlinear kinetics in or near the therapeutic dosing range, and the rate and extent of absorption are both important.

Providing that a drug met one or more of these six criteria, a bioequivalence requirement would be established. The requirement could be either an in vivo or an in vitro requirement, as specified by the FDA. The types of bioequivalence requirements include the following [25]:

1. An in vivo test in humans.
2. An in vivo test in animals, other than humans, that has been correlated with human in vivo data.
3. An in vivo test in animals, other than humans, that has not been correlated with human in vivo data.
4. An in vitro bioequivalence standard (i.e., an in vitro test that has been correlated with human in vivo bioavailability data).
5. A currently available in vitro test (usually a dissolution rate test) that has not been correlated with human in vivo bioavailability data.

The 1977 regulations state that in vivo testing in humans would ordinarily be required if there is well-documented evidence that pharmaceutically equivalent drug products intended to be used interchangeably meet one of the first three criteria used to establish a bioequivalence requirement:

1. The drug products do not give comparable therapeutic effects.
2. The drug products are not bioequivalent.
3. The drug products exhibit a narrow therapeutic ratio (as described in the foregoing).

The following in vivo approaches, in descending order of accuracy, sensitivity and reproducibility, are acceptable for determining the bioavailability or bioequivalence of a drug product, according to the 1977 regulations [26]:

1a. In vivo testing in humans in which the concentration of the active drug ingredient or therapeutic moiety or its metabolite(s), in whole blood, plasma, serum, or other appropriate biological fluid, is measured as a function of time.
1b. In vivo testing in humans in which the urinary excretion of the active drug ingredient or therapeutic moiety or its metabolite(s) is measured as a function of time.
2. In vivo testing in humans in which an appropriate acute pharmacologic effect of the active drug ingredient or therapeutic moiety, or metabolite(s),

A U.S. Regulatory Perspective

is measured as a function of time, if such effect can be measured with sufficient accuracy, sensitivity, and reproducibility.
3. Well-controlled clinical trials in humans that establish the safety and effectiveness of the drug product in comparison with the reference drug product.
4. Any other in vivo approach approved by FDA (e.g., in vivo testing in a suitable animal model, rather than in humans, or using a radioactive or nonradioactive isotopically labeled drug product).

In the hierarchy of different approaches to bioequivalence testing, in vivo testing in humans, in which the active drug ingredient or therapeutic moiety is measured in the systemic circulation, is preferable, if possible and practicable. These studies are normally conducted as single-dose investigations in healthy human volunteers.

An important feature of the 1977 bioavailability and bioequivalence regulations is the provision for waiver of in vivo bioequivalence study under certain circumstances. A firm may request the FDA to waive in vivo requirements provided the firm submits the request with the NDA or ANDA and documents that the drug meets the criteria for waiver specified in the regulations. Justification for the waiver must be provided by the applicant, and the FDA must concur that the waiver is justified. The regulations permit waiver of in vivo bioavailability or bioequivalence study if the drug product meets one of the following criteria [27]:

1. The drug product is a solution intended solely for intravenous administration and contains the active drug ingredient in the same solvent and concentration as an intravenous solution that is the subject of an approved full NDA.
2. The drug product is a topically applied preparation intended for local therapeutic effect.
3. The drug product is an oral dosage form not intended to be absorbed.
4. The drug product is administered by inhalation as a gas or vapor and contains the active drug ingredient in the same dosage form as a drug product that is the subject of an approved full NDA.
5. The drug product is an oral solution, elixir, syrup, tincture or similar other solubilized form that contains an active drug ingredient in the same concentration as a drug product that is the subject of an approved full NDA and contains no inactive ingredient that is known to significantly affect absorption of the active drug ingredient.
6. The drug product is a solid oral dosage form (other than enteric-coated or controlled-release dosage form) that has been determined to be effective for at least one indication in a DESI notice and is not included in the FDA list of pharmacological classes and drugs within a class for which in vivo bioequivalence testing is required.
7. The drug product is a parenteral drug product that is determined to be effective for at least one indication in a DESI notice and is shown to be identical, in both active and inactive ingredients formulation, with a drug product

that is currently approved in an NDA. The regulations exclude certain parenteral products (suspensions and sodium phenytoin powder for injection) from the waiver provision.

This section of the regulations also permits waiver if:

1. The drug product is one for which only an in vitro bioequivalence requirement has been imposed by the FDA.
2. The drug product is in the same dosage form, but in a different strength, and is proportionally similar in its active and inactive ingredients to another drug product made by the same manufacturer and the following conditions are met:
   a. The bioavailability of this other product has been demonstrated
   b. Both drug products meet an appropriate in vitro test approved by the FDA
   c. The applicant submits evidence showing that both drug products are proportionally similar in their active and inactive ingredients.
3. The drug product is shown to meet an in vitro test that assures bioavailability (i.e., an in vitro test that has been correlated with in vivo data).
4. The drug product is a reformulated product that is identical, except for color, flavor, or preservative, with another drug product made by the same manufacturer and both of the following conditions are met:
   a. The bioavailability of the other product has been demonstrated.
   b. Both drug products meet an appropriate in vitro test approved by the FDA.

THE DRUG PRICE COMPETITION AND PATENT TERM RESTORATION ACT OF 1984 (THE WAXMAN-HATCH AMENDMENTS)

The passage of the *Drug Price Competition and Patent Term Restoration Act of 1984* (the Waxman-Hatch Amendments of 1984) was an important milestone in United States drug regulation history. (The act amended the *Federal Food, Drug, and Cosmetic Act*, thus will be referred to in this chapter as the 1984 amendments.) The new law [22] consists of two titles. Title I (*Abbreviated New Drug Applications*) gives the FDA statutory authority to accept ANDAs for approval of generic new drugs, and Title II (*Patent Extension*) authorizes extension of patent terms for approved new drugs. The two parts of the bill were intended to strike a careful balance between promoting competition among brand name (pioneer) and generic drugs and encouraging research and innovation.

Title I amends the *Federal Food, Drug, and Cosmetic Act* to expand the universe of drugs for which the FDA would accept ANDAs. Before the enactment of the new law, ANDAs were permitted under FDA regulations for duplicates [i.e., drug products that were the same as the already-approved drug product in dosage form, route of administration, kind and amount of active ingredient, and indication(s)] of drugs originally approved between 1938 and 1962 on the basis of safety and, subsequently, determined to be effective as a result of a DESI review. The regulations permitted ANDAs for "similar" and "related" products only if FDA had made a separate finding, following a manufacturer's petition, that an ANDA was appropriate for that product. Title I provides for the submission of ANDAs for duplicates of post-1962 drugs listed in the approved drug product list published by the agency [1], the patents of which have expired. Title I retains the provision for approving ANDAs for similar and related products by the manufacturer's petition procedure. The requirement of premarketing approval of the ANDA ensures that generic products will be as safe and effective as their brand name counterparts, but without the submission of duplicative safety and effectiveness data.

Title I also makes the existence of a patent for an approved drug a factor in the approval of generic versions of that drug. It establishes a system—the so-called exclusivity provisions—for rewarding research associated with significant innovation by providing for a delay in the submission or in the effective approval date of certain generic applications.

Title II of the new law provides for the extension of drug patent terms beyond the normal 17 years, to reflect a portion of the period of patent life lost during FDA's review of safety and effectiveness data for the drug. These extensions of the normal 17-year term of a patent apply to a product, a method of using a product, or a method of manufacturing a product. They are intended to encourage the innovation necessary for the development of important new drug products by increasing the period during which innovator products are protected from competition.

The *Drug Price Competition and Patent Term Restoration Act* thus endeavors to

1. Speed up the approval process of generic drug products, resulting in greater competition in the marketplace, thereby reducing health care costs.
2. Make therapeutically equivalent and high-quality generic versions of brand name drugs more widely available to consumers.
3. Eliminate the costly, unnecessary, and ethically questionable duplication of preclinical and clinical studies required to support the safety and efficacy of generic versions of post-1962 drugs.
4. Assure and encourage the continuing development of new drugs (new chemical entities) through special incentives, which include periods of patent term restoration and market exclusivity.

In addition to extending the ANDA process to generic versions of post-1962 drugs, another important aspect of this act is the absence of authority to defer the requirement of demonstration of in vivo bioequivalence of a generic product. Previously, bioequivalence requirements were imposed, but were sometimes deferred. The new law requires that an ANDA for any new drug shall contain information to show that the new drug is bioequivalent to the listed drug (i.e., deferrals are no longer granted). Evidence of bioequivalence, either in vivo, in vitro, or both, is required for all dosage forms: topical ointments and creams, transdermal patches, ophthalmics, injectables, tablets, capsules, suspensions, solutions, and so on.

Before the 1984 amendments, most of the concern and interest about bioequivalence was focused on systemically available solid oral dosage forms— conventional-release tablets and capsules and controlled-release products. The 1977 regulations, therefore, dwelt mostly on the bioavailability and bioequivalence of these dosage forms. The testing procedures used for those drugs were generally based on measurement of the active drug ingredient or therapeutic moiety in the systemic circulation. These procedures were adequate for such dosage forms and have been a valuable tool in implementing the new law of 1984. Recently, patents have expired for certain nonsystemically absorbed drugs; additional patents will expire in the next few years. Consequently, bioequivalence evaluation of nonsystemically absorbed drugs has become very important to the FDA. Blood levels of these drugs are either nonexistent or of no relevance to therapeutic effect. Orally administered drugs such as bile acid-binding resins or antiulcer drugs (colestipol HCl, sucralfate) and drugs used as metered-dose inhalers for treatment or prophylaxis of asthma (albuterol, cromolyn sodium) require bioequivalence testing based either upon an acute pharmacologic effect or upon clinical trials. Traditional blood level studies are inappropriate.

The new law [22] describes bioequivalent drugs as follows:

A drug shall be considered to be bioequivalent to a listed drug if either

1. The rate and extent of absorption of the drug do not show a significant difference from the rate and extent of absorption of the listed drug when administered at the same molar dose of the therapeutic ingredient under similar experimental conditions in either a single dose or multiple doses, or
2. The extent of absorption of the drug does not show a significant difference from the extent of absorption of the listed drug when administered at the same molar dose of the therapeutic ingredient under similar experimental conditions in either a single dose or multiple doses, and the difference from the listed drug in the rate of absorption of the drug is intentional, is reflected in its proposed labeling, is not essential to the attainment of effective body drug concentrations on chronic use, and is considered medically insignificant for the drug.

On 10 July 1989, the FDA proposed regulations [16] to implement Title I of the 1984 amendments, which amends section 505 of the *Federal Food, Drug, and Cosmetic Act*. The proposed regulations would (1) reorganize and revise 21 *Code of Federal Regulations (CFR) Part 314 (Applications for FDA Approval to Market a New Drug or an Antibiotic Drug)* to incorporate the new requirements and procedures imposed upon applicants by the 1984 amendments and (2) revise 21 *CFR* Part 320 (*Bioavailability and Bioequivalence Requirements*). Revision of Part 320 was necessitated by the bioequivalence requirements of the 1984 amendments, as well as FDA's follow-up to the bioequivalence hearing held 29 September through 1 October 1986 [28] and current agency policy.

The following are some of the important changes or revisions the FDA proposed to 21 *CFR* Part 320 [29]:

1. Revise the definition of "bioavailability" to add a reference to drugs that are not intended to be absorbed systemically; restate the definition of "bioequivalence;" and remove the definition of "bioequivalence requirement."
2. Restate the requirements for submission of bioavailability and bioequivalence data.
3. Restate the waiver provision and remove the automatic waiver of evidence of in vivo bioavailability for topically applied preparations and oral dosage forms not intended to be absorbed systemically.
4. Remove the list of "bioproblem" drugs from existing bioavailability/bioequivalence regulations and provide notice of in vivo or in vitro study requirements through the list. The FDA will continue to waive in vivo studies for the DESI oral dosage forms that FDA determines do not pose an actual or potential bioequivalence problem.
5. Modify the provision to clarify that deferral of a requirement for submission of evidence of in vivo bioavailability is applicable only to full NDAs. Under the 1984 amendments, there is no authority to defer a showing of bioequivalence for drug products approved through ANDAs.
6. Add a new paragraph in 320.22 to state that FDA for good cause may require evidence of in vivo bioavailability for any product if the agency determines that any difference between a proposed drug product and a listed drug may affect the bioavailability of the proposed drug product.
7. State the methods that may be used to meet an in vivo or in vitro testing requirement.
8. Clarify when an Investigational New Drug Application (IND) is required for an in vivo bioavailability or bioequivalence study.
9. Amend the current regulations under subpart C by removing the subpart heading and those regulations that apply to establishing a bioequivalence requirement, and revise the remaining regulations to delete any reference to establishing a bioequivalence requirement.

The proposed regulations implementing the 1984 amendments state [30] that the following in vivo and in vitro approaches, in descending order of accuracy, sensitivity and reproducibility, are acceptable for determining the bioequivalence of a drug product:

1a. An in vivo test in humans in which the concentration of the active ingredient or active moiety and its active metabolites, in whole blood, plasma, serum, or other appropriate biological fluid is measured as a function of time.

1b. An in vitro test that has been correlated with and is predictive of human in vivo bioavailability data.
1c. An in vivo test in animals that has been correlated with and is predictive of human bioavailability data.
2. An in vivo test in humans in which the urinary excretion of the active moiety and its active metabolites are measured as a function of time.
3. An in vivo test in humans in which an appropriate acute pharmacologic effect of the active moiety and its active metabolites are measured as a function of time if such effect can be measured with sufficient accuracy, sensitivity, and reproducibility.
4. Appropriately designed comparative clinical trials, for purposes of demonstrating bioequivalence.
5. Any other approach deemed adequate to establish bioequivalence by the FDA.

The proposed regulations state that the in vivo test in humans based on blood levels is particularly applicable to dosage forms intended to deliver the active moiety to the systemic circulation. Although the in vivo test in humans based upon urinary excretion may be applicable to some drugs, it is only appropriate when urinary excretion is a significant mechanism of elimination. The in vivo test in humans based upon an acute pharmacologic effect is particularly applicable to dosage forms that are not intended to deliver the active moiety to the systemic circulation. Clinical trials in humans may be appropriate for dosage forms intended to deliver the active moiety to the systemic circulation only when analytical methods or other tests cannot be developed to permit use of one of the foregoing listed approaches 1–3. Clinical trials may also be appropriate for determining the bioequivalence of dosage forms intended to deliver the active moiety locally (e.g., topical preparations for the skin, eye, and mucous membranes; nonsystemically absorbed oral dosage forms; and bronchodilators administered by inhalation if the onset and duration of pharmacological activity are defined).

BIOEQUIVALENCE PRACTICES, CRITERIA, AND ISSUES

The bioequivalence regulations and proposed regulations discussed in the foregoing provide the framework for FDA review and determination of bioequivalence of generic products. In the following sections, current practices in the conduct of in vivo bioequivalence studies, the submission of study data, and criteria for bioequivalence evaluation are discussed. In addition, some important bioequivalence issues, including logarithmic transformation, outliers, in vitro dissolution testing, and waivers of in vivo study, are discussed. These discussions are restricted to primarily regulatory issues associated with conventional-release solid oral dosage forms of drugs that are systemically absorbed.

Study Design

The most frequent type of bioequivalence studies are those performed on solid oral dosage forms of drugs that are absorbed into the systemic circulation. Studies may be either single dose or multiple dose, with the former more common. Single-dose studies generally should include the following major elements [31]:

1. The comparison of test and reference products should be conducted in healthy adult human volunteers.
2. The test and reference products should be administered to subjects in the fasting state (i.e., overnight fast for at least 10 hr, plus 2 hr after administration of the dose) unless some other approach is more appropriate for valid scientific reasons.
3. A two-way crossover study design, which minimizes variability not attributable to the drug products should normally be used. The sequence of administration of drug products should be determined in advance, and subjects should be randomly assigned to sequences. Other designs may be acceptable if they are more appropriate for valid scientific reasons.
4. Each phase of the crossover study should be conducted to encompass a drug elimination period that is at least three times the half-life of the active drug ingredient or therapeutic moiety or its metabolite(s) measured in blood or urine.
5. Blood samples should be taken with sufficient frequency to
    a. Define adequately the ascending and descending parts of the concentration–time curve
    b. Permit an estimate of the peak concentration (C_{max}) in the blood of the active drug ingredient or therapeutic moiety or its metabolite(s)
    c. Permit an estimate of the total area under the drug concentration–time curve (AUC) for a period of at least three times the half-life of elimination of the active drug ingredient or therapeutic moiety or its metabolite(s).
6. When bioequivalence is to be based on urinary excretion, samples of urine should be collected with sufficient frequency to permit an estimate of the rate and extent of urinary excretion of the active drug ingredient or therapeutic moiety or its metabolite(s).
7. The washout period (i.e., the interval between two treatments or study periods) should be at least five times the half-life of the active drug ingredient or therapeutic moiety or its metabolite(s).

For some drug products, multiple-dose bioequivalence studies may be appropriate and required. Typical requirements are summarized in the current regulations, which describe five circumstances under which a multiple-dose study may be required [32]:

1. When there is a difference in the rate of absorption, but not in the extent of absorption.

2. When there is excessive variability in bioavailability from subject to subject.
3. When the concentration of the active drug ingredient or therapeutic moiety or its metabolite(s) in the blood, resulting from a single dose, is too low for accurate determination by the analytical method.
4. When the drug product is a controlled-release dosage form.
5. When the drug exhibits nonlinear kinetics.

To conduct a well-controlled bioequivalence study, the following additional features should be part of the protocol:

1. Blinding of volunteers and immediate investigators with respect to identity of the drug products administered; blinding of the analyst with respect to identity of the treatments administered.
2. Standardization of physical characteristics of the subjects (such as age, height, weight, and health).
3. Standardization of all meals and fluid intake during the study.
4. Standardization of physical activity and posture during the study; subjects should be ambulatory as far as possible and should not engage in strenuous physical activity.

Subjects

Subjects in a bioequivalence study should normally be healthy, adult human volunteers. When women are included, there should be appropriate testing to ensure that they are not pregnant during the study. The selection and characterization of subjects is an important element of a protocol for a bioequivalence study. A major objective of the subject selection criteria is a reduction in pharmacokinetic variability ascribed to subject characteristics. Subjects must be well characterized as to their demographics (age, sex, height, weight, race, or other), health, mental condition, habits, and such. This will necessarily involve a physical examination (including electrocardiogram or radiological testing, or both, for some drugs), assessment of medical history, and evaluation of clinical laboratory tests. The medical supervisor or his designee must ensure that the subjects are well informed about the objective(s) and benefits (if any) of the study, procedures involved, and possible adverse reactions that could be encountered. A written informed consent must be obtained from each volunteer participating in the study. Subjects should be available to participate in all legs of the study. To accommodate dropouts during the study, extra subjects should be included. Reasons for withdrawal or removal of a subject from a study should be well documented, and analytical results of all samples (including those from subjects withdrawn or removed) must be included in the study report.

Sampling Times

For analysis of concentrations of drug absorbed systemically, blood (rather than urine) is the sample medium of choice. Usually, plasma or serum is harvested for analysis. However, analysis of whole blood may be appropriate under special circumstances, such as substantial drug binding to erythrocytes. When blood (plasma or serum) concentrations cannot be measured with a great deal of certainty, urine may be employed as the biological fluid for sampling if urinary excretion is the major pathway of elimination and a significant portion of the administered drug is eliminated unmetabolized.

As mentioned before, blood samples should be taken with sufficient frequency to adequately characterize the ascending and descending parts of the concentration–time curve (absorption, distribution, and elimination). This usually entails collection of 10–15 blood samples from each volunteer for each dose in a single-dose, two-way crossover study. Care should be taken not to exceed taking 1 pt (about 475 mL) of blood in a bioequivalence study in a 1-month period. When more than 1 pt of blood is expected to be drawn, prior permission from the Institutional Review Board (Ethics Committee) must be obtained and the hematocrit should be monitored before, during, and after the study.

The duration of blood sampling should cover a drug elimination period of at least three times the half-life of elimination of the drug. This should be sufficient to account for over 80% of the absorbed drug.

The Reference Product

Selection of the proper reference product is a critical component of a protocol. Normally, the proper reference product is one that has been approved on the basis of clinical studies in a full NDA (i.e., the innovator product). However, there are cases in which the agency must designate a specific product from among two or more possible products [e.g., Proventil Tablets, 4 mg (Schering), not Ventolin Tablets, 4 mg (Allen & Hanburys), is the reference product in bioequivalence studies of albuterol sulfate tablets (conventional release)].

For studies conducted in foreign countries, the generic firm must document that the reference product is the one marketed in the United States. Frequently, an innovator firm may market a formulation in international markets different from the one it markets in this country. The best approach in such cases is to purchase the reference product in the United States. In view of the unacceptability of a bioequivalence study conducted with an inappropriate reference product, consultation with the agency on this point is important, should there be any doubt.

Validation of the Analytical Procedure

A well-validated, specific, precise, and accurate analytical method is a sine qua non for confidence in the bioequivalence data. The analytical method validation is, therefore, a critical component of a bioequivalence study. Inadequate validation of the method is one of the major causes of a deficient submission.

Acceptable assay validation requires that each of the following validation parameters be characterized adequately:

1. Stability of stored samples
2. Range
3. Linearity
4. Accuracy (relative recovery)
5. Precision
6. Sensitivity limit (limit of quantitation)
7. Specificity

The *United States Pharmacopeia (USP)* has defined the foregoing listed validation parameters that are pertinent to compendial assay methods [33]. A systematic approach to analytical method validation has recently been described [34]. Both monographs describe validation parameters from the viewpoint of quality assurance and quality control. The validation of methods for the analysis of drugs in biological fluids has been discussed [35,36], and a practical description of the analytical validation process has been presented [37].

General Comments on Analytical Validation Parameters

To minimize assay variation as a source of intrasubject variability, assay of all clinical samples (test and reference) from a given subject on a single day is recommended. The number of days required to assay all samples will depend upon the complexity of the assay. However, a standard curve should be determined on each assay day. Also during each assay, quality control (QC) samples should be run. The QC samples are samples of known concentration prepared by spiking drug-free biological fluid with drug. These samples should be prepared in low, medium, and high concentrations. To avoid possible confusion between QC samples and standard solutions (calibrators; drug-free biological fluid spiked with the drug) during the review process, preparation of QC samples at concentrations different from those used for the calibrators is recommended. The desirable concentrations of the QC samples are:

Low QC sample: two to three times the sensitivity limit
Medium QC sample: 25–50% of the highest standard
High QC sample: about 80% of the highest standard

A QC sample should be assayed following the assay of every eight to ten clinical

A U.S. Regulatory Perspective

samples [38]. Whereas a standard curve is often determined only at the beginning of each assay day, each of the three QC samples is assayed several times during the day. The QC samples provide the following benefits:

Intraday accuracy and precision of the analytical system may be estimated.
Unlike calibrators, QC samples are not used in the determination of the standard curve. Therefore, their accuracy and precision should be more representative of those of the clinical samples.

Comments on Individual Analytical Validation Parameters

Stability of stored samples. Stability of the drug in the biological fluid should be demonstrated for the time that will elapse between the clinical and analytical phases of a study and for the conditions of storage (often $-20\,°C$). During method development, stability may be established by spiking drug-free biological fluid with drug. Validation of stability should also be established by periodic assay of several authentic clinical samples stored for a period of not less than the actual storage period [39]. Stability data should include freezing-and-thawing cycles representative of actual sample handling.

Range and linearity. The range of the standard solutions (calibrators) should extend from the lowest to the highest concentration samples that are anticipated in the study. There should be no fewer than six calibrators over the range.

The regression line to fit the linear (straight line) standard curve may be based on unweighted or weighted least squares analysis (see following paragraph). When the standard curve is curvilinear, the regression line may be based on a power equation, or the data may be divided into high and low standard curves, each of limited range and each approximated by a straight-line plot. Aarons has discussed the inappropriateness of the correlation coefficient as an indicator of linearity and has suggested a superior test [40]. Logit-log plots are routinely used to linearize radioimmunoassay data.

Assay calibration has, in general, received inadequate attention by analytical laboratories. A weighted least squares (WLS) fit is common, using a weight equal to the reciprocal of the concentration squared. Aarons and co-workers have discussed and applied three least squares methods to cases of nonuniform variance in assay calibration [40,41]. The application of these or other regression methods to calibration data has relevance for improved precision, particularly at low concentrations. Since the sensitivity limit is based upon acceptably low precision, improved regression methods may lower the sensitivity limit, thereby allowing drug to be measured for a longer period after administration.

Accuracy (relative recovery) and precision. *Accuracy* applies to both absolute recovery and relative recovery. An assay with a high absolute recovery should have improved precision and a lower sensitivity limit [37]. Since each of these latter two parameters must be validated, submission of absolute recovery data is optional. Relative recovery must be validated. For each of the six or more calibrators and for each of the three QC samples, the firm should tabulate the back-calculated concentrations for each assay day. As an example, if the laboratory required 18 days to complete the assay, it would have 18 standard curves and 18 sets of QC samples. For each of the calibrators, the mean concentration, the standard deviation, and the coefficient of variation should be reported. Similarly, these parameters should be determined over all individual QC samples at each concentration. Mean concentrations should be reported in both concentration units and as percentages of the known concentrations of each standard solution. Intra-day accuracy and precision of QC samples should also be determined.

Sensitivity limit (limit of quantitation). The sensitivity limit is frequently the most troublesome component of the assay validation. To quantitate drug levels through at least three biological half-lives, there may be a tendency by the investigator to demand greater sensitivity of the method than it is capable of.

The distinction between *limit of detection* (the lowest concentration of drug that will yield an assay response significantly different from that of a sample blank [34]) and *sensitivity limit* (the lowest concentration of drug that can be determined with acceptable precision and accuracy under the stated experimental conditions [33]) is emphasized. The sensitivity limit should be based upon the lowest calibrator possessing an acceptable coefficient of variation. This is the approach used by the agency for all assays, including radioimmunoassays. A common alternative approach, setting the limit at some low multiple (e.g., 3) of the background noise of the assay is not acceptable; it provides no measure of variance. Moreover, the acceptable percentage coefficient of variation is not set at a predetermined value for all drugs and analytical methods, but is considered on a case-by-case basis. Only those concentration values should be used in which there is considerable confidence [40]. Since the assay is assumed to possess unacceptably high error at all concentrations below the sensitivity limit, any unknown sample with a concentration lower than this limit must be reported as zero.

Specificity. Specificity in the presence of endogenous compounds, drug metabolites, or coadministered drugs is essential. Documentation of specificity with radioimmunoassays can be difficult, particularly for a drug with incompletely defined metabolism. In some cases, the literature reports a metabolite in humans, with no indication of its quantitative importance. In other cases, a metabolite is reported in a different species. Furthermore, these metabolites may not be available for determination of cross-reactivity. For such drugs, an alternative analytical method with improved specificity is preferred, providing it possesses adequate sensitivity.

Statistical Requirements for Bioequivalence

The statistical outcome of a bioequivalence study is the primary basis of the decision for or against a determination of therapeutic equivalence. Other factors that also may be considered in the bioequivalence review process are the biopharmaceutic and pharmacokinetic characteristics of the drug and drug products, the therapeutic range (if known), and the indications for the drug. Factors including conformity with compendial or other standards, labeling, and compliance with Current Good Manufacturing Practices are important, but these issues are reviewed by the Division of Generic Drugs or the Division of Scientific Investigations, not by the Division of Bioequivalence.

Decision rules for approval of generic drugs have evolved from the 1970s to the present. In the early 1970s, approval was based on mean data. Mean AUC and C_{max} values for the generic product had to be within $\pm 20\%$ of those of the innovator product. In addition, plasma concentration-time profiles for conventional-release products had to be reasonably superimposable (plasma concentrations not significantly different at most or all individual sampling times). Beginning in the late 1970s, the *75/75* (or *75/75-125*) *rule* was incorporated into the review process, along with mean product performance. According to the 75/75 rule, the relative AUC and C_{max} for the test product (i.e., test/reference ratio) must be within 0.75-1.25 for at least 75% of the subjects. The rule was an attempt to consider the individual variability in the rate and extent of absorption. In the early 1980s, the *power approach* [42] was applied to AUC and C_{max} parameters. The power approach consisted of two statistical tests: (1) a test of the null hypothesis of no difference between formulations using the F test and (2) the evaluation of the power of the test to detect a 20% mean difference in treatments [43]. The power approach was often used in conjunction with the 75/75 rule. In addition, plasma concentration-time profiles had to be reasonably superimposable. Statistically, the power approach and the 75/75 rule have poor performance characteristics [42,44-46]. Bioequivalence study evaluation based on these methods was discontinued by the Division of Bioequivalence in 1986. [An alternative method for assessing individual bioequivalence, that is, bioequivalence based upon a within-subject comparison of the test product and reference product ratios for the particular parameter (e.g., AUC), has recently been published [46].]

Since 1986, the division has used a decision rule termed the *two one-sided tests procedure*, also referred to as the 90% confidence interval approach [42]. The power approach tested the hypothesis of no difference—that is, it was a test of whether test and reference treatments were *identical* in their AUCs, C_{max}s, and other parameters. As pointed out by Westlake, this approach is an inappropriate tool, insomuch as the two treatments, although they may be close, will not be identical in these parameters. In fact, if two batches of the same reference product were compared, differences would be anticipated [47,48]. Therefore, it is more appropriate to recognize that there *will* be a difference in mean values between treatments and to use a test that provides reasonable assurance that the mean differences are acceptable [48]. The 90% confidence interval approach was adopted with the recognition that in general no two treatments will have *exactly* the same AUC and C_{max} values. By custom and by regulatory precedent, mean treatment differences of 20% or less are generally assumed to be of no clinical significance. Therefore, the current statistical test asks the question "Is the *difference* between the test and reference means not more than 20% from the reference treatment mean?"

The confidence interval (CI) for the difference of two means has the form [42,43]:

$$\mu_{T,obs} - \mu_{R,obs} \pm t_{0.95(\nu)} \, s\sqrt{2/n} \tag{1}$$

where

$\mu_{T,obs}$ = observed mean for the test treatment

$\mu_{R,obs}$ = observed mean for the reference treatment

ν = the degrees of freedom associated with the "error" mean square

$t_{0.95(\nu)}$ = the point that isolates probability of 0.05 in the upper tail of the Student's *t* distribution with ν degrees of freedom

s = the square root of the "error" mean square from the crossover design analysis of variance

n = the total number of subjects participating in the crossover design

$s\sqrt{2/n}$ = standard error of the estimate

The two one-sided tests procedure consists of a pair of ordinary one-sided *t*-tests. Since the nominal confidence level of each one-sided test is $\alpha = 0.05$, the two one-sided tests procedure is operationally equivalent to the ordinary (shortest) $1 - 2(\alpha)$ (or 90%) confidence interval. By this procedure, if test and reference products are not bioequivalent (i.e., means differ by more than 20%), there is a 5% (not a 10%) chance of concluding that they are bioequivalent.

The foregoing confidence interval equation (Eq. 1) applies to a balanced crossover study [42] in which

1. There is an equal number of subjects in each treatment–administration sequence.
2. There are no missing observations from any subject.

It is a frequent occurrence in a two-treatment, two-period crossover study that n_1 subjects have received the test formulation in period 1 and the reference

A U.S. Regulatory Perspective

formulation in period 2, and n_2 subjects have received the treatments in the opposite order ($n_1 \neq n_2$). For this unbalanced study design the confidence interval is [42]:

$$\mu_{T,ls} - \mu_{R,ls} \pm t_{0.95(\nu)} \, s \, \sqrt{\frac{1}{2}\left(\frac{1}{n_1} + \frac{1}{n_2}\right)} \tag{2}$$

where

$\mu_{T,ls}$ = least squares mean for the test treatment

$\mu_{R,ls}$ = least squares mean for the reference treatment

$s \sqrt{\frac{1}{2}\left(\frac{1}{n_1} + \frac{1}{n_2}\right)}$ = SE = standard error of the estimate

and other terms have been defined in Eq. (1).

In an unbalanced study, neither the estimated least squares means nor their difference are, in general, equal to the observed values. The least squares means, their difference and the standard error of the estimate are obtained from a computer routine. [Analysis of variance is routinely performed using the SAS Proc GLM (General Linear Models Procedure) with the least-squares means option [49], although any program providing equivalent information is acceptable]. Confidence intervals are readily calculated from such analyses using the general form of the equation:

$$\mu_{T,ls} - \mu_{R,ls} \pm t_{0.95(\nu)} \, SE \tag{3}$$

Example: Compute the 90% confidence interval (two one-sided tests procedure) for the difference of the test and reference C_{max} means given the following information. A two-treatment, two-period, single-dose crossover design study was conducted with 24 subjects. The study was balanced, meeting both criteria stated earlier (i.e., 12 subjects participated in each treatment-administration sequence and there were no missing observations from any subject).

The following data were obtained following analysis of variance performed using the SAS Proc GLM (General Linear Models Procedure).

$\mu_{T,obs}$ = 24.7 ng/mL

$\mu_{R,obs}$ = 23.7 ng/mL

ν = 22

$t_{0.95(22)}$ = 1.7171

s = 5.693

n = 24

$s\sqrt{2/n}$ = 5.693 $\sqrt{2/24}$ = 1.643

Solution: The first of the two confidence interval equations (Eq. 1) may be applied. Substituting the foregoing data into this equation:

24.7 − 23.7 ± 1.7171(1.643) ng/mL

1.0 ± 2.82 ng/mL

−1.82 ng/mL; 3.82 ng/mL

Therefore, the 90% confidence interval extends from −1.82 ng/mL below to +3.82 ng/mL above the observed reference treatment mean value. As indicated earlier, confidence interval (CI) approval criteria are based upon percentage differences from the reference treatment mean value (taken as 100%). Thus, converting to percentages:

$$\text{The lower CI limit} = \frac{23.7 - 1.82}{23.7} \times 100 = 92.3\%$$

$$\text{The upper CI limit} = \frac{23.7 + 3.82}{23.7} \times 100 = 116\%$$

As required for approval, the 90% confidence interval for the difference of the C_{max} means falls entirely within the range of 80–120% of the reference treatment mean value; thus, it meets the bioequivalence requirement for peak concentration. In general, this 90% confidence interval (two one-sided tests procedure) is asymmetric, insomuch as it is centered about the test/reference ratio of the observed means, which in the foregoing example is 1.04. Note also that, for a balanced study, the confidence interval based upon analysis of least squares means is identical with that based upon analysis of observed means.

Logarithmic Transformation and Outliers

An analysis of variance (ANOVA) may be performed on untransformed data, with the assumption that AUC and C_{max} values are normally distributed. Alternatively, an ANOVA may be performed on log-transformed data, with the assumption that AUC and C_{max} values are log normally distributed. The agency recommends the former approach, and in practice, submissions routinely include the statistical analysis performed on untransformed data. Only if the study fails to meet the 90% confidence interval criterion for either AUC or C_{max} will the firm consider an analysis based on log-transformed data. However, confidence intervals based on log-transformed data will be considered by the agency only when the normal distribution assumption on the untransformed data is not justified. Although other tests could be used, the agency recommends that the firm perform the Box–Cox analysis [50] to demonstrate that log transformation is preferred.

Although log transformation of AUC and C_{max} data before statistical analysis is of only secondary importance in FDA's bioequivalence evaluation process, it does have merit as the primary approach to analysis. The scientific basis for this approach is the following:

1. Clearance and volume of distribution are subject effects related in a multiplicative way to area and concentration, respectively. A log transformation makes these relationships additive, rather than multiplicative, which is consistent with the ANOVA model [48].
2. Some studies may include data from two or more subpopulations, as, for example, a bimodal distribution because of rapid and slow acetylators [51]. Here, a single normal distribution is not representative of the data.
3. Whether the distribution of a bioequivalence parameter from the study is "skewed," for instance, owing to clearance or volume of distribution effects, or is "contaminated," as with a few subjects belonging to a subpopulation, the log transform may have the effect of pulling in long tails in the distribution, resulting in an essentially log normal distribution [45].

Rather than assuming a normal or log normal distribution, a more thorough data analysis could be performed both with and without log transformation; residual plots would be used in the determination of the more appropriate analysis [48]. Alternatively, testing for normality of the distribution, rather than assuming normality, has been recommended [52,53]. With the small sample sizes typically used in bioequivalence studies, however, it may be very difficult to determine the true distribution.

Outliers are relatively small or large values that are considered to be different from, and not belong to, the main body of data [43]. Outliers may be divided into three groups:

1. Values resulting from a true error.
2. Values from a "skewed" population.
3. Values from a "contaminated" data set, as the foregoing bimodal distribution indicated.

Although groups 2 and 3 do not represent errors, as a result of the inability to determine the underlying distribution of the data set, as indicated, it may not be possible to determine to which of the three groups the outlier belongs.

A relatively frequent source of outliers is the chemical analysis of the samples. A result for a particular sample may be inconsistent with other assay data. When this occurs, the common practice is to reassay the sample one or more times. To avoid an arbitrary selection of the "correct" value, the firm should have a clearly defined standard operating procedure (SOP) that describes the criteria for reassay, as well as the criteria for discarding an assay result. Excessive reassays with large differences between results are an indication of analytical problems that should be minimal in a properly validated assay.

Outliers may also be observed in AUC or C_{max} parameters. Providing the clinical report documents an administration error, such as failure of the subject to swallow the medication, dosage with the wrong number of units, or premature expulsion of a rectal suppository, the aberrant value is a true error and should be discarded. For reasons other than a documented clinical problem or analytical error, outliers should not be discarded. They may be representative of a more complex parameter distribution than was realized. Providing the Box–Cox criterion is met, statistical analysis of the entire data set may be based on log-transformed data. There may be alternative statistical approaches also. For instance, the literature may document polymorphic metabolism, for which multivariate analysis may be appropriate. However, the value may not arbitrarily be discarded simply to narrow the AUC or C_{max} confidence interval(s).

Dissolution Testing and Waiver Requests

Comparative dissolution testing of solid oral dosage forms, as well as certain other dosage forms, is a required component of the bioequivalence section of an ANDA. Testing must be performed on the same lots of test and reference products used in the in vivo study. Following approval, dissolution testing is used as a quality control procedure to assure process and batch-to-batch consistency [54].

When applicable, comparative dissolution testing is used as one element of the requirements for waiver of in vivo study:

1. For those pre-1962 drugs with no actual or potential bioequivalence problems (i.e., those conventional release solid oral dosage forms rated AA in the *Orange Book*) approval from a bioequivalence point of view may be granted on the basis of in vitro (i.e., comparative dissolution) data.
2. For those drugs with multiple strengths and for which in vivo bioequivalence has been demonstrated for one strength, waiver may be granted for up to three additional strengths, providing that the formulations of the additional strengths are proportional to the strength tested in the in vivo study and that these additional strength products meet dissolution requirements.
3. For those drug products with an in vitro test that has been correlated with and is predictive of in vivo bioavailability, waiver may be granted on the basis of comparative dissolution data [25]. As a result of the in vitro–in vivo correlation established under FDA contract, the FDA accepts dissolution data as evidence of bioequivalence of prednisone tablets.

Comparative dissolution testing is a valuable tool in the formulation development process for a generic product. Once the test product has been formulated, it is recommended that the generic firm perform dissolution testing on several lots of the reference product; a representative reference lot should then be selected for in vivo study. Dissolution profiles should be obtained (generally at three or four equally spaced sampling times up to and including the time stated in the dissolution specification) for the test and reference products, using the dissolution conditions recommended by FDA. For those cases in which the FDA and *USP* dissolution conditions or specifications differ, the profile should be determined by the FDA method. However, the firm's product must meet both FDA and *USP* criteria. For those cases in which no FDA or *USP* dissolution test is available, the sponsor of the ANDA should contact the Division of Bioequivalence for advice concerning appropriate dissolution testing conditions and specifications.

The policy of the Division of Bioequivalence is to require testing of 12 dosage units each of the test and reference products. For conventional-release dosage forms, this corresponds to stage S_2 of the *USP XXII* acceptance table [55]. Therefore, the mean dissolution at the time indicated in the dissolution specification must be equal to or greater than Q, and no unit must be less than $Q - 15\%$. For controlled-release dosage forms, dissolution (drug release) testing specifications are established at three or more sampling times [56]. At each of the sampling times, the 12 dosage units must meet the requirements of level L_2 of *USP* Acceptance Table 1 [55]. The mean drug release lies within each of the stated ranges and is not less than the stated amount at the final test time; none is more than 10% of the labeled content outside each of the stated ranges; and none is more than 10% of labeled content below the stated amount at the final test time. The testing of 12 dosage units applies only to the bioequivalence section submission. It does not apply to the finished product release and stability program, which (at stage S_1 or level L_1 of *USP* testing) requires only six dosage units (i.e., dissolution or drug release testing by the *USP* three-stage procedure [55]).

Content and Format of the Bioequivalence Section of an ANDA

The regulations do not provide detailed guidance on content and format of the bioequivalence section of an ANDA. Such information has been briefly described in a February 1987 guideline [57]. In addition, a description of an ideal bioequivalence study submission has also been published [38].

The most comprehensive document [58] available that outlines the content and format of an in vivo bioequivalence study submission was prepared by the Division of Bioequivalence. The introduction to this draft document states:

> This proposed format and content write-up is prepared for submission of bioequivalency study involving both plasma/serum level and urinary excretion data. This is arranged in discrete sections in a sequence that is intended to give the reviewer a clearer and comprehensive picture of the study. Each section is intended to be complete and self-sufficient, thus allowing the reviewer a relatively easy and quick access to the required information for speedy and comprehensive review.

Table 3 is adapted from the document and lists the necessary components of a bioequivalence study submission. As indicated, the submission includes not only in vivo data, but comparative dissolution and other in vitro data, as well as formulation and batch record information.

The Division of Bioequivalence has issued a guidance [59] describing the submission of in vivo data on a floppy disk. At the present time, this electronic submission is made in addition to the hard-copy submission and is intended to facilitate confirmatory analysis or additional statistical evaluation by the reviewer without requiring the tedious manual reentry of data into the computer.

Bioequivalence Testing Laboratories and Compliance

Most bioequivalence studies are performed by contract bioequivalence testing laboratories, which are generally equipped to conduct both the clinical and analytical phases of a study. Most often, the two study phases are conducted by the same laboratory, although (because of scheduling, special analytical expertise, desire of the pharmaceutical manufacturer to conduct the analytical portion of the study in-house) they may be conducted by different laboratories. There are several firms in the United States, Canada, Europe, and Australia that possess extensive experience in the conduct of such studies. The sponsor is urged to rigorously evaluate the candidate contract laboratory(ies) before initiating the study. The evaluation should include examination of assay validation data obtained from pilot or other studies. In general, those contract laboratories with frequent dealings with the FDA understand the level of sophistication of current assay validation requirements. For those contract laboratories with infrequent dealings with the FDA, consultation with the agency prior to conducting the analysis is recommended.

The clinical studies must be conducted in compliance with Institutional Review Board (IRB) requirements [60] and with informed consent requirements [61]. For acceptance of data from any laboratory, foreign or domestic, it is important that the laboratory meet good laboratory practices and procedures. It must have a qualified staff and must keep good records of the procedures undertaken and the results obtained. Monitoring by the sponsor of each phase of the study, including validation of the assay method, protocol design, subject selection, collection and storage of the blood or urine samples, and pharmacokinetic and statistical analyses of the data, is recommended [38]. The FDA has issued a guideline discussing acceptable approaches to the monitoring of clinical investigations [62]; this guideline is generally applicable to bioequivalence studies.

To assure sound approval decisions and to investigate those instances in which gross problems are suspected, the FDA utilizes its In Vivo Bioequivalence Compliance Program. Inspections of both clinical and analytical facilities conducting bioequivalence studies may be made on an "expedited audit" basis or on a "for

Table 3 Proposed Format and Contents of an In Vivo Bioequivalence Study Submission and Accompanying In Vitro Data

Title Page

Study title
Name of sponsor
Name and address of clinical laboratory
Name of principal investigator(s)
Name of clinical investigator
Name of analytical laboratory
Dates of clinical study (start; completion)
Signature of principal investigator (and date)
Signature of clinical investigator (and date)

Table of Contents

I. Study Resume
   Product information
   Summary of bioequivalence study
   Summary of bioequivalence data
      Plasma
      Urinary excretion
   Figure of mean plasma concentration–time profile
   Figure of mean cumulative urinary excretion
   Figure of mean urinary excretion rates

II. Protocol and Approvals
   Protocol
   Letter of acceptance of protocol from FDA
   Informed consent form
   Letter of approval of Institutional Review Board
   List of members of Institutional Review Board

III. Clinical Study
   Summary of the study
   Details of the study
   Demographic characteristics of the subjects
   Subject assignment in the study
   Mean physical characteristics of subjects arranged by sequence
   Details of clinical activity
   Deviations from protocol
   Vital signs of subjects
   Adverse reactions report

IV. Assay Methodology and Validation
   Assay method description
   Validation procedure
   Summary of validation

Continued

Table 3 *(Continued)*

IV. *Continued*
   Data on linearity of standard samples
   Data on interday precision and accuracy
   Data on intraday precision and accuracy
   Figure for standard curve(s) for low/high ranges
   Chromatograms of standard and quality control samples
   Sample calculation

V. Pharmacokinetic Parameters and Tests
   Definition and calculations
   Statistical tests
   Drug levels at each sampling time and pharmacokinetic parameters
   Figure of mean plasma concentration-time profile
   Figures of individual subject plasma concentration-time profiles
   Figure of mean cumulative urinary excretion
   Figures of individual subject cumulative urinary excretion
   Figure of mean urinary excretion rates
   Figures of individual subject urinary excretion rates
   Tables of individual subject data arranged by drug, drug/period, drug/sequence

VI. Statistical Analyses
   Statistical considerations
   Summary of statistical significance
   Summary of statistical parameters
   Analysis of variance, least squares estimates and least squares means

VII. Appendices
   Randomization schedule
   Sample identification codes
   Analytical raw data
   Chromatograms of at least 20% of subjects
   Medical record and clinical reports
   Clinical facilities description
   Analytical facilities description
   Curricula vitae of the investigators

VIII. In Vitro Testing
   Dissolution testing
   Dissolution assay methodology
   Content uniformity testing
   Potency determination

IX. Batch Size and Formulation
   Batch record
   Quantitative formulation

cause" basis. The *expedited audit* is directed at studies currently under review and on which no decision of approvability has yet been made. The *for cause* audit is directed at studies, whether approved, disapproved, or pending, in which gross problems or inadequacies are suspected. The laboratory facility and its records, therefore, must be available for inspection if the agency deems this necessary.

CONCLUSION

This chapter provides a historical perspective on current bioequivalence regulations in the United States. The development of these regulations is discussed in terms of the convergence of several related factors: greatly improved analytical methodology, growth in the sciences of drug metabolism and pharmacokinetics and the increased awareness of bioavailability problems with many marketed drugs. The development and key provisions of the landmark *Bioavailability and Bioequivalence Regulations* of 1977 and *Drug Price Competition and Patent Term Restoration Act of 1984* are discussed. In addition, current bioequivalence practices and criteria are discussed, with emphasis on conventional-release solid oral dosage forms of drugs that are systemically absorbed. Bioequivalence aspects of controlled-release solid oral dosage forms have been previously considered [56]. The chapter does not address requirements for nonsystemically absorbed dosage forms (for which clinical trials may be required), nor does it address requirements for transdermal dosage forms (which are currently under consideration by the FDA).

REFERENCES

1. U.S. Department of Health and Human Services, Food and Drug Administration. *Approved Drug Products with Therapeutic Equivalence Evaluations*, 10th ed. U.S. Government Printing Office, Washington, D.C., pp. 1-1, 3-389, 3-390, 3-391, and monthly cumulative supplements (1990).
2. Bioequivalence of solid oral dosage forms. A Presentation to the U.S. Food and Drug Administration Hearing on Bioequivalence of Solid Oral Dosage Forms, September 29–October 1, 1986. Pharmaceutical Manufacturers Association, Washington, D.C., (1986) Appendix IV.
3. D. Melnick, M. Hochberg, and B. L. Oser. Physiological availability of the vitamins. I. The human bioassay technique. *J. Nutr.* 30:67-79 (1945).
4. A. B. Morrison, D. G. Chapman, and J. A. Campbell. Further studies on the relation between in vitro disintegration time of tablets and the urinary excretion rates of riboflavin. *J. Am. Pharm. Assoc. Sci. Ed.* 48:634-637 (1959).
5. A. B. Morrison and J. A. Campbell. The relationship between physiological availability of salicylates and riboflavin and in vitro disintegration time of enteric coated tablets. *J. Am. Pharm. Assoc. Sci. Ed.* 49:473-478 (1960).

6. E. J. Middleton, J. M. Davies, and A. B. Morrison. Relationship between rate of dissolution, disintegration time, and physiological availability of riboflavin in sugar-coated tablets. *J. Pharm. Sci. 53*:1378–1380 (1964).
7. G. Levy. Comparison of dissolution and absorption rates of different commercial aspirin tablets. *J. Pharm. Sci. 50*:388–392 (1961).
8. G. Levy. Effect of dosage form properties on therapeutic efficacy of tolbutamide tablets. *Can. Med. Assoc. J. 90*:978–979 (1964).
9. J. Doluisio. Historical Perspectives of Bioavailability. A Presentation at the Symposium on Bioavailability and Bioequivalency of Psychotropic Drugs, Dallas, Texas. May 19, 1985.
10. A. P. Melikian, A. B. Straughn, G. W. A. Slywka, P. L. Whyatt, and M. C. Meyer. Bioavailability of 11 phenytoin products. *J. Pharmacokinet. Biopharm. 5*:133–146 (1977).
11. P. J. Tannenbaum, E. Rosen, T. Flanagan, and A. P. Crosley, Jr. The influence of dosage form on the activity of a diuretic agent. *Clin. Pharmacol. Ther. 9*:598–604 (1968).
12. A. J. Glazko, A. W. Kinkel, W. C. Alegnani, and E. L. Holmes. An evaluation of the absorption characteristics of different chloramphenicol preparations in normal human subjects. *Clin. Pharmacol. Ther. 9*:472–483 (1968).
13. M. C. Meyer. *The Therapeutic Equivalence of Drug Products—A Second Look.* College of Pharmacy, University of Tennessee Center for the Health Sciences, Memphis (1985).
14. H. M. Abdou. *Dissolution, Bioavailability and Bioequivalence.* Mack, Easton, Pa., Chap. 27 (1989).
15. Food and Drug Administration. Human drugs: Proposed rulemaking. *Fed. Reg. 40*:26142–26171 (1975).
16. Food and Drug Administration. Abbreviated New Drug Application regulations; Proposed rule. *Fed. Reg. 54*:28872–28942 (1989).
17. Food and Drug Administration. Part 130—new drugs: Abbreviated applications. *Fed. Reg. 35*:6574–6575 (1970).
18. Drug bioequivalence. A report of the Office of Technology Assessment Drug Bioequivalence study panel. U.S. Government Printing Office, Washington, D.C., (1974).
19. Scientific commentary: Drug bioequivalence. *J. Pharmacokinet. Biopharm. 2*:433–466 (1974).
20. Food and Drug Administration. Bioequivalence requirements and in vivo bioavailability procedures. *Fed. Reg. 42*:1624–1653 (1977).
21. Bioavailability and bioequivalence requirements. 21 *CFR* 320.
22. *Drug Price Competition and Patent Term Restoration Act of 1984.* Public Law 98-417, 98 Stat. 1585–1605, September 24, (1984).
23. B. E. Cabana. Bioavailability/bioequivalence. *Food Drug Cosm. L. J. 32*:512–526 (1977).
24. Criteria and evidence to establish a bioequivalence requirement. 21 *CFR* 320.52.
25. Types of bioequivalence requirements. 21 *CFR* 320.53.
26. General approaches for determining bioavailability. 21 *CFR* 320.24.
27. Criteria for waiver of evidence of in vivo bioavailability. 21 *CFR* 320.22.

28. Report by the Bioequivalence Task Force on recommendations from the bioequivalence hearing conducted by the Food and Drug Administration (September 29–October 1, 1986). Food and Drug Administration, Rockville, Md (1988).
29. Food and Drug Administration. VI. Conforming amendments. In, *Abbreviated New Drug Application Regulations*; proposed rule. *Fed. Reg.* 54:28911–28912 (1989).
30. Food and Drug Administration. Types of evidence to establish bioavailability or bioequivalence (21 *CFR* 320.24) in Abbreviated New Drug Application regulations; proposed rule. *Fed. Reg.* 54:28940–28941 (1989).
31. Guidelines on the design of a single-dose in vivo bioavailability study. 21 *CFR* 320.26.
32. Guidelines on the design of a multiple-dose in vivo bioavailability study. 21 *CFR* 320.27.
33. *U.S. Pharmacopeia*, 22nd rev. U.S. Pharmacopeial Convention, Rockville, Md., pp. 1710–1712 (1990).
34. D. R. Williams. An overview of test method validation. *BioPharm (Nov)* 1:34–36, 51 (1987).
35. V. P. Shah. Analytical methods used in bioavailability studies: A regulatory viewpoint. *Clin. Res. Pract. Drug Regul. Affairs* 5:51–60 (1987).
36. H. T. Karnes, G. Shiu, and V. P. Shah. Validation of bioanalytical methods. *Pharm. Res.* (accepted for publication).
37. M. A. Brooks and R. E. Weinfeld. A validation process for data from the analysis of drugs in biological fluids. *Drug Dev. Ind. Pharm.* 11:1703–1728 (1985).
38. S. V. Dighe. Current bioavailability and bioequivalence requirements and regulations. *Clin. Res. Pract. Drug Regul. Affairs* 2:401–421 (1984).
39. J. A. F. de Silva. Validation of bioanalytical procedures: An example. In, *Drug Determination in Therapeutic and Forensic Contexts*. (E. Reid and I. D. Wilson, eds.) Plenum, New York, pp. 385–392 (1984).
40. L. Aarons, S. Toon, and M. Rowland. Validation of assay methodology used in pharmacokinetic studies. *J. Pharmacol. Methods* 17:337–346 (1987).
41. L. Aarons. General approach to handling nonuniform variance in assay calibration. *J. Pharm. Biomed. Anal.* 2:395–402 (1984).
42. D. J. Schuirmann. A comparison of the two one-sided tests procedure and the power approach for assessing the equivalence of average bioavailability. *J. Pharmacokinet. Biopharm.* 15:657–680 (1987).
43. S. Bolton. *Pharmaceutical Statistics: Practical and Clinical Applications*, 2nd ed. Marcel Dekker, New York, pp. 153, 187, 354–355 (1990).
44. J. D. Haynes. FDA 75/75 rule: A response. *J. Pharm. Sci.* 72:99–100 (1983).
45. C. M. Metzler and D. C. Huang. Statistical methods for bioavailability and bioequivalence. *Clin. Res. Pract. Drug Regul. Affairs* 1:109–132 (1983).
46. S. Anderson and W. W. Hauck. Consideration of individual bioequivalence. *J. Pharmacokinet. Biopharm.* 18:259–273 (1990).
47. W. J. Westlake. Use of confidence intervals in analysis of comparative bioavailability trials. *J. Pharm. Sci.* 61:1340–1341 (1972).
48. W. J. Westlake. Bioavailability and bioequivalence of pharmaceutical formulations. In, *Biopharmaceutical Statistics for Drug Development*, Chap. 7 (K. E. Peace, ed.) Marcel Dekker, New York (1988).

49. SAS Institute Inc. SAS/STAT *User's Guide*, Release 6.03 ed. SAS Institute Inc., Cary, NC, Chap. 20 (1988).
50. G. E. P. Box and D. R. Cox. An analysis of transformations. *J. R. Stat. Soc. Ser. B* 26:211–252 (1964).
51. C. M. Metzler. Equivalence of bioavailability and efficacy in drug testing. In, *Pharmacokinetics: Mathematical and Statistical Approaches to Metabolism and Distribution of Chemicals and Drugs*. (A. Pecile and A. Rescigno, eds.) Plenum Press, New York, pp. 215–225 (1988).
52. E. G. Boyce and J. M. Nappi. Is there significance beyond the t-test? *Drug Intell. Clin. Pharm.* 22:334–335 (1988).
53. J. Zuidema and H. J. A. Wynne. Data-reduction problems in biopharmaceutics and pharmacokinetics. *Pharm. Weekbl. Sci. Ed.* 11:76–82 (1989).
54. PMA's Joint Committee on Bioavailability. The role of dissolution testing in drug quality, bioavailability, and bioequivalence testing. *Pharm. Technol.* 9(6):62, 64, 66 (1985).
55. *U.S. Pharmacopeia*, 22nd rev. U.S. Pharmacopeial Convention, Rockville, Md., Chaps. 711 and 724, pp. 1578–1583 (1990).
56. S. V. Dighe and W. P. Adams. Bioavailability and bioequivalence of oral controlled-release products: A regulatory perspective. In, *Pharmacokinetics: Regulatory-Industrial-Academic Perspectives*, Chap. 8 (P. G. Welling and F. L. S. Tse, eds.) Marcel Dekker, New York (1988).
57. U.S. Department of Health and Human Services, Food and Drug Administration. Guideline for the format and content of the human pharmacokinetics and bioavailability section of an application. U.S. Government Printing Office, Washington, D.C. (1987).
58. R. N. Patnaik. Proposed format and contents of submission of bioequivalency study and dissolution testing sections of ANDA. Division of Bioequivalence, Food and Drug Administration, Rockville, Md. (1987).
59. M. R. Hamrell. Informal guidance on the submission of data for bioequivalence studies in computer format. Division of Bioequivalence, Food and Drug Administration, Rockville, Md. (1987).
60. Institutional Review Boards. 21 *CFR* 56.
61. Protection of human subjects. Informed consent of human subjects. 21 *CFR* 50 (Subpart B).
62. Guideline for the monitoring of clinical investigations. Division of Compliance Policy, Bioresearch Program Coordinator, Food and Drug Administration, Rockville, Md, Docket No. 82D-0322 (1988).

13
Bioequivalence: A Canadian Regulatory Perspective

Iain J. McGilveray
Health Protection Branch
Bureau of Drug Research
Ottawa, Ontario, Canada

INTRODUCTION

During the late 1960s an unusual juxtaposition of scientific research and political direction in Canada led to the first use of (what later would be defined as) bioequivalence data in the approval of drug products. It was, without question, controversial. Some of the legislative background in that era has been discussed by Cook [1,2]. Essentially, following the report of a Parliamentary Committee chaired by H. C. Harley [3] concerning drug costs within the Canadian health care system, the government adopted policies to attempt to provide drugs at reasonable costs. Most disputed were the amendments to the Patent Act (June 1969), which simplified procedures for obtaining a compulsory license. Although the Compulsory Licensing Amendment was revised in 1988 to extend patent protection, from 1969 many generic New Drug products were marketed in Canada under the arrangements devised by Harley. However, the recommendations also delegated additional responsibilities to the Drugs Directorate of the Department of National Health and Welfare, to ensure that *requirements* of the food and Drug Act and Regulations were met. These call for the manufacturer to file a New Drug Submission (NDS), similar to the U.S. New Drug Application (NDA) that must provide evidence of safety, efficacy, and consistency of quality for New Drugs, essentially those marketed after 1962 (but which may be applied to older agents if presented for new claims or in new dosage forms or strength). As well as requiring increased in vitro testing and promulgation of information on product quality, the responsibility for comparative efficacy assessment was made a priority.

As it developed, after the early description of "physiological availability" for vitamins by Oser in 1945, in the 1950s and 1960s scientists in the department (particularly the Nutrition Division) had been involved in research into bioavailability.

J. M. Campbell and A. B. Morrison and their associates contributed a seminal series of scientific articles and reviews, mainly for vitamins, but also including some drugs such as salicylates [4] and *p*-aminosalicylic acid [5]. They had been searching for improved quality control procedures that would reflect "physiological availability," having found the *United States Pharmacopeia (USP)* or *British Pharmacopoeia (BP)* disintegration tests deficient [6]. In fact, Pernarowski, who worked in this group, later developed the rotating basket prototype for the USP dissolution apparatus I [7]. Thus, when the responsibility for comparative efficacy assessment was delegated to the department, Morrison, by now a senior official, was attuned to the potential for bioavailability comparisons. Hence, the new program, (the Quality Assessment of Drugs Program; QUAD), integrated pre- and postmarketing surveillance, including a component to generate comparative bioavailability data. Obviously, there were other documentary aspects of the program (which will not be described in detail) including drug master files, in vitro testing to stated standards, and so forth, and the provision of information to the provincial departments of health and the health professions.

[It is important to note that in Canada, as with the individual states in the United States, the ten provinces and two territories have the responsibility for health care and licensing of health professions. Various "Pharmacare" programs are administered by provincial jurisdictions, mainly by formulary systems. Many of these formularies have pharmacy and therapeutic committees of external academic consultants who consider items for the formulary and, particularly, aspects of interchangeability, which has not been a direct federal concern. It is thus possible for a new drug product to be allowed on the market by the federal agency, but, because of some concern in the responsible provincial committee, not be listed (e.g., disputing that the evidence of bioequivalence is sufficient to allow substitution for a critical drug).]

The remainder of this chapter will review the measures taken to implement this first regulatory program to apply bioequivalence (as it was later defined by the United States) and the guidelines now developed.

BIOAVAILABILITY: CANADIAN DEFINITION AND ADVISORY COMMITTEE

Definition and Standard

One of the first tasks toward the use of comparative bioavailability data as evidence of comparative efficacy was to define bioavailability and to set a standard to be attained for acceptance.

The definition of *bioavailability* published in 1973 [8] stated.

> Bioavailability of a drug product is determined by rate and extent (efficiency) of absorption and distribution of the active substance to the site of action in the body in relation to the substance's rate of loss.

It was also noted, however, that

> In practice [relative] bioavailability is usually estimated as the ratio of areas under the drug concentration curves in time–serum concentration profiles for the test formulation and reference, to the same group of subjects according to a statistically sound design. It may also be based on similar comparisons of drug excreted in the urine.

An initial arbitrary standard of, at least, 80% extent of biovailability relative to a reference formulation was announced. This was decided by senior officials, in part, because official [8] in vitro drug content standards (as well as those professed in NDSs) commonly gave tolerances of 90–110% for oral dosage forms, whereas content uniformity usually allowed a range of 85–115% for individual units. The announcement led to scrutiny of the total program by various groups, notably the Canadian Medical Association and the Pharmaceutical Manufacturers Association of Canada, between 1971 and 1974.

Expert Advisory Committee

This resulted in yet another report of a Special Advisory Committee to the Health Protection Branch [9] which, as well as refining the definitions and indicating that improved limits should be set, suggested that there be a permanent Expert Advisory Committee (EAC) on Bioavailability. This was struck in 1974. From the onset the chairman has been Dr. John Ruedy, originally from McGill University School of Medicine, but presently at the University of British Columbia, St. Paul's Hospital, Medical School.

There have been about 20 different committee members rotated, representing various medical specialties, as well as faculties of pharmacy. They have advised on specific drug problems as required, but most recently have been preparing guidelines that will be summarized later in this chapter.

EARLY LABORATORY WORK

Background

In 1969, no other country was using comparative bioavailability in regulatory efficacy assessment. Aside from early research, such as cited under Campbell and Morrison and also reviewed in Wagners 1971 book [10], there were no experimental protocols for bioavailability comparisons. Neither were there established data treatments including statistical analyses. The laboratory arm of the Drugs Directorate (now the Bureau of Drug Research), therefore developed plans to undertake pilot studies, as well as larger-scale studies of multisource drugs to develop a suitable data base.

It should be noted, however, that there had been previous generic drug products available in most countries. These were formulations of older agents, such as aspirin and quinidine, which were multisource and regulated only with pharmacopeial in vitro standards. As the provision of adequate safety and efficacy information for New Drug products (essentially, post-1962) to be introduced under compulsory license was the responsibility of the manufacturers under the new drug regulations [11] mandate, old drug formulations were studied in the department laboratory. The criteria developed for the choice of drugs to study included medical use, criticality of dose, available methodology, and potential for poor bioavailability (such as described in the literature). Although larger studies were contracted out, many of the studies were carried out in-house, with civil servant volunteers. Before any experiment, all protocols had to be approved by the Branch Human Studies Committee (i.e., The Institutional Ethical Review Board). They provided strict reviews, for example, they would not allow griseofulvin to be studied, even with a "single-dose, crossover" protocol involving about six single-doses, because the drug is mutagenic. Erythromycin estolate was also withdrawn from a study because of a few reports of hepatotoxicity during therapeutic use.

Drugs Under Study

The number of drugs and products studied over 14 years is given in Table 1. This chapter will not review all the studies, but will focus on a few in which the discussions of Health Protection Branch (HPB) officials and the EAC led to the development of standards. In addition to the bioequivalence assessment, an early goal was the desirability of establishing correlations between the in vitro results and dissolution or even dissolution–permeation data. The search for in vitro predictive tests for bioequivalence was largely abandoned, as described later using published and unpublished information.

Early studies with nitrofurantoin and hydrochlorothiazide used colorimetric assays of cumulative urinary excretion. The experiments were designed in Latin squares (such as 7 × 7) and volunteers were water-loaded to enable production

Table 1 Comparative Bioavailability Studies Completed by the Bureau of Drug Research

Drug	Dosage form	Number of products tested
Acetaminophen	Tablets	10
Allopurinol	Tablets	6
Ampicillin	Capsules	7
Aminophylline	Tablets	2
Betamethasone	MR tablets	1[a]
Chlordiazepoxide	Capsules	14
Chlordiazepoxide	Tablets	2
Diazepam	Tablets	2
Digoxin	Tablets	18
Erythromycin base	Tablets	2
Erythromycin stearate	Tablets	2
Erythromycin ethyl succinate	Tablets	2
Hydrochlorothiazide	Tablets	32
Ibuprofen	Tablets	3
Isoniazid	Tablets	3
Lithium carbonate	Capsules	2
Metronidazole	Tablets	8
Nitrofurantoin	Tablets	16
Oxtriphylline	Tablets	2
Phenylbutazone	Tablets	21
Phenylbutazone	Capsules	1[b]
Phenytoin	Capsules	6
Phenytoin	Tablets	1
Prednisone	Tablets	2
Quinidine sulfate	Tablets	8
Quinidine gluconate	Tablets	2
Qunidine polygalacturonate	Tablets	1
Sulfamethizole	Tablets	4
Sulfisoxasole	Tablets	13
Tetracycline HCl	Capsules	16
Tetracycline HCl	Tablets	12
Tetracycline w/phosphate	Capsules	9
Warfarin sodium	Tablets	3
Warfarin potassium	Tablets	1[c]
Zinc aminochelate	Tablets	2
Zinc citrate	Tablets	1
Zinc gluconate	Tablets	1
Zinc oratate	MR tablets	1
Zinc sulfate	Capsules	1[d]

[a]Reference: conventional tablet
[b]Reference: innovator tablet
[c]Reference: innovator warfarin sodium
[d]Reference: for all zinc products

of frequent urine samples. The statisticians implemented analysis of variance (ANOVA) methods appropriate for the design. Multiple comparison tests, such as those of Dunnett [12] or Tukey [13], were employed to ensure an experiment-wide error rate of 5% when comparing means from different products.

Major Study: Phenylbutazone

However, it was a large study of phenylbutazone products in 1974 [14] that was pivotal in rationalizing the parameters to be examined and the statistical approach; therefore, this study will be described and examined in detail.

There were 22 solid oral dosage form products, including reference innovator lot (Butazolidin, 100-mg tablets) and a solution. These formulations were given in single (2 × 100-mg) doses to groups of overnight-fasted volunteers, following randomization into a crossover design, with blood collected up to 192 hr (8 days) after each dose and a minimum washout period of 3 weeks. There were ten groups of nine subjects to whom the reference and two different products per group were given, according to a design comprising three, 3 × 3 Latin squares. One group involved eight volunteers, to whom reference, solution (200 mg in 200 mL, pH 7.4 buffer), and two tablet products were given, following duplicate 4 × 4 Latin squares. In all cases plasma phenylbutazone was estimated with an ultraviolet absorption procedure [15], validated against gas chromatographic and high-performance liquid chromatographic procedures [14].

Typical results are shown as the average profiles for the eight subjects who received reference and solution and two other products (Fig. 1). This study was probably the first time such a large data base on bioavailability comparison with one drug had been collected, and some important data management concerns were soon realized.

Drug Content Correction

When the results were being examined, an early decision was to "normalize for dose," recognizing that, if no drug content corrections were made, manufacturers submitting bioequivalence studies could select lots almost 10% higher in content than reference (according to usual pharmacopeial tolerances). The FDA currently calls for lots tested in comparisons to be within 5% in label assay to accomplish a similar end [16]. In any event, the phenylbutazone and subsequent studies, as well as evaluations at the HPB, required correction for test and reference content.

Parameters

It was found that concentration–time curves could be sufficiently compared by three parameters: extent of absorption by area under the curve (AUC) calculated with the trapezoidal rule to the last blood collection point (AUC_{192}); rate of absorption by peak concentration (C_{max}); and time to attain C_{max}, t_{max}. The terminal

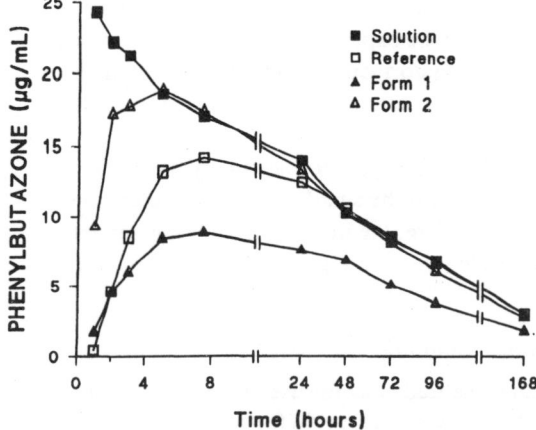

Figure 1 Mean plasma concentration profiles obtained after single-dose, crossover administration of 2 × 100-mg tablets (refererence, formulation 1 and 2) of phenylbutazone to eight normal volunteer subjects. A solution (200 mg in 20 mL of pH 7.4 buffer) was also administered.

half-life ($t_{1/2}$) was also calculated; however, the latter is not used in comparisons, as this is generally a function of the drug, not the formulation.

Study Design

The crossover design was quite useful, because volunteers tended to show less variation within themselves than between themselves or, expressed in another way, the intrasubject variance component was much smaller than the *inter*subject variance component. This meant that fewer subjects could be used than would be required in parallel studies.

Logarithmic Transformation

The usefulness of logarithmic (log) transformation for concentration-based measures proved invaluable because of the large *inter*subject variation. The rationale for effecting the log transformation is based on the common formula

$$\log (T/R) = \log T - \log R$$

The ratio (T/R) (e.g., relative AUC) can be obtained by analyzing the logs and transforming the difference of the means of the logs back into the original scale.

As more data on more drugs was collected within the branch, the evidence for the use of the log transformation grew. Ormsby [17] noted that for 70% of the studies submitted to the HPB since 1985, the log transformation gave a smaller error variance than did the same analysis on the raw scale. This result indicates that differences between formulations may be expressed in a multiplicative manner within a subject. The use of the transformation converts a multiplicative response into an additive one, such that the assumption of additivity is assured in the ANOVA.

It was also noted that tests such as Box–Cox [18] for normality have very little power in discriminating distributions with the small sample sizes common in comparative bioavailability studies. Therefore, the individual study cannot determine the scale to use, and it was decided that the log transformation should be used a priori [19].

Hypothesis Testing and Confidence Intervals

It was also noted from the phenylbutazone study that the use of the null hypothesis test of no difference from the ANOVA as a decision rule for bioequivalence was not appropriate. It is inappropriate for two reasons. First, when there is high variability, the hypothesis test would fail to reject the null hypothesis of no difference because the power of the test is very low. Second, when there is small variation, a statistically significant difference, of say 10%, may be declared, which is of no clinical relevance for many drugs. It was decided that the decision rule would be based on the classic 95% confidence interval (CI) because, by definition, the interval gave what was desired (i.e., there is a 95% chance that the interval contains the true value). All that was then needed was to define a bioequivalence interval within which the CI should fall, such that bioequivalence could be declared. Therefore, limits were needed to quantitate how much the test formulation could differ from the reference formulation to have little clinical difference. The ± 20% difference was derived logically from the earlier 80% standard described previously. Since the log transformation was used, the bioequivalence interval (BI) was set at 80–125%. This asymmetry about 100% is due to transforming back into relative percentage.

The result of using the combination of the CI and the BI as a decision rule is illustrated in Figure 2. The two curves give the probability that the CI will fall within the BI, thus accepting the test formulation for a given set of parameters. The greatest chance of passing occurs when the true means are the same (i.e., 100%), but the chances fall off quite rapidly as the true ratio deviates from 100%. With a coefficient of variation (CV) of 30%, common for drugs with complicated kinetics, the chance that a study will pass has a maximum of only around 0.20. Curves calculated in this way are particularly useful in determining how many subjects to include in a proposed study.

The adoption of the classic 95% CI along with the BI was an attractive way to examine results from different studies. This is illustrated by the tablulation of the AUC findings for all the phenylbutazone products (Table 2).

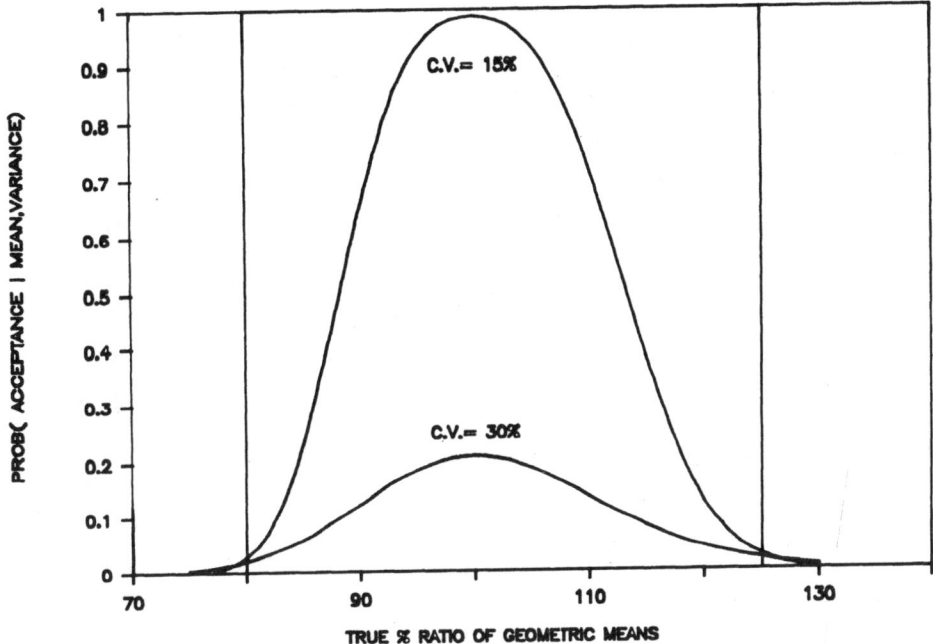

Figure 2 Probability of acceptance of a test formulation given the true ratio of geometric means for intrasubject CVs of 15 and 30%. Probabilities are based on a 20-subject, two-period crossover design; analysis on the log scale; the 95% CI for the ratio of geometric means; and a bioequivalence interval of 80–125%.

The results for formulations 1, 7, 8, 19, and 20, which gave mean AUCs less than 80%, led to withdrawal of these products from the market. Although action against products with 95% CIs outside the 80–125% range was considered, for this study it was deferred.

About the time of this phenylbutazone study, literature started appearing on decision rules for bioequivalence data. Westlake [20] proposed the use of the classic confidence interval and later [21] proposed a different interval symmetric about 100%, not around the point estimate as in classical CI. The FDA continued with hypothesis testing, with the added requirement that the study had to have 80% power to distinguish a 20% difference [22]. Later the 75/75 rule was used, until it was shown to be biased when the reference formulation was more variable [23]. Continuing in the hypothesis framework, Schuirmann [24] of the FDA, proposed the two one-sided test, which appears to be the one the FDA now applies. It should be noted that the two one-sided test of an α of 5% leads to the identical decisions on

Table 2 Phenylbutazone 2 × 100-mg Tablet Formulations. Extent of Bioavailability vs Reference Ranked by % AUC ratio

Formulation	AUC ratio (%)[a]	95% CI
1	58	(49, 70)
19	63	(55, 73)
8	67	(57, 78)
7	73	(63, 86)
20	78	(68, 89)
15	82	(76, 88)
6	83	(75, 93)
3	90	(83, 98)
21	97	(86, 109)
12	97	(92, 103)
13	97	(93, 101)
2	98	(82, 118)
17	100	(91, 110)
18	101	(92, 112)
22	102	(91, 115)
4	104	(95, 113)
14	105	(101, 110)
Solution	105	(88, 126)
5	106	(95, 117)
11	108	(103, 113)
16	108	(101, 116)
10	112	(103, 121)
9	116	(107, 127)

[a]AUC entries are AUC_{192}, corrected for potency, with 95% classic confidence intervals.

bioequivalence that a 90% CI does when the same BI is used. Most recently, Hauschke et al. [25] have proposed a nonparametric CI that takes into account the period effect in the crossover nature of the data collection.

Possibly the major advantage of the confidence interval is that it summarizes the quality of the data quantitatively for the nonstatistician, and it was used in subsequent studies, such as metronidazole [26] and phenytoin [27]. Indeed, major medical journals have recently asked that most data be presented with confidence intervals [28].

Statisticians defer the decision on what should be acceptable, either with a hypothesis test or a confidence interval, to the clinical pharmacology or medical specialist. However, this option has not been well developed because of the uncertainties in the relationship between the plasma concentration–time course of most drugs and their quality and duration of effects. Comparison of confidence intervals of several studies, in fact, provides the reviewer with a perception of the range of variation of a particular drug. The idea of a flexible bioequivalence interval for drugs with high intrinsic variation, has been discussed, but has not been adopted. Currently, more subjects have to be used.

Solution Standards

The phenylbutazone study and earlier studies attempted to use a "baseline" standard formulation of a solution or suspension. However, this idea was largely abandoned, partly because the clinical trial work to prove claims had been completed with an originator's solid dosage form and partly because the solution was usually so unpalatable that it led to nausea and vomiting. Also, if it were not a marketed formulation, ethics committees were skeptical of its relevance versus safety and comfort of the subjects, and often solutions exhibited pharmacokinetic properties different from the marketed formulation. Many of these caveats are also relevant to the intravenous formulation used as absolute reference. Nonetheless, in many cases, solutions have a role in early developmental work. Suspensions are more difficult to use, since, for poorly soluble drugs, particle size can cause problems.

Problem of Absorption Rate in Bioequivalence

Rate consideration, with pharmacokinetic modeling, was considered for equivalence evaluation of *rate* of absorption. It was soon apparent that even with simple models, which may be inappropriate, all data from all subjects could not be fitted.

An example is given with a calcium channel antagonist in Figure 3; the mean profile could be fitted readily, but not the individual data in which fluctuation occurred. Also, in examining the statistics for absorption rate, it was difficult to formulate a decision rule, as the clinical significance of differences was obscure, and usually, there were too few data points or within-subject variability was high, resulting in poor discrimination. Usually, to obtain reliable estimates of absorption rate variables, administration of a solution or even an intravenous dose was required, and this was rarely acceptable.

For phenylbutazone, the absorption rate indicator, C_{max}, as well as concentration at 2 hr was exained and five formulations were significantly higher or lower than that of the innovator. However, since the drug is given in multiple-dose courses, the Advisory Committee decided that only the extent criterion (i.e., AUC) would be applied to these formulations.

Warfarin Study and Rate

Another single-dose bioequivalence study completed with warfarin in the 1970s, again resulted in intensive statistical consideration. The trial involved three formulations of test and a reference tablet (A, B, C, and R, respectively). The

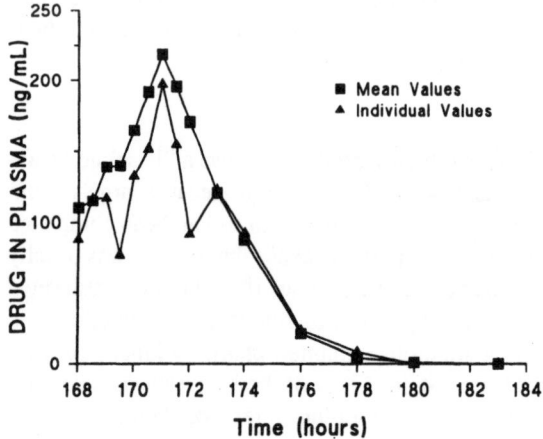

Figure 3 Plasma concentration profiles of a calcium channel antagonist drug at the end of steady-state dosing (q6h). The mean values of 24 subjects are compared with those from an individual subject for the same manufacturer's formulation.

study was completed with eight volunteers, according to a duplicated 4 × 4 Latin square design [29]. The overall results are shown in Table 3.

It is evident from the AUC ratios that one formulation, C, although above 80% in geometric mean, was significantly less absorbed than the reference, but the confidence interval is narrow. The committee was concerned about the C_{max} ratio for this drug, which exhibits nonlinear response. Two of the formulations, C and D, gave significantly lower C_{max} values than the reference, and all three gave 95% confidence lower limits below 80%.

The advice rendered was that, although individually the products were considered satisfactory, ". . . they showed sufficiently different bioavailability

Table 3 Warfarin 5-mg Tablet (Four Tablet) Formulation Bioavailability Results

Formulation	AUC%[a] 95% CI	C_{max} %[a]	95% CI
B	97 (88, 107)	89	(78, 102)
C	87 (79, 95)	78	(68, 70)
D	101 (91, 111)	86	(75, 98)

[a]AUC_{96} and C_{max} vs reference expressed as % ratio geometric mean of three formulations B, C, D, to reference, 95% classic confidence interval in parenthesis.

characteristics that interchange or substitution of one product for another was not recommended without retitration of the patient" [30]. The HPB reviewers were thus encouraged to use an 80–125% interval decision rule.

Add-on Study Concerns

In 1978, a protocol for a single-dose, comparative 12-subject study of a combination, antihypertensive generic product versus innovator was submitted for review. Although warned that the variation from the *non*-thiazide component could be as high as 40%, according to the literature and, thus, that 12 subjects would be unlikely to provide the required confidence, the study was completed.

The AUC results are listed in Table 4 and did not meet the 80–125%, 95% CI requirement. The manufacturer subsequently sponsored a study with 22 subjects, and this again did not meet the interval. The statisticians, however, agreed that the studies could be combined and the results were thought to be clinically acceptable (combined results also in Table 4). Two points were established following this decision. It is expected that the 95% CI limit for AUC should be kept within 80–125% and that different studies may be combined. The concept of an "add-on" study is not accepted by all statisticians; however, recently Karpinski has formalized the branch position [31], and, provided tests of consistency are acceptable, this approach may be used. However, it is *not* a mechanism to permit pilot study data to be combined with those from larger studies to influence a major bioequivalence decision. The add-on design is one possible mechanism for study of drugs with high intrinsic variability.

Importance of C_{max} in Assessment of Short-Term Use Drugs

For most drugs used in long-term therapy, unless the kinetics are unusual, it is the extent of bioavailability represented by AUC that determines the steady-state profile attained. The single-dose, fasted subject, comparative blood or serum level study is relatively efficient at providing a reasonable estimate that provides a proxy measure of efficacy relative to a standard. There are complications perturbing this simple model, such as patients with disease states who may react differently from the volunteers tested. The most obvious limitation of the extent criterion

Table 4 Antihypertensive Combination. AUC_t ratio of one component. Geometric mean vs reference with 95% CI and *intra*subject CV%

	AUC%	95% CI	CV%
Study 1, n = 12	91	(70, 119)	29
Study 2, n = 22	110	(91, 132)	31
Combined 1 and 2	103	(89, 120)	30

is with drugs used acutely, the action onset time of which may be related to rate of input. For these, some measure of absorption rate is needed.

The branch experience with several formulations of ibuprofen demonstrates the problem. Although manufacturer data cannot be presented, the bureau undertook a comparative study of two generic formulations, designated A (sugar-coated) and B (film-coated), 200-mg tablets of ibuprofen versus innovator (Motrin). This was an 18-subject, three-period crossover design, under fasting conditions.

The overall results are given with the mean profiles in Figure 4. The two test formulations are more slowly absorbed, although not different in extent.

Results are shown in Table 5. The geometric means of AUC_{12} ratios 95.4 and 98.2% were also well within the 80–125% ratio for a 95% CI. The C_{max} ratios, however, are not within either a mean ratio or the 95% CI tolerance of 80–125%. Some manufacturer studies, however, did have results that were marginally acceptable for C_{max}. Thus, some other area ratios were examined, such as AUC to 2 hr (AUC_2) and AUC ratio to the time of the reference t_{max} (AUC_{IT}). Although the variation was high for AUC_2, it could be used with a bioequivalence interval in several studies. Although AUC_{IT} appears reasonable for this study, it was often too variable with CV > 100% when several sets of manufacturer's data were examined.

DISSOLUTION AND BIOEQUIVALENCE

Dissolution Study Objectives

When the program of bioequivalence studies was initiated, one objective, also examined by other investigators, was to attempt to correlate in vivo plasma concentration results with in vitro dissolution. Some of the experiments were completed before the *USP* had official apparatuses and some after these were introduced. Overall, as others have found, the dissolution results from this laboratory could not reliably predict in vivo behavior. A few relative successes are cited, along with some reasons for other failures.

Successful Dissolution Correlations

Phenylbutazone: Dissolution and Bioavailability

A relatively successful correlation between extent of bioavailability and mean time for 60% of drug to be dissolved was obtained with the phenylbutazone study described earlier [32]. Of two apparatuses (the *USP* rotating basket and a reciprocating basket akin to the *USP* disintegration test) with two sets of conditions, the reciprocating basket, with pH 7.2 phosphate buffer, provided the most discriminating conditions. All but one of the formulations with 80% or greater AUC ratio and only one of the less-than-80% bioavailable formulations were more

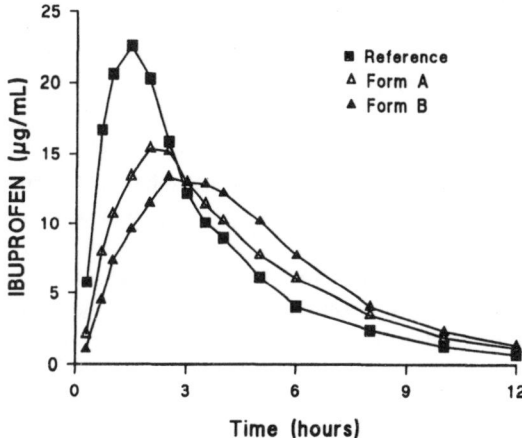

Figure 4 Mean plasma concentrations obtained after single-dose crossover administration of 300 mg ibuprofen tablets (reference, formulations A and B) to 18 normal volunteers.

than 60% dissolved at 50 min, and the correlation coefficient (r) was 0.84. Pretreatment of tablets with pH 1.2 hydrochloric acid before the phosphate buffer did not improve the correlation. The *USP* rotating basket, with pH 7.2 phosphate, was less discriminating, which may be accounted for by differences in the intensity of agitation between the apparatuses. The comparisons with C_{max} and t_{max} are unreported in the publication, but were no better than the AUC results.

Tetracycline: Dissolution and Bioavailability Comparison

Perhaps the most successful correlation obtained in our laboratories was with a study of nine brands of tetracycline tablets [33], which were compared in 12

Table 5 Comparative Bioavailability Parameters of Sugar-Coated (A) and Film-Coated (B) vs Reference Ibuprofen, 200-mg Tablets

Parameter	Form A	Form B
AUC_2 ratio (%)	50 (32, 77)	28 (18, 44)
AUC_{12} ratio (%)	95 (89, 106)	98 (89, 109)
$AUC_{IT}{}^a$ ratio (%)	38 (20, 71)	19 (10, 37)
C_{max} ratio (%)	70 (65, 78)	62 (57, 69)
t_{max} diff (hr)	1.15 (0.5, 1.8)	1.71 (1.0, 2.4)

[a] AUC_{IT} is the area under the plasma level curve to the t_{max} of the innovator.

volunteers, with solutions (given three times) assaying both whole blood tetracycline concentrations and urinary excretion. Again the *USP* rotating basket at 100 rpm and the reciprocating basket just described were operated in pH 1.2 hydrochloric acid. The in vivo results were bimodal in distribution, with most tablets having AUC ratios of 80% or greater, compared with solution and urinary excretion of 75–100% of the solution doses. Two products had AUC ratios of 25–35% and cumulative urinary excretion of 25 and 42% of that solution. Although an excellent $r^2 > 0.95$ was obtained between the in vivo percentage bioavailability and time to 60% dissolution, the bimodal nature of the relationship was felt to be misleading. Nonetheless, both dissolution procedures gave good rank order correlations, significant at $p < 0.05$, discriminating the very poorly absorbed formulations. Examination of the scatter of formulations with AUC ratios from 74–95%, versus the time to 60% dissolution, indicated that the test was less sensitive in predicting over this range.

Less Successful Dissolution Correlations

Background Problem

Several of the studies in the later 1970s, such as isoniazid [34], gave plasma profiles (in this case, of two test versus reference tablets) that were virtually superimposable (AUC ratio 100–105%, CV 11%), and the dissolution results with the *USP* rotating basket showed more differences than in vivo, with the mean time for 60% to be dissolved ranging from 1 to 11 min between formulations. However, two examples are provided when there were in vivo differences that were not detected by dissolution.

Allopurinol. Six tablet formulations of allopurinol (300 mg) were studied in 12 subjects according to a duplicated 6 × 6 Latin square design for single-dose bioavailability comparison, with innovator as reference. The lots were chosen for study on the basis of differences in dissolution. Plasma profiles of allopurinol and the major metabolite oxipurinol were obtained up to 72 hr after each dose. The results are summarized in Table 6. Absorption rates and mean residence times were also derived.

The dissolution conditions applied to these tablets involved *USP* apparatus 1 and 2, with water, or pH 1.2 hydrochloric acid at 50 and 100 rpm. Different volumes (900 and 1800 mL) were also used, and the amounts dissolved at 15, 30, 45, and 60 min were observed. Summary results for dissolution are given in Table 7.

No useful correlation was obtained predictive of bioavailability. The highest coefficient of determination was obtained between amounts dissolved in 15 min (*USP* paddle, water = at 100 rpm) and t_{max} of oxipurinol ($r^2 = 0.95$), but the differences in t_{max} were neither significant, nor did they reflect bioavailability!

Table 6 Comparative Bioavailability Parameters of Five Allupurinol Products (B,C,D,E,F) vs Reference (observed means with 95% CI in parentheses)

Parameter	Formulations				
	B	C	D	E	F
%AUC_t ratio (AL)	104 (77, 140)	84 (62, 113)	88 (65, 119)	112 (83, 151)	100 (74, 135)
%AUC_t ratio (OX)	98 (87, 111)	81[a] (72, 92)	101 (89, 114)	110 (97, 124)	101 (89, 114)
%C_{max} ratio (AL)	95 (71, 111)	55[a] (41, 74)	87 (65, 117)	120 (89, 161)	102 (76, 137)
%C_{max} ratio (OX)	93 (80, 109)	77[a] (66, 90)	90 (77, 105)	106 (91, 124)	93 (79, 108)
t_{max} (AL) (hr)	1.11	1.61	1.36	1.23	1.45
t_{max} (OX) (hr)	3.84	4.61	5.32	3.77	4.68

[a]Significant at $\alpha = 0.05$.
AL, allopurinol; OX, oipurinol.

Table 7 Dissolution Times of Allopurinol 300-mg Tablet Products[a]

Formulation	Medium	Time (min)			
		15	30	45	60
Reference	W	82	89	92	94
	A	95	96	98	97
B	W	99	100	100	100
	A	96	97	97	98
C	W	67	84	90	93
	A	62	84	92	95
D	W	8	11	14	17
	A	82	94	95	97
E	W	103	103	104	104
	A	103	103	103	103
F	W	35	52	62	70
	A	13	35	53	64

[a]% Dissolved in time (min) *USP* apparatus 2 at 100 rpm water (W) or 0.1 N hydrocholoric acid (A).

Only one product (C) gave significantly reduced extent and rate of bioavailability (80%) (see Table 6). Unfortunately, product C was in the midrange of dissolution with two other lots D and F giving slower dissolution in the conditions used (see Table 7).

Ibuprofen. The second drug in which a significant in vivo difference could not be predicted was ibuprofen, for which in vivo data are given in Table 5. Dissolution studies were undertaken, under a variety of conditions, using *USP* apparatuses 1 and 2 to test the dissolution of the three lots of ibuprofen 300-mg tablets, compared in a bioavailability study described earlier. Because of the pK_a of the drug, very little drug dissolved from the tablets in pH 5.0 acetate buffer (10–20% in 1 hr) and about only 10% in 1 hr with distilled water. Thus, only results at pH 7.2 are compared with some key pharmacokinetic parameters in Table 8.

There is no significant difference in AUC among products, but the C_{max} and t_{max} means were significantly different from reference ($p < 0.05$), indicating slower absorption from the two test products. However, there is almost an inverse correlation with C_{max} and t_{max} for the two conditions tested. The findings are in agreement with those reported by Albert [35], and dissolution of ibuprofen does not appear predictive of bioavailability.

Overview of Dissolution Limitations

Thus, overall, although correlations among pharmacokinetic and dissolution parameters may be obtained for specific formulations, the general applicability of the dissolution test as a predictor of bioavailability should not be assumed. There are certainly cases (as the *USP* preamble indicates [36]) when

Table 8 Dissolution and Pharmacokinetic Parameters of Three Ibuprofen 300-mg Formulations. R (Reference), A, and B

	Reference	Test A	Test B
AUC_∞ (µg · h/mL)	85	81	84
C_{max} (µg/mL)	25	18[b]	16[b]
T_{max} (h)	1.2	2.3[b]	2.9[b]
A-30, USP%	84.2	97	90
A-45, USP%	94.1	100	99
A-30, MOD%	65	80[b]	85[b]
A-45, MOD%	69	84[b]	92[b]

[a]Dissolution conditions, USP, rotating basket, pH 7.2 phosphate buffer at 150 rpm; MOD, modified, paddle, pH 7.2 phosphate buffer at 50 rpm; A-30 and A-45, amount dissolved in 30 and 45 min, respectively.
[b]Significantly different from reference $\alpha = 0.05$.

formulations of adequate bioavailability fail the dissolution criteria. The foregoing examples of allopurinol and ibuprofen indicate that there are situations when products that could be considered to have undesirable bioavailability characteristics can have superior dissolution characteristics compared with adequately bioavailable products. Drugs must be considered on their merits, and dissolution testing should be considered a sensitive in vitro quality control procedure, rather than an in vivo predictor.

CANADIAN GUIDELINES AND STANDARDS

The Expert Advisory Committee: Objectives of Guidelines

In discussion with HPB reviewers and scientists, the EAC (chaired by Dr. J. Ruedy) has prepared a report for the Health Protection Branch, Drugs Directorate, entitled *Guidelines and Standards for Bioavailability of Oral Dosage Formulations of Drugs Used for Systemic Effects* [19]. These are being published for comment (expected date August 1990), and most of their recommendations are likely to be adopted. The guidelines are based on consideration of the results from the work in the HPB reviewed in the foregoing, as well as from experience of review of several hundred manufacturers' submissions. The major features of the guideline for "uncomplicated" drugs and secondly for modified-release formulations of uncomplicated drugs are reviewed. The term *uncomplicated* refers to drugs that do not have complicated or variable pharmacokinetics or other special characteristics complicating the evaluation of bioavailability; these will be discussed later in this chapter. Except for such situations, it is considered that many drugs share enough common characteristics to permit formulation of guidelines for bioavailability studies and declaration of standards of bioequivalence. The bioavailability attributes of drugs with uncomplicated characteristics are usually determined from single-dose experiments.

Bioavailability Guidelines

Introduction

The introduction to the guidelines considers the concept of bioavailability as ". . . an important attribute of oral dosage formulations of drugs used for systemic effects." It is usually assessed by serial measurement of the drug or its metabolites in the systemic circulation, to provide a plasma (serum or whole blood) profile from which pharmacokinetic parameters can be calculated: AUC, C_{max}, and t_{max}. The AUC provides an estimate of extent of absorption, whereas the t_{max} reflects rate. C_{max} is a more complex function that, together with t_{max}, reflects the rate of absorption. The guidelines note that for most drugs *absolute* bioavailability is estimated from comparison of the AUCs after oral versus intravenous administration of an equivalent dose. *Comparative* bioavailability is estimated from comparison of the plasma (serum or whole blood) concentration-time curve for a *test* oral formulation with that of the standard oral product of a particular drug. Acceptable bioavailability of the test product is declared by means of appropriate statistical assessment, from which products containing identical drug products in identical dose may be declared "bioequivalent." As defined, bioequivalence is assessed from measurement of drug or its metabolites, or both, in plasma (serum or whole blood). However, urinary excretion may be employed. In the absence of suitable analytical methodology for measurement of drug or metabolites in plasma or urine, therapeutic equivalence should be determined by clinical trials. It is noted that urinary and clinical trial assessments are generally less sensitive than the plasma (serum or whole blood) estimate of equivalence.

The Study Objective

This should be clearly stated, and there *must be information to justify the inclusion of the drug in the category of drugs with "uncomplicated" characteristics.*

There are sections of the guidelines dealing with Good Ethical-Clinical Practice and others with Good Laboratory Practice, such that all investigators and facilities should be identified, with the suitability of the latter being demonstrated. The guidelines used in ethical review by institutional ethical review boards must be identified, such as the *Guideline on Research Involving Human Subjects* (1987) of the Medical Research Council of Canada [37].

Subjects

A major section of the guidelines describes the mandatory and desirable aspects of subject selection and characterization. Mostly, uncomplicated drugs in conventional formulations would be tested in normal, healthy volunteers. If women are included, there should be suitable assurance that they are neither pregnant nor likely to become pregnant until after the study. Some studies may have to be carried out with subjects having special characteristics, such as the elderly.

It is emphasized that a major goal in selection of subjects is to reduce variability in pharmacokinetics attributed to subject characteristics. The supervising physician must ensure that the subjects are physically and psychologically fit to participate in, and comply with, the restrictions of the study. This will involve physical examination, along with assessment of medical history and appropriate biochemical test results. The subjects must be available for all legs of the study *without coercion* (ethical guidelines), and it is recommended that extra subjects be included in studies to allow for potential withdrawal or removal. Reasons for withdrawal or removal from a study must be reported, and the subject's plasma (or blood) concentration data provided (i.e., results of all samples measured must be included in the study report). The measures to identify adverse drug reactions (ADRs) and side effects are an important part of planning. In some cases, formulation ingredients or characteristics, and not the active ingredient, may cause the ADR. The same observer and format for identifying and recording ADRs should be used for all subjects. This observer should be unaware of the identity of the formulation given on a particular day of study ("blinded"). The incidence, severity, and duration of ADRs and side effects observed must be reported. The investigator should comment *whether or not* an adverse effect is drug induced and justify the decision.

Study Design and Environment

The study design and the environment represents another major section in the guidelines prefaced by the statement: "The design of a bioavailability study should minimize variability which is not attributable to the drug and eliminates bias as much as possible." A crossover design should be used (i.e., each person is given reference product and at least one of the test products, if there are more than one). The sequences of administration of reference and test products should be specified in advance, and subjects are randomly assigned to sequences. Other designs may be accepted after consultation, but the statistical appropriateness should be justified. Every effort should be made to standardize the conditions in all legs of the study, notably diet and exercise. Nonsmokers are preferred; volunteers should not be taking any drugs (prescription, nonprescription, or nonmedical); and previous use should be evaluated to determine if enzyme inducers, inhibitors, or other interfering agents have been taken. If an emergency drug, such as acetaminophen, is taken during the study, it should be reported. The elimination of the results of any subject who has not followed the protocol should occur *before* statistical analysis, but results should be included in the report.

If possible, double-blinding of volunteer and immediate investigator should be a protocol feature. The person monitoring ADRs and the persons involved in analysis of biological samples *must* not know the identity of the treatments. Codes should not be broken until analysis is completed. Unless it is a special study, bioequivalence and bioavailability of uncomplicated drugs should be studied with a fasting protocol (i.e., overnight 10-hr fast, up to 250 mL of water permitted up to 2 hr before drug administration). The dose should be taken at the same time in each phase with a standard volume of water, such as 150 mL, at the same temperature. No further fluid should be taken until 2 hr after dosing, when 250 mL of xanthine-free fluids are permitted. All meals should be standardized and repeated on each study day, with the first being given 4 hr after drug dosing. This regimen also refers to intravenous phases, when oral formulations are being compared with that route of administration. It should be noted that when drugs are commonly given with food (e.g., to avoid side effect in the gastrointestinal tract), studies with standard meals should be included.

The pattern of posture and physical activity should be standardized in all phases of the study. In most cases, volunteers would be ambulatory, but for drugs that can cause dizziness, sitting may be necessary in the first hour or so postdosing. This standardization is intended to reduce effects on gastrointestinal motility or blood flow. The interval between treatments (in single-dose crossover studies) should be long enough to allow elimination of virtually all the previous dose from the body. To take into account subjects exhibiting long half-lives, a period 10 times that of the *mean* terminal half-life of the drug is recommended.

Sampling Times

Blood is the sampling medium of choice, and usually, plasma or serum should be harvested for analysis of drug concentrations. Sometimes, however, analysis on whole blood may be more appropriate because of binding characteristics (e.g., to erythrocytes). If blood (plasma) drug concentrations cannot be quantitated, then urine may serve as the biological fluid to be sampled if $>$ 40% of the drug is eliminated unmetabolized.

Although better correlations with effect are sometimes obtained with drug profiles in other fluids, such as synovium, because drug must first be absorbed, it remains appropriate to estimate bioavailability from drug blood concentrations. Samples must be processed and stored in a standard manner that should not cause significant degradation of analytes.

Usually, 12–18 blood samples are obtained from each volunteer for each dose to allow calculation of pharamcokinetic parameters. Thus, accurate estimation of C_{max}, AUC (to 80% of the known "infinity" value), and terminal disposition rate (λ) should be possible. Preferably four or more blood collection points should be spaced in the terminal log-linear phase of the profile. When urinary excretion is being used, then enough samples must be obtained to permit rate and extent of renal excretion to be estimated.

An important requirement is that the duration of blood sampling in a study should be sufficient to account for at least 80% of the known AUC to infinity (usually three to four times the half-life of the medication).

Drug and Reference Drug Products

The products must be of acceptable quality, as defined by New Drug Submission Standards, such as identity, purity, drug content and uniformity, stability, and dissolution.

The dose of drug in each formulation in a bioequivalence study should be the molar equivalent, and production batches must be used. For uncomplicated drugs, when different strengths are formulated in which the proportion of excipient to drug is unaltered and dissolution characteristics are the same, bioequivalence testing of one strength (usually the highest) will suffice. The reference preparation in bioequivalence studies must be that marketed by the innovator in *Canada*, or if there is no recognized innovator, the market leader. This requirement has led to disputes. Although the regulatory agency may know that the innovator's product is identical in two countries, it is confidential information. Thus, generic manufacturers usually have to conduct a study with a representative lot from the Canadian innovator. In bioavailability studies of new chemical entities (NCEs), usually an intravenous solution comparison would be advised, but when not possible, an oral solution should be used.

Measurement Methodology and Analytical Validation

Precise and accurate estimation of the active ingredient or its metabolite(s) in a biological fluid, as a function of time, is a key element in bioavailability determination. Usually, measurement of parent drug (absorbed species) will suffice, but determination of active metabolite(s) may also be required, depending on their relative activity and concentration. For a prodrug, the active component should be determined.

The analytical procedures to measure the drug or major active metabolites in blood, plasma, or other biological matrix must be validated for specificity, sensitivity, precision, and accuracy, sufficiently to provide satisfactory, reproducible results. This validation should be shown to provide an adequate method *before* initiating the bioavailability study. Validation of certain operating parameters during the analysis of unknown samples will also be required. As noted, under the earlier section on sampling times, the stability of analytes in the biological matrix and extracts, over the time of storage and during the analytical process should be documented.

The *selectivity* of the assay should be established, such that parent drug, metabolites, and potential endogenous interferences will not interfere with the assay method.

The *recovery* of the analyte(s) from any extraction process must be known to be precise at the low, medium, and high concentrations of the expected range. In procedures for which an internal standard is used, this should also be tested at the appropriate concentration.

Standard curves should be established over the expected range of concentrations before the study, and within- and between-day variability should be reported as the coefficient of variation (CV%) at each concentration. These attributes will be used to determine the acceptability of the standard curve, and they should be obtained on each analytical day when unknown study samples are being evaluated. The *limit of quantitation* (or lowest quantifiable concentration) is established from the standard curve. At this low end *but not over the whole calibration range* the limit is established when *within*-day CV% is no greater than 15% and *between*-day is <20%. Precision and accuracy of the assay are also determined from the standard curve at the low, medium, and high concentrations of the range. At midrange and high end, CV% values of 10% should be the maximum allowed.

Quality control must be assessed with analyst-blinded samples, spiked with reference standard analyte, as well as replicate unknown analysis. For stable analytes, quality control samples must be prepared in the matrix of study (e.g., plasma), at concentrations representative of the low, middle, and high range of the calibration range. These "blinded" samples should be stored under the same conditions and over the same time as the study samples, and sets must be analyzed with each batch of unknown samples each analytical day, and the results must be reported in full. For less stable analytes, daily or weekly quality control samples may be prepared, but again, they must be treated as for the study samples.

Another quality control measure is the use of *replicate study samples* in which all metabolites would be present. At least 15% of the samples must be randomly selected from the whole group in a study for duplicate analysis and be reported separately. The guidelines also have a section on reassay of samples, indicating that there should be a standard protocol for situations when there have been analytical problems, such as poor chromatography, when reanalysis should be carried out before breaking the analytical code. After the analytical code has been broken, the circumstances for reassay are more restricted—perhaps to confirm a double peak. It is noted that if the original and repeat samples are within 15% of each other [i.e., (high − low value)/low value in percent], then these would be acceptable, and the average should be used. If there is >15% difference, then a third analysis should be done. When three analytical results suggest that one is spurious, the average of the other two should be used. In any event, the criteria used in selecting results for inclusion in calculations must be stated.

Note: Several decision rules remain to be elaborated for analytical validation, and it is expected that these will be finalized in early 1991.

Presentation of Data

This section of the guidelines indicates the format in which data should be presented and the method of analysis. It is accompanied by a detailed example (Appendix I).

There should be a tabulation of the concentration of the drug in plasma (or other matrix) for each subject, sampling time, and formulation displayed, as observed and corrected (as noted in the foregoing), for measured content of the dosage form. There should be footnotes, as necessary, in those tables, to note and identify any deviations from the protocol, such as missed or late collection of samples. This data should also be presented in computer-readable form. Graphs of the results should also be provided, including a linear and semilogarithmic plot of drug concentrations as a function of time. There should be graphs for each formulation with each subject, and mean values for each formulation tested. When appropriate, the semilog plots should indicate the regression lines fitted to estimate the terminal disposition rate constant, λ. The pharmacokinetic parameters that should be tabulated for each subject with each treatment are as follows. AUC_t, which is the area up to the last quantifiable concentrations (as established above) and AUC_∞, which is the AUC_t plus the estimated additional area extrapolated to infinity by using λ. AUC_t/AUC_∞ should be calculated for

Bioequivalence: Canadian Regulatory Position

each subject, and the ratio should be >0.8. C_{max}, t_{max}, and λ should also be included in tables. If additional pharmacokinetic parameters are presented, the methods/assumptions used in their estimation should be described in full.

Statistical Analysis

Analysis of variance appropriate to the study design and execution should be presented. The tables of ANOVA should include statistical tests of all effects in the model and should include all *data for all subjects*. Other selected analyses with particular subjects or data points excluded may be presented, but exclusions *must be justified*. It is indicated that if more than 5% of the subjects, or 10% of the data for a single subject or formulation, are omitted (even with justification), the study may not be accepted. The ANOVA should be completed for the logarithmically transformed (ln) AUC_t, AUC_∞, and C_{max} data and on the observed data for t_{max} and λ. Tabulations are to contain means and CVs across subjects for each product, mean squared error, associated degrees of freedom, and the derived intrasubject CV. Additionally, for AUC_t and C_{max}, the ratio of geometric means for test versus reference products and their 95% CIs should be given.

Standards for Bioequivalence

For uncomplicated drugs with conventional (immediate-release) formulations the Canadian standards for bioequivalence comprise an AUC_t and C_{max} component, as discussed earlier.

1. AUC_t: The 95% CI for the percentage ratio of the test/reference formulation AUC_t geometric means should be within 80–125%.
   [An example of the calculation from a set of data is given in the Appendix I]
2. C_{max}: The percentage ratio of test/reference C_{max} geometric means should be between 80 and 125%.

These standards are applied to the differences in means and their confidence intervals transformed back into the original scale. It is important to note that the classic and *not* Westlake confidence interval is applied. It is noted that "This AUC standard is a refinement of that used by the Health Protection Branch for 20 years." It is augmented by a criterion for C_{max} indicative of absorption rate:

> The *combination* of AUC and C_{max} criteria serve as limit on difference in rate of absorption for (uncomplicated) drugs since t_{max} is usually related to these parameters. The parameter t_{max} is often difficult to establish accurately and the significance of differences varies from drug to drug.

"The standards are not intended to be used for determination of bioinequivalence." For example, if the AUC_t, 95% CI interval of test/reference ratio is within 80–125% (the bioequivalence interval) then the formulation is bioequivalent (provided the C_{max} mean ratio is within the interval). If the lower AUC_t 95% CI is below 80%, the test formulation is not bioequivalent. However, *bioinequivalence* can be declared only when both lower and upper 95% CIs are below (or above) the 80–125% interval.

DRUGS WITH COMPLICATED CHARACTERISTICS

Introduction

The major examples of drugs with complicated characteristics for which the modified guidelines, methodology, and standards would likely be required are given in Table 9.

Except for modified-release (MR) formulations, for which summary guidelines are given later, Canadian guidelines have not been established and, thus, *the opinions are those of the author.*

Drugs With Complicated or Variable Kinetics

Bioavailability or bioequivalence standards for drugs with high intrasubject variability, such as those with high first pass, are a challenge to investigators. Although some reduction of variability may be achieved by standardized treatments of volunteers with close monitoring, variability of >30% (within subject CV) occurs (e.g., verapamil). In such cases, even with 40 subjects, the likelihood of meeting the bioequivalence interval of 80–125% (despite attaining a mean AUC ratio of 100%) remains poor (see Fig. 2). Some authorities have suggested multiple-dose protocols, but as well as risk to volunteers, these add to the expense of studies, often without markedly lowering the variation.

Table 9 "Complicated" Drugs Requiring Modified Guidelines

1. Modified-release dosage forms
2. Drugs with complicated or variable pharmacokinetics, e.g.,
    Nonlinear kinetics: first pass >40%
    Variable kinetics: e.g., genetic phenotype
    Chiral effects: e.g., in vivo inversion
    Long $t_{1/2}$ (>72 hr)
3. Drugs for which time of onset or rate of absorption is important
4. Highly toxic drugs or with narrow therapeutic range
5. Drugs for which measurement methodology is inadequate (require to measure three half-lives)
6. Combination products
7. Biologicals

There has been resistance to widening the bioequivalence interval, but, according to the therapeutic risk with the drug, such measures may have to be considered. The use of two reference treatments, to confirm that the variation is characteristic of the drug and not a particular product, has also been discussed [38].

Genetic phenotypes in drug metabolism, such as acetylation, although increasing the intersubject variation, have less implication in a crossover design, and mainly such drugs can be accommodated with the uncomplicated standards. There is debate concerning the suggestion of separate studies in slow- and fast-metabolizer groups. Slight changes in rate of absorption would show up to a greater degree in fast metabolizers.

Chiral effects, when there is little change in profile shape, would likely not require use of selective methodology in normal bioequivalence studies. For ibuprofen, which exhibits 80% chiral inversion from R to S, Cox et al. [39] showed that very similar results were found in bioequivalence of a formulation with slower absorption, using both selective and nonselective procedures. However, for new chemical entities, there should be pivotal studies of bioavailability that use stereoselective procedures. Also, for modified-release or change of route of administration, such studies would be required.

Drugs with long and very long-half-lives present a problem for crossover designs. Parallel designs may have to be used, but would involve many more subjects. In addition, innovative sampling protocols may be used.

Drugs for Which Time of Onset of Effect or Rate of Absorption Is Important

Drugs, such as short-term use analgesics and hypnotics or even those such as nifedipine, for which change of input rate has been shown to directly increase heart rate [40], will require some tighter definition of absorption rate. As Gibaldi and Perrier wrote in 1982 [41] "Pharmacokinetic theory is well developed and generally accepted for the determination of the extent or relative extent of absorption of a drug from a dosage form. Unfortunately similar agreement does not exist with respect to characterizing the absorption rate of a drug." And such agreement is not found today. Many of the "absorption rate" calculations require administrations of intravenous drug. Also, as seen in Figure 3, for some drugs, although the mean profile can be fitted reasonably with a pharmacokinetic model, data from some individual subjects present difficulty owing to fluctuations in concentrations. Such devices as partial area analysis (e.g., ratio of AUC to the t_{max} of the reference product, or ratio of AUC to an early time point such as 2 hr) encounter the high variation (e.g., *intra*subject CVs > 100%!) of individual subjects caused by variation in gastrointestinal transit. Certainly, a prescribed confidence interval on C_{max} would provide some extra control. Depending on the drug, some limit on t_{max} difference may also be considered.

However, as previously noted, this parameter is difficult to estimate with accuracy and precision.

Drugs With a Narrow Therapeutic Range

These are typically drugs for which therapeutic drug monitoring is applied with a reasonably established "therapeutic window." Again, the problem of limiting differences in rate of absorption becomes important.

In addition, if interchangeability (substitution) is intended, application of a narrower bioequivalence interval on AUC_t, such as 90–112%, could be examined. However, if the intrasubject CV is 15% or above, this requirement probably would not be realistic (see Fig. 2).

Highly Toxic Drugs

The highly toxic category presents a different problem in bioequivalence; healthy volunteers cannot be administered such drugs in bioavailability studies. Patient studies with antineoplastic agents are difficult to arrange with proper study design. Also, the disease status of the patient in a crossover study may change from dose to dose. So far, animal models have been rejected in replacement of human bioequivalence studies [42]. However, a protocol in which formulations are tested in two animal models, before going on to a limited clinical trial, may be worth investigating.

Drugs for Which Measurement Methodology is Not Reliable

Drugs, such as albuterol inhalation, which is not evaluable by plasma or urinary excretion, may have to be studied by pharmacodynamic measures (i.e., respiratory function in asthmatics). However, such assessments tend to have less precision than direct pharmacokinetic parameters.

Combination Products

Unless there is synergism, these can often be evaluated by applying the bioequivalence standard to each component. For some antimicrobials or other synergistic combinations, the ratios of components over time may have to be examined.

Biological Products

By their nature, the new, mainly protein, products of the biotechnology revolution will present challenges, both in development of delivery systems and in the evaluation of their bioavailability [43].

MODIFIED-RELEASE FORMULATIONS

Introduction

The EAC, in a separate guideline [44], defines *modified-release* (MR) dosage forms as ". . . drug formulations which differ in the rate of release of drug from that of conventional formulations."

Examples of modified-release include enteric-coated (to delay drug degradation or diminish the likelihood of gastrointestinal adverse effects) products, as well as products to provide effective drug concentrations after a single-dose for a longer period, to minimize fluctuations in drug concentrations during the dosage interval, and even to provide multiple peaks and troughs to mimic repeated conventional doses.

It was considered that different guidelines are required for MR dosage forms because of greater chance of increased intersubject variability and dose dumping. In addition, there is a possibility of greater accumulation when the drug is given in repeated doses at the recommended dosage intervals. The MR guidelines were developed for *uncomplicated* drugs. There are different requirements for MR formulations developed in different situations, such as first market entry, with or without previous marketing of a conventional product, second or subsequent entry, and so on.

Factors in Modified-Release Study Objectives

Although bioavailability data must be obtained for all MR dosage forms, factors considered in the standards are whether or not the introduction of a new chemical entity is involved, whether it is the first MR, when there is already a conventional formulation, or the second or subsequent MR. The extent of accumulation expected of the drug after repeated dosing would also influence evaluation methodology. Claims for effectiveness and safety of MR formulations must be supported by adequate clinical studies.

As well as the objectives of the bioavailability study, the therapeutic rationale of the MR formulations should be stated and the pharmacokinetic objectives clearly defined. The submission should also provide information to justify the inclusion of the drug in the category of MR drugs without complicated or variable kinetics (i.e., not included in Table 10).

Occasionally, it may be possible to rely on plasma concentrations alone as the basis of approval of an MR product, when there is a well-defined relationship between plasma concentrations of drug or active metabolite and quantitative response of one or more pharmacologic effects.

For first market entry MRs, appropriate safety and efficacy data must be provided, with sufficient pharmacokinetic studies to indicate consistency of formulation. If the formulation is the first market MR, following a convetional formulation,

Table 10 Summary of Proposed Canadian Bioavailability and Bioequivalence Standards for MR Products

---

I. No accumulation, i.e., $AUC_x/AUC_\infty{}^a \geq 0.8$, single-dose, crossover fasted and fed vs reference.
   A. *Bioavailability Standard* (reference = conventional or solution for 1st entry)
      1. Percentage ratio AUC_t between 80 and 125%, fasted and fed;
      2. And % ratio C_{max} not exceed 125, fasted and fed.
      3. Pharmacokinetics support label claim.
   B. *Bioequivalence Standard* (reference = 1st MR or conventional)
      1. 95% CI of % ratio AUC_t and AUC_x between 80 and 125% fasted and fed.
      2. And % ratio of C_{max} between 80 and 125 fasted and fed.
      3. Pharmacokinetics support label claim.

II. Accumulation likely. $AUC_x/AUC_\infty{}^a < 0.8$. (1) single-dose, fasted and food; (2) multiple-dose steady state. Both crossover.
   A. *Bioavailability Standard* (reference = conventional or solution for 1st entry) For single-dose no standard, but food challenge studies are required.
      1. Steady-state % ratio of AUC_τ between 80 and 125.
      2. And % ratio of C_{max} not exceed 125.
   B. *Bioequivalence Standard* (reference = 1st MR *or* conventional).
      1. Single-dose 95% CI of % ratio of AUC_t and AUC_x between 80 and 125, fasted and fed.
      2. And % ratio of C_{max} between 80 and 125, fasted and fed.
      3. At steady state, the 95% CI of % ratio of AUC_τ should be between 80 and 125.
      4. The % ratio C_{max} should be between 80 and 125.
      5. And the % ratio C_{min} should be between 80 and 125.
      6. The pharmacokinetics should support the label claim.

AUC_t = AUC to the last measurable concentration.
AUC_x = AUC over the usual dosage interval (most common).
AUC_∞ = AUC_t with extrapolation to infinity
AUC_τ = AUC over a dosage interval at steady state (i.e., MR dose interval).
[a] All *ratios* are test/reference *geometric means*.

comparative bioavailability studies must be performed against the conventional product. The standards depend on whether or not accumulation is likely to occur in single-dose studies.

The decision on this is based on the ratio of AUC_x to AUC_∞ over the dosing interval zero to x, where x is the usual interval. If this ratio is equal to or greater than 0.8 then it is considered nonaccumulating, and single-dose studies will suffice. If the AUC_x/AUC_∞ value is less than 0.8, single- *and* multiple-dose studies will be required.

Note that second-entry modified-release products may be accepted on the basis of bioequivalence information when there is an originator MR product already on the market. If compared at the same dose level and frequency, then it may be acceptable without clinical evidence of efficacy. For both bioavailability and bioequivalence, the standards must be met after single-dose testing in the same subjects, both in the fasted condition, as well as administered following an appropriate meal at a specified time before taking the drug.

From single-dose studies, the following pharmacokinetic parameters will be obtained: AUC_x, AUC_t, AUC_∞, and C_{max}, and λ (for MR the terminal slope is not likely to be the true elimination rate constant of the drug); from steady-state studies: AUC (area under the curve over a steady-state dosage interval), C_{max}, C_{pd} (concentration prior to a dose at steady-state), and C_{min} (observed C_{min}. [Note, C_{pd} will often be C_{min}, but lag time sometimes occurs resulting in higher C_{pd}.] An attempt to give a summary of the bioavailability and bioequivalence standards is given in Table 10.

The bioavailability standards are different for drugs that are unlikely to accumulate in the dosage regimen used than for those that would accumulate.

Bioavailability Standards

No Accumulation

For this decision the criterion of AUC_x/AUC_∞ < or > 0.8 is applied. Single-dose studies alone are accepted for the nonaccumulating drugs, and the *bioavailability standards* versus the conventional reference determined over the dosage interval of the MR formulation in the fasting state and following an appropriate food challenge are the following:

1. The percentage ratio of AUC geometric *means* (i.e., AUC_x and AUC_t), of the MR compared with the conventional formulation should be between 80 and 125%, both in the fasted and food-challenge conditions.
2. The percentage ratio of test to reference C_{max} geometric means under these conditions should not exceed 125%.
3. The pharmacokinetic characteristics should support the labeled claim of the manufacturer.

This latter phrase is intended to focus the study objective (e.g., if the strategy is to mimic repeated dosing of two conventional doses the data should support this claim).

Accumulating Drugs

For accumulating drugs, the comparison should also be made at steady state over a single-dose interval of the MR formulation versus the doses of the conventional formulation that it is intended to replace, which are administered according to the conventional dosing regimen. The *bioavailability standards* to be met are the following:

1. The percentage ratio of the MR versus conventional product AUC_τ geometric means over dosing interval at steady state should be within 80–125%.
2. The percentage ratio of C_{max} geometric means at steady state MR versus conventional formulation should not exceed 125%.
3. The pharmacokinetic characteristics should support the labeled claim.
4. In addition, food challenge studies should be carried out with single-dose studies of test and reference product, (i.e., crossover with both food and fasted, with both dosage forms).

The foregoing bioavailability standards are *for guidance*. If a manufacturer has satisfactory clinical trial data to indicate that, despite not meeting the bioavailability standard, the drug is effective to meet the claims, then it would be acceptable. The food challenge study is for information to provide dosing instructions for safer use of the drug and to demonstrate that increase (dose dumping) or decrease in plasma drug profiles does not occur with food–formulation interactions.

Bioequivalence for Modified-Release Drugs

For most drugs, bioequivalence would be acceptable only as evidence of efficacy when the MR product is the second or subsequent MR entry, and comparisons would thus be with the innovator MR product with which bioequivalence is claimed.

Exceptions to this would be when there is a well-defined relationship between plasma concentrations and clinical effects for which comparisons could be made with a conventional reference. However, manufacturers choosing the bioequivalence route would first have to characterize their product for *bioavailability* and test for dose dumping with single-dose (and, when appropriate, multiple-dose) studies in comparison with a "conventional" reference product. The foregoing bioavailability standards would have to be met.

Bioequivalence of Nonaccumulating Drugs

Bioequivalence for *nonaccumulating* drugs would be tested in single-dose comparisons both *with fasted subjects and with a food challenge*, and the following standards should be met:

1. The 95% CI for the percentage ratio of test/reference geometric means, for both AUC_x and AUC_t, should be within 80–125%.
2. The percentage ratio of test/reference C_{max} geometric means should be between 80–125%.

3. The pharmacokinetic characteristics should support the labeled claims.

Thus if there were differences between the formulations in the effect of food, bioequivalence could not be claimed, and clinical trial proof of efficacy would be required for the second MR product.

Bioequivalence of Accumulating Drugs

For MR products of drugs *that accumulate*, bioequivalence may be claimed after testing against a previously marketed MR product (or conventional product) at single dose and steady state. The steady-state dosage interval should be the same for both products. The bioequivalence standards are the following:

1. The 95% CI for the percentage ratio of test/reference, geometric means for both AUC_x and AUC_t should be within 80–125% when compared after a single MR dose interval in both fasted and appropriate food challenge experiments.
2. The percentage ratio of test/reference C_{max} geometric means, under the conditions in (1) should be within 80–125%.
3. The 95% CI of the test to reference formulation AUC_τ geometric means (at steady state) should be within 80–125%.
4. Under the conditions of (3) the percentage ratio of C_{max} geometric means should be within 80–125%.
5. At steady state, the percentage ratio of test/reference C_{min} geometric means should be within 80–125%.
6. The pharmacokinetic characteristics should support the labeled claims of the manufacturer.

The practical experience in reviewing drug submissions indicates that both bioavailability and bioequivalence standards for MR products may be difficult to achieve. However, as noted previously, with adequate clinical trials, the failure to meet the bioavailability standard can be overruled. When bioequivalence cannot be demonstrated, the clinical trial option can again be followed.

Study Design and Statistical Considerations in Bioavailability in Bioequivalence of Modified-Release Products

The remainder of the MR guideline discusses similar protocol and reporting requirements as described in the foregoing for conventional uncomplicated drug bioavailability. Particular features occur under "Design" and "Administration of Food."

It is suggested that a three-period crossover design (reference drug fasting, test-drug fasting, test drug after food) may be adequate for comparative bioavailability studies to establish the bioavailability of the MR formulation. To establish bioequivalence, two two-period crossover (or one four-period crossover) would be mandatory to allow the fasted and food conditions to be compared with test and reference. (However, there may be two references conventional and innovator MR).

Also outlined is general advice on the food challenge: Conditions and diet should be chosen based on the physicochemical and pharmacokinetic characteristics of the drug and its formulation. "The purpose is to select a test meal which has the greatest potential to demonstrate altered bioavailability."

There is also advice on steady-state sampling, which follows the usual pharmacokinetic convention of requiring three C_{min}, or more likely C_{pd}, to demonstrate steady state at *the same time* of day. "Sufficient samples must be obtained to provide information required to sustain labeled claims, identify C_{max}, and calculate AUC over the dosing interval."

The foregoing guidelines for uncomplicated drugs will be adapted and modified to accommodate the aforementioned "complicated" drugs.

CONCLUSION

Although the bioavailability guidelines for conventional drugs are only now being formalized in Canada, in-house studies and extensive review experience indicate that they are workable for evaluation of bioequivalence for a large majority of drugs. Although criticisms of the 80–125% interval were made to suggest that (as originally applied) drugs with 80% AUC are acceptable, this does not survive examination.

Even though the width of the interval in each trial will vary, such that for less variable drugs an *actual* mean of AUC of 90% may be acceptable, for more variable drugs, even slight departure from true 100% would be likely to cause rejection (see Fig. 2). Evaluation of formulations of such drugs remains a major problem, even for major manufacturers, who may have occasion to reformulate.

There has been much less experience with modified-release dosage forms, and strategies for assessing bioequivalence of other forms, such as transdermals or suppositories, remain to be developed.

ACKNOWLEDGMENTS

The author wishes to express appreciation to Dr. John Ruedy and the Expert Advisory Committee on Bioavailability to the Health Protection Branch whose recommended guidelines are quoted; the Director of the Bureau of Drug Research, Dr. Keith Bailey, who edited the guidelines, the many scientists who completed the in-house bioequivalence assessments cited in the text and Mr. Eric Ormsby who edited the statistical section and whose example is quoted in part in Appendix I.

APPENDIX I (STATISTICAL ANALYSIS)

The following example summarizes the analysis of AUC_t required by the Canadian Health Protection Branch. The AUC_t data for this example was generated from a two-period two-formulation crossover study in which $n_1 = 8$ volunteers were randomised to sequence Test:Reference and $n_2 = 8$ volunteers to sequence Reference:Test. AUC_t values estimated are listed in the raw and natural log scales, as well as relative Test:Reference AUC_t.

Table A1 AUC_t Data

		Raw Scale			Log Scale	
ID	Sequence	Test AUC_t	Reference AUC_t	Relative AUC_t (%)	Test ln (AUC_t)	Reference ln (AUC_t)
1	TR	365	375	97	5.90	5.93
2	RT	405	595	68	6.00	6.39
3	RT	703	471	149	6.55	6.16
4	TR	233	190	123	5.45	5.25
5	RT	247	257	96	5.51	5.55
6	TR	178	175	102	5.18	5.17
7	RT	246	382	65	5.51	5.94
8	TR	408	361	113	6.01	5.89
9	RT	315	218	144	5.75	5.39
10	TR	140	92	153	4.94	4.52
11	TR	165	269	61	5.11	5.59
12	RT	88	106	83	4.48	4.66
13	RT	183	290	63	5.21	5.67
14	TR	122	230	53	4.81	5.44
15	RT	68	144	47	4.22	4.97
16	TR	275	344	80	5.62	5.84
Mean		259	281	94	5.39	5.52
SD		158	136	35	0.61	0.51
CV		61	48	37		

Table A2 ANOVA for ln (AUC_t)

Source	df	SS	MS	F	PR>F
SEQ	1	0.0535	0.0535	0.09	0.770
Subject	14	8.4375	0.6027	8.26	<0.001
Period	1	0.0241	0.0241	0.33	0.574
Form	1	0.1373	0.1373	1.88	0.192
Residual	14	1.0211	0.0729		

Intrasubject CV $\sim 100 \times$ (MS residual)$^{0.5}$
$\sim 100 \times (0.0729)^{0.5} = 27\%$

Table A3 Calculations Based on ln (AUC$_t$)

$$\overline{Y}_{TEST} = \frac{\Sigma Y_{T1}/n_1 + \Sigma Y_{T2}/n_2}{2} = \frac{5.38 + 5.40}{2} = 5.39$$

$$\overline{Y}_{REFERENCE} = \frac{\Sigma Y_{R1}/n_1 + \Sigma Y_{R2}/n_2}{2} = \frac{5.45 + 5.59}{2} = 5.52$$

Difference = $\overline{Y}_{TEST} - \overline{Y}_{REF}$ = 5.39 − 5.52 = − 0.13

$$SE_{DIFFERENCE} = (\frac{n_1 + n_2}{2\ n_1\ n_2}\ MS\ Residual) = 0.0955$$

Ratio of geometric means = $e^{DIFFERENCE} \times 100\%$ = 88%

95% Confidence limits

Lower, upper = $e^{(DIFFERENCE\ \pm\ t_{\alpha/2, n_1+n_2-2}\ \times\ SE_{DIFFERENCE})} \times 100\%$

Lower = $100 \times e^{(-0.13\ -\ 2.145\ \times\ .0955)} \times 100\%$ = 72%

Upper = $100 \times e^{(-0.13\ +\ 2.145\ \times\ .0955)} \times 100\%$ = 108%

REFERENCES

1. D. Cook. *Pharmacology* 8:190 (1972).
2. D. Cook. *Drug Absorption* (L. F. Prescott and W. S. Nimmo, eds.) ADIS Press, New York, p. 324 (1981).
3. Second (final) report of the Special Committee of the House of Commons on "Drug Costs and Prices" (chairman H. C. Harley) Queen's Printer and Controller of Stationery, Ottawa, p. 17 (1967).
4. A. B. Morrison and J. A. Campbell. *J. Am. Pharm. Assoc. Sci. Ed.* 49:473 (1960).
5. D. G. Chapman, R. Crisafio, and J. A. Campbell. *J. Am. Pharm. Assoc. Sci. Ed.* 45:374 (1956).
6. A. B. Morrison and J. A. Campbell. *J. Pharm. Sci.* 54:1 (1965).
7. R. O. Searl and M. Pernarowski. *Can. Med. Assoc. J.* 96:1513 (1967).
8. A. B. Morrison, D. Cook, and W. G. B. Casselman. *Can. Med. Assoc. J.* 109:800 (1973).
9. J. Ruedy, R. O. Davies, J. Brodeur, N. A. Hinton, I. R. Innes, A. Natel, and J. M. Parker. *Can. Med. Assoc. J.* 109:920 (1973).
10. J. G. Wagner. *Biopharmaceutics and Relevant Pharmacokinetics*. Drug Intelligence Publications, Hamilton, Ill., p. 82 (1971).
11. Government of Canada. *Food and Drug Act and Regulations*: Division 8, New Drugs, p. 126B (1981).
12. C. W. Dunnett. *J. Am. Stat. Assoc.* 50:1096 (1955).
13. G. W. Snedecor. *Statistical Methods*. Iowa State College Press, Ames, p. 251 (1956).

14. I. J. McGilveray, N. Mousseau, and R. Brien. *Can. J. Pharm. Sci.* *13*:33 (1978).
15. E. Jänchen and G. Levy. *Clin. Chem.* *18*:984 (1972).
16. L. A. Ouderkirk. Guidance for In-Vivo Bioequivalence Studies for Tolmetin Sodium Tablets and Capsules. Division of Bioequivalence, FDA, April 20 (1989).
17. E. Ormsby. *Proceedings of Bio'International 1989: Issues in the Evaluation of Bioavailability Data.* Trimel, Toronto, p. 158 (1990).
18. G. E. D. Box and D. R. Cox. *J. R. Stat. Soc. Ser. B* *26*:211 (1964).
19. Expert Advisory Committee Report. Guidelines and Standards for Bioavailability of Oral Dosage Formulations of Drugs Used for Systemic Effects. Health and Welfare, Canada (1990).
20. W. J. Westlake. *J. Pharm. Sci.* *61*:1340 (1972).
21. W. J. Westlake. In *Current Concepts in Pharmaceutical Sciences: Dosage Form Design and Bioavailability* (J. Swarbrick, ed.) Lea & Febiger, Philadelphia, p. 149 (1973).
22. M. R. Hamrell, M. N. Martinez, S. V. Dighe, and P. D. Parkman. *Drug Intell. Clin. Pharm.* *21*:362 (1987).
23. J. D. Haynes. *J. Pharm. Sci.* *70*:673 (1981).
24. D. J. Schuirmann. *J. Pharmacokinet. Biopharm.* *15*:657 (1987).
25. D. Hauschke, V. W. Steinijens, and E. Diletti. *Int. J. Clin. Pharmacol.* *28*:72 (1990).
26. I. J. McGilveray, K. K. Midha, J. C. K. Loo, and J. K. Cooper. *Int. J. Clin. Pharmacol.* *16*:110 (1978).
27. S. Sved, R. Hossie, I. J. McGilveray, N. Beaudoin, and R. Brien. *Can. J. Pharm. Sci.* *14*:67 (1979).
28. I. C. Bailar and F. Mosteller. *Ann. Intern. Med.* *108*:266 (1988).
29. I. J. McGilveray, K. K. Midha, and J. K. Cooper. *Can. J. Pharm. Sci.* *13*:9 (1978).
30. J. Ruedy, R. O. Davies, M. A. Gagnon, W. A. McLean, W. G. Thompson, T. G. Vitti, and T. W. Wilson. *Can. Med. Assoc. J.* *115*:105 (1976).
31. K. Karpinski. In *Proceedings of Bio'International 1989: Issues in the Evaluation of Bioavailability Data.* Trimel, Toronto, p. 138, 1990.
32. E. G. Lovering and C. A. Mainville. *Can. J. Pharm. Sci.* *12*:48 (1977).
33. E. G. Lovering, I. J. McGilveray, I. McMillan, W. Tostowaryk, T. Matula, and G. Marier. *Can. J. Pharm. Sci.* *10*:36 (1975).
34. S. Sved, I. J. McGilveray, and N. Beaudoin. *J. Pharm. Sci.* *66*:1761 (1977).
35. K. S. Albert. Transcript of The FDA Bioequivalence Hearing, Food and Drug Administration, Rockville, Md, p. 177 (1986).
36. *United States Pharmacopeia XXII 1990*. USP Pharmacopeial Convention, Rockville, Md, p. xliii (1989).
37. Medical Research Council of Canada. Guidelines for Research Involving Human Subjects.
38. Report by the Bioequivalence Task Force on recommendations from the bioequivalence hearing conducted by the Food and Drug Administration Sept. 29–Oct. 1, 1988, p. 26; 27 (January 1988).
39. D. R. Cox, M. A. Brown, D. J. Squires, E. A. Murrill, D. Lednicer, and D. W. Knuth. *Biopharm. Drug Dispo.* *9*:539 (1988).
40. C. H. Kleinbloesem, P. Van Brummelen, M. Danhof, H. Faber, J. Urquart, and D. D. Breimer. *Clin. Pharm. Ther.* *41*:26 (1987).

41. M. Gibaldi and D. Perrier. *Drugs and the Pharmaceutical Sciences*, vol. 15; *Pharmacokinetics*, 2nd ed. Marcel Dekker, New York, p. 145 (1982).
42. P. G. Welling and J. P. Skelly, eds. *Proceedings of a Pharmaceutical Manufacturers Association/Food and Drug Administration Workshop*. Pharmaceutical Manufactures Association, Washington, D.C. (1990).
43. L. M. Sanders. *Eur. J. Drug Metab. Pharmacokinet.* 15:95 (1990).
44. Expert Advisory Committee. Report on Bioavailability Guidelines and Standards for Bioavailability of Oral Modified Release Dosage Formulations of Drugs Used for Systemic Effects. Health and Welfare Canada (1990).

14

Bioequivalence: A European Community Regulatory Perspective

A. G. Rauws
*National Institute of Public Health and Environmental Protection
Bilthoven, The Netherlands*

INTRODUCTION

It can be taken for granted that European perspectives, whether in landscape, culture, or in politics, present a patchwork picture, in comparison with the large vistas of, for instance, the Americas. Medical tradition, until World War II, was very nationalistic, medical examinations in most countries being state examinations. After the war, the influence of Anglo-Saxon medicine has spread, but one can still discern an Anglo-Saxon/Nordic, a German/Central European, and a Romance or Southern European complex in medicine.

These complexes mould, with other influences, the local concepts on the use and limitations of medicinal products. Moreover, differences in the practice of pharmacy and production of pharmaceuticals have led to large differences among countries in price setting. In countries with relatively low drug prices there has been little incentive for marketing generic products. In countries, like the Netherlands, where drug prices are relatively high, generic products compete for a large segment of the market. So the problems of bioequivalence were considerable in some countries, whereas in other countries they were almost unknown.

Until recently, reimbursement policies seem to have had little influence on generic substitution, unlike the situation in the United States. But, now, under strong pressures to reduce public spending on health care, there is a tendency in every country to introduce some incentive for generic substitution into reimbursement schemes. In the Federal Republic of Germany this leads to rather radical interventions in the freedom of choice, not only for brand, but also for active substance! So the politicalization of the pharmaceutical market is now also a fact in Western Europe, at least.

Meanwhile, the European Community (EC) has been developing since the 1950s toward European integration. Its efforts to build up a system of common rules for many years involved the laborious procedure of reaching unanimity. Thereby each member-state contributed its own administrative, legal, and technical proclivities, not always ready to appreciate those of other states. This situation often led to legislation and directives bearing the mark of weary compromise. Now that the year 1992 is approaching rapidly and frontiers have to open for free exchange of people, services, and goods, a certain "élan," spirit, is taking possession of those cooperating to shape the future of the EC. One feels that now things are going to happen! Especially the European Commission—the executive body of the EC—puts great pressure on those preparing legislation and directives to make clear decisions, instead of postponing difficulties—and there are many—until the next meeting.

THE MACHINERY OF EUROPEAN COMMUNITY REGULATION ON MEDICINAL PRODUCTS

In the EC, part of national competences is transferred to community institutions, such as the Council of Ministers, the European Parliament, the European Commission, and the European Court of Justice. The European Commission prepares draft directives. These draft directives are discussed in the European Parliament and in the Economic and Social Committee. In their final form, they are approved by the Council of Minsters. Decisions are made by a qualified majority, the votes of the member states reflecting, in an attenuated way, the size of their populations. In case of conflict, EC directives prevail over national law, and the latter has to be adapted. In this way, the community works toward one European system of legislation, administration, and jurisdiction.

Several bodies of the European Commission are charged with regulatory tasks in the area of medicinal products [1]. The Pharmaceutical Committee, consisting of officials of the European Commission and of the health ministries of the member states, is more politically oriented and discusses the proposals of the European Commission; for example, a central registration procedure for biotechnologic products and a multistate registration procedure for more conventional products. The proposals of the European Commission and the Pharmaceutical Committee are finally laid down in draft directives by the European Commission. These are prepared for approval as described in the foregoing.

However, because of the rather differing administrative traditions in the different member states, procedural unity does not guarantee unity in administrative practice. To promote standardization of evaluation, and to stimulate parallel thinking among the national authorities, guidance documents on many subjects of importance are formulated. This is done by the Committee on Proprietary Medicinal Products (CPMP) and the Committee on Veterinary Medicinal Products (CVMP). These bodies consist of officials of the European Commission and one representative from each member state. Decisions are made on a one person–one vote basis. Other tasks of these committees are the preparation of "opinions" on submissions for biotechnologic or "high-tech" products, and also formulation of "opinions" on multistate applications and pharmacovigilance: evaluation of and proposals for decisions on side effects of drugs. Thus, these committees work on a scientific–technical level, based on the procedures laid down in the directives concerned and in internal rules. The procedures are discussed regularly in the Operational Group of the CPMP.

Guidance by the CPMP is prepared by working parties on Quality, on Safety, and on Efficacy. Outside experts, mostly from national authorities, may be invited to take part in the work. The working party "Efficacy" has prepared the Note for Guidance, *Investigation of Bioavailability*, which was completed in 1984.

BIOAVAILABILITY GUIDANCE IN THE EUROPEAN COMMUNITY

Within the European Community, needs for regulatory action on the issue of bioavailability and bioequivalence are vastly different. These depend on the structure of the pharmaceutical market, the share of generic products in it, and on the degree of regulatory sophistication. For instance, the situation in the Netherlands, with relatively expensive proprietary pharmaceutical products, leaves room for inexpensive generic products. In member states, like France and Italy, entirely different market structures and regulatory practices prevail.

However, the evolution toward a common market requires a common base for granting marketing authorizations. Therefore–on the basis of the directives concerned [2,3]–a first version of the EC recommendation was drafted in the early 1980s by the Working Party, Efficacy of Drugs, of the Committee for Proprietary Medicinal Products (CPMP). This became official in March 1987 [4]. After some definitions and very general remarks on design and conduct of studies, the guideline puts emphasis on the regulatory aspect. It distinguishes between Applications with Full Clinical Documentation (mostly new active substances) and Applications Without Full Documentation (mostly generic products). It enumerates situations in which bioavailability studies are especially needed, and those in which bioavailability studies may be omitted. The whole is rendered in brief in Figure 1, which necessarily lacks the nuances of the full text.

In the patchwork quilt of national European regulation the EC guidance is promulgated to serve as a standard, albeit somewhat vague, for decision-making and to induce more uniformity among the member states of the community. At that time, it was not possible to reach unanimity on more concrete requirements.

Regulatory policy should not operate below this standard, nor, on the other hand, too far above it, to prevent unequal justice. National guidance, if any, should understandably be compatible with it. It was hoped that this guide would contribute to the gradual convergence of the rather divergent ways of thinking on this matter in Europe. It is difficult to judge if the document has met the expectations. Probably, nobody in the overburdened national authorities has had time to make international comparisons on practices that may be based on this recommendation.

The lack of requirements at the technical level is remarkable. In this, it is to be expected that the guidance documents in the United Kingdom and in the Netherlands and the nonofficial guidance by the "Arbeitsgemeinschaft für

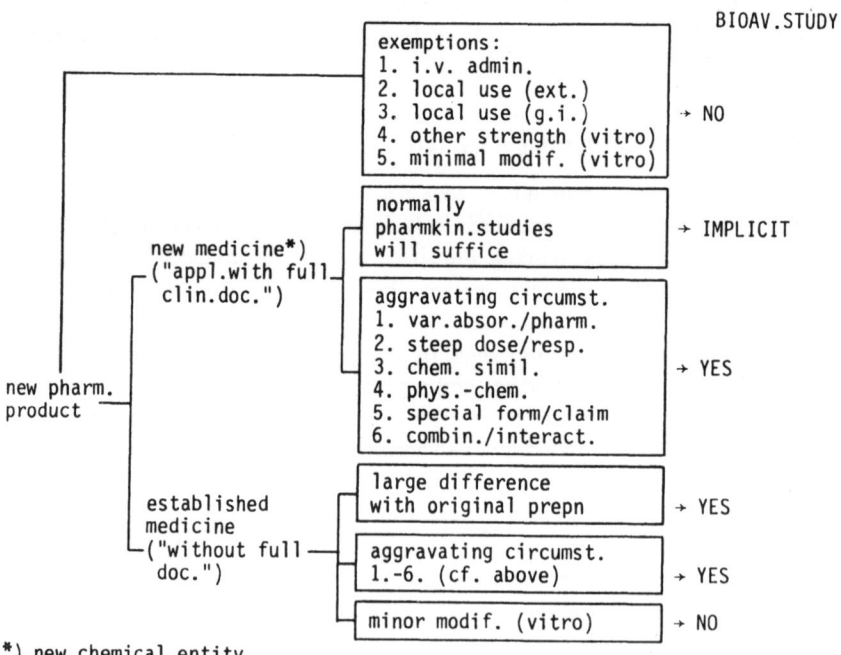

*) new chemical entity

Figure 1 Recommendation for the European Communities.

Pharmazeutische Verfahrenstechnik" (APV, International Association for Pharmaceutical Technology) in the FRG will have had more impact on raising the quality of the bioequivalence studies during the 1980s. In contrast with other guidance outlines [5], no quantitative norm has been stated for the bioequivalence requirement. Also lacking are recommendations for the bioequivalence problems that arise with products containing new active substances, for instance, when the experimental forms used in the clinical studies, especially the dose-finding studies, differ from those of the final product to be marketed. Other guidelines pay more attention to this problem [5,6].

NATIONAL GUIDANCE IN EUROPEAN COMMUNITY MEMBER STATES

The EC Note for Guidance, *Investigation of Bioavailability*, has been influenced by existing and emerging practices in several member states including the United Kingdom and the Netherlands. This applies especially to the revised version, to be finalized in the spring of 1990. This guidance has been influenced by the experience gathered in about 10 years of tightened-up evaluation of generic products, especially in the German Federal Republic, the Netherlands, and the United Kingdom. Therefore, it seems appropriate to briefly review, in chronologic order of their guidance-taking effect, the relevant developments within these member states that have been confronted most with the problems of generic products.

United Kingdom

The first guidance in Europe on bioavailability and bioequivalence was set forth by the UK Government [7] (Fig. 2), allowing abridged applications to be made for generics (pharmaceutical equivalents), other dosage strengths, or chemical forms (salts, esters, or other) of active substances (pharmaceutical alternatives), or products in special formulations (e.g., suppositories, modified-release products, and such).

From the text, it appears that a requirement for in vivo studies is more related to safety considerations, "significant hazard to the patient." Unfavorable substance properties, such as low solubility or poor absorption, lead to the requirement for in vitro tests, unless a safety hazard (narrow therapeutic margins or lack of efficacy) requires studies in vivo.

The United Kingdom guidance [8] has a structure quite different from the others, described later, and thereby reflects a quite different way of administrative thinking: The typically Anglo-Saxon reliance on jurisprudence, rather than attempts at exhaustive regulation. The latter is a continental habit that we owe to the Prussian kings and to Napoleon. The British attitude will necessitate incidental choices in the course of handling a submission. This requires much wisdom in judgment by the officials and a good memory, or better—a careful

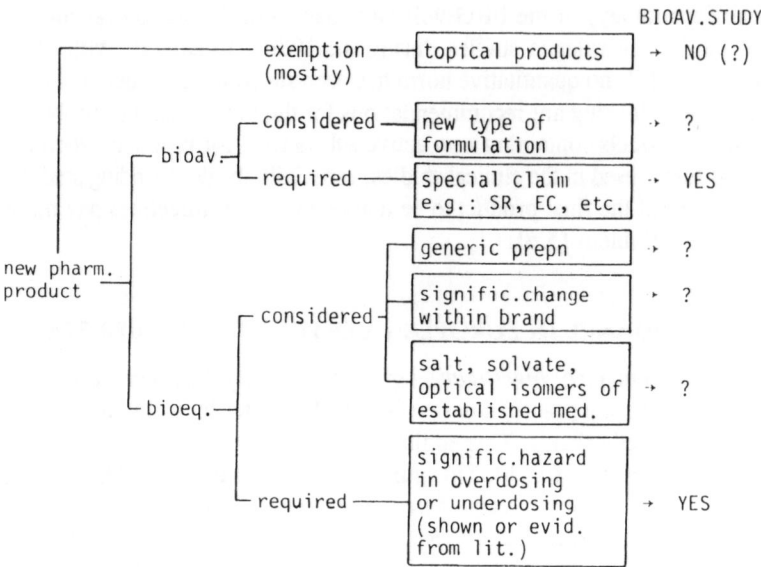

Figure 2 Recommendation for the United Kingdom.

documentation of precedents. It also shows the British reliance on fair play between applicant and authority, rather than on watertight regulation.

The Netherlands

Before 1978, generic products in the Netherlands were certified on the basis of a pharmaceutical dossier by the Medicines Inspectorate. From 1978 onward, generic products had to be evaluated by the "College ter Beoordeling van Geneesiddelen" (Committees for Evaluation of Medicines) on an abbreviated submission containing a pharmaceutical part; a clinical pharmacologic part, with the bioequivalence studies or arguments for not having them executed; and the summary of product characteristics (SPC, Appendix IB). On several occasions, the authorities attention has been drawn, from outside, to the problem of bioequivalence (e.g., Breimer [9]). In early 1978, a preliminary set of requirements for internal use had already been formulated to aid in reaching consistency in assessments. On the basis of experience accumulated in the early 1980s and in a structured consultation with academia and the pharmaceutical industry, a recommendation for conventional generic products was written, which became official in 1985 [10] (Fig. 3). This recommendation was used in harmony

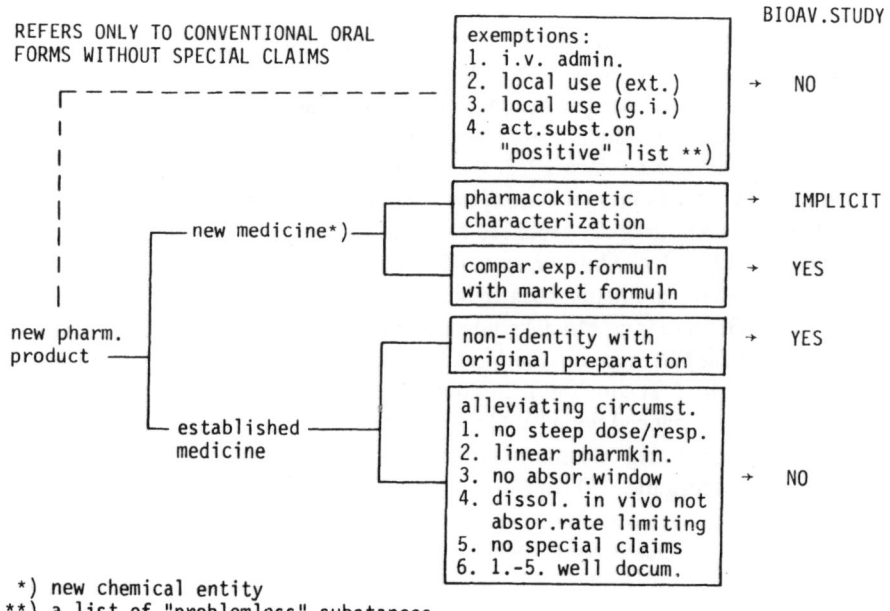

Figure 3 Recommendation for the Netherlands.

with the EC recommendation, the latter being more general and vague in its formulation.

The Dutch recommendation always asks for studies of bioequivalence unless arguments are given to prove that these studies are not necessary: namely, if there are (1) no steep dose–effect relationship, or small margin of safety; *and* (2) linear pharmacokinetics; *and* (3) no influence of (realistic) formulation variables on bioavailability from conventional forms; *and* (4) no claims related to release pattern in vivo. The Committee even decided to institute a list of substances obviously satisfying these conditions, the so-called positive list.

Furthermore, the Dutch recommendation contained a considerable amount of reasoned technical requirements in an attempt to improve the—at that time often rather low—quality of studies submitted. In the 1987 revision, some requirements were clarified or extended, especially those on reporting. The ease with which changes appeared to be made in reports, of which the photocopied versions were submitted, led to the sentence; "The Committee for Evaluation of Medicines may question the textual integrity of unauthorized copies of reports" [10].

Federal Republic of Germany

The pharmaceutical market in the Federal Republic of Germany is characterized by a multitude of separate products. An important section of it consists of older generic products of widely diverging pharmaceutical quality. A retrospective evaluation of these products seems hardly possible with the present evaluating capacity. Nevertheless, since 1978, the Institut für Arzneimittel des Bundesgesundheitsamtes (Medicines Institute of the Federal Health Office; BGA) has, aided by 14 review commissions, produced standard monographs on some thousands of products [11]. Meanwhile, in spite of overload and backlog, bioequivalence requirements have gradually been tighened in the second half of the 1980s.

In the FRG, there is no official guidance on the subject. However, the Arbeitsgemeinschaft für Pharmazeutische Verfahrenstechnik (International Association for Pharmaceutical Technology), in cooperation with industry, academia, and authorities, has produced the APV Guideline *Studies on Bioavailability and Bioequivalence*, containing recommendations on design, conduct, evaluation, and reporting of such studies [6]. In German-speaking countries the APV Guideline is now considered as a standard (Fig. 4). The technical requirements of the APV Guideline and the Dutch recommendation [10] are much the same.

It is more difficult to define in which cases in vivo studies are necessary.

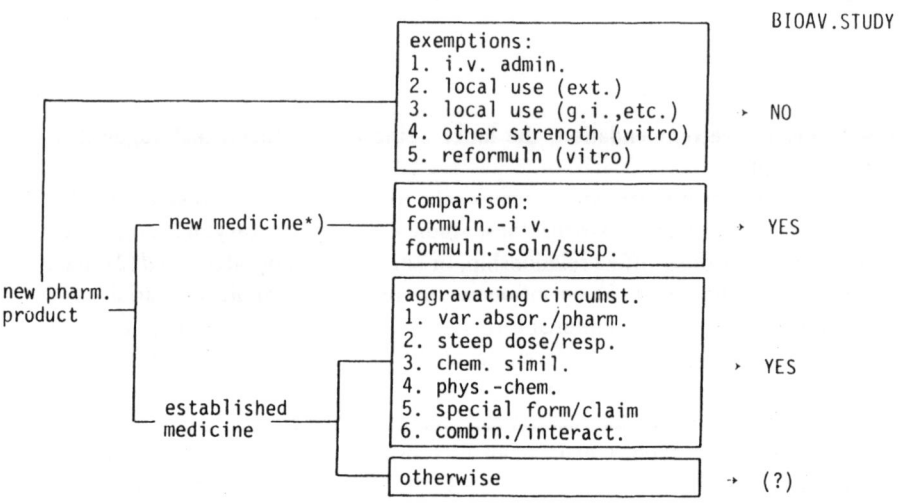

*) new chemical entity

Figure 4 APV Recommendation.

The approach by the BGA is as follows: For conventional oral products a sequence of criteria has been drawn up.

1. Critical therapeutic categories
2. Unfavorable pharmacokinetic and physicochemical properties
3. Structural analogy with problematic substances
4. Substances with documented bioavailability problems

Working parties are systematically considering all active substances on the market, according to these criteria.

For all substances exhibiting narrow therapeutic ranges or used for serious indications, such as infections and cardiac disease (criteriun 1), bioequivalence must be proved. Substances outside these therapeutic groups are evaluated according to criteria 2, 3, and 4, in a standardized format, taking into account low solubility, slow absorption, nonlinear kinetics, and so forth. This may lead to the conclusion that bioequivalence of pharmaceutical equivalents or alternatives has to be shown. In cases of insufficient information, the onus of proof resides with the applicant. In all other cases, appropriate dissolution studies in vitro will suffice.

An initial list of active substances considered to present bioavailability and, thus, bioequivalence problems, was published in 1988. Additional lists were published in 1990. For modified-release products or products administered by a nonoral route, but intended to exert a systemic action, studies in vivo are always required.

THE REVISED EUROPEAN COMMUNITY RECOMMENDATION: INVESTIGATION OF BIOAVAILABILITY AND BIOEQUIVALENCE

Developments both outside and inside the European Community in the area of bioavailability and bioequivalence (e.g., new methods of statistical evaluation [12-14] and the growing body of knowledge on design of studies) underscored the need for a revision of the old 1984 guidance. On the basis of the experience gained in the last years the Efficacy Working Party has carried out this task.

What are the differences between the 1984 recommendation and the 1990 version? They are many. Apart from the necessary updating, an attempt has been made to eliminate some vagueness in the old recommendation and to add an amount of technical detail analogous to the Dutch and the APV guidance. The new version will be discussed in the form that was finalized by the Efficacy Working Party, in July 1990. Its content still has to be officially approved (for an overview, the reader is referred to Table 1).

Table 1 Comparison of Old and New EC Recommendations

Investigation of Bioavailability	Investigation of Bioavailability and Bioequivalence

1. *General Remarks*
   a. Studies during development of new product
   b. Comparison between existing and new formulations
	1. *Introduction*
	   Explication of background

2. *Definitions*
   Definition of bioavailability and comment
	2. *Definitions*
	   2.1 Pharmaceutical equivalents
	   2.2 Pharmaceutical alternatives
	   2.3 Bioavailability
	   2.4 Bioequivalents
	   2.5 Essentially similar products
	   2.6 Therapeutic equivalents

3. *Parameters*
   General remarks, no detailed rules
   a. Remarks on design: crossover
   b. Gastrointestinal factors: fasting, meals
	3. *Design and Conduct of Studies*
	   Reference to pharmacokinetic basis
	   3.1 Design
	   3.2 Subjects
	   3.3 Variables to be measured
	   3.4 Chemical analysis
	   3.5 Reference and test product
	   3.6 Data analysis
	   3.7 Reporting

4. *Applications with Full Clinical Documentation*
   Studies especially needed if
   a. Formulation effects on absorption
   b. Risk for patient (inefficacy or toxicity)
   c. Structural relation with problem substance
   d. Unfavorable physicochemical/pharmacokinetic properties
   e. Special in vivo release characteristics
   f. Fixed combination product with possible absorption interaction
	4. *Applications for Products Containing New Active Substances*
	   4.1 Bioavailability (systemic)
	   4.2 Bioequivalence (versus formulations used in clinical trials)

5. *Applications Without Full Documentation*
   Essential question: bioequivalence?
   a. Substantial departure from original formulation or problems
	5. *Applications for New Products Containing Approved Active Substances*
	   Comply with Directive 87/21/EEC concerned with protection of

Continued

Table 1 (Continued)

Investigation of Bioavailability	Investigation of Bioavailability and Bioequivalence

5. *Continued*
  as outlined in 4.a–f: bioequivalence study
  b. Minor modification in existing product: comparison of in vitro dissolution rate
	5. *Continued*
	 product information. Situations requiring in vivo studies:
	  1. Unfavorable physicochemical properties
	  2. Structurally similar to problem substance
	  3. Formulation effects on absorption
	  4. Risk for patient (inefficacy or toxicity)
	  5. Nonoral route of administration
	  6. Special in vivo release characteristics
	  7. Fixed combination product with possible absorption interaction
	 5.1 Bioequivalence studies
	  1. If risk of bioinequivalence
	  2. If risk of inefficacy or toxicity
	 5.2 Exemptions
	  1. Other strength (conditional)
	  2. Minor modification in existing product
	  3. Parenteral solution (IM, SC)
	  4. Oral solution (conditional)
	  5. In vitro/in vivo correlation shown
	 5.3 Suprabioavailability

6. *Situations in Which Biological Availability Need Not Be Studied*
  a. Product only for intravenous use
  b. Product only for local use (except safety)
  c. Product only for internal nonsystemic use
  d. Other strength (conditional)
  e. Minor modification in existing product
	6. *Situations in Which Bioavailability Study Is Not Relevant*
	  1. Product only for intravenous use
	  2. Product only for local (external or internal) nonsystemic use (does not preclude eventual safety studies)

Definitions

Paragraph 2 in the definitions has been extended, with an attempt to align these as much as possible with those already existing, especially, with FDA documents [15] and those of the Office of Technology Assessment [16]. It is now important to aim for a coherent body of terminology on bioavailability and bioequivalence that can be used in international harmonization on this subject.

1. *Pharmacuetical equivalents*: Medicinal products are pharmaceutical equivalents if they contain the same amount of the same active substance(s) in the same dosage forms that meet the same or comparable standards.
2. *Pharmaceutical alternatives*: Medicinal products are pharmaceutical alternatives if they contain the same therapeutic moiety, but differ in the salt or ester of that moiety or in dosage form or strength.
3. *Bioavailability*: Bioavailability means the rate and extent to which the active ingredient or therapeutic moiety is absorbed from a pharmaceutical form and become available at the site of action.
4. *Bioequivalents*: Two medicinal products are bioequivalents if they are pharmaceutical equivalents or alternatives and if their bioavailabilities (rate and extent) after administration in the same molar dose are similar to such degree that their effects, with respect to both efficacy and safety, will be essentially the same.
5. *Essentially similar products*: A medicinal product will be regarded as essentially similar to another product if it has the same qualitative and quantitative composition in terms of active substance(s), and the pharmaceutical form is the same, and, where necessary, bioequivalence with the first product has been demonstrated by appropriate bioavailability studies carried out.
6. *Therapeutic equivalents*: A medicinal product is therapeutically equivalent with another product if it contains the same active substance or therapeutic moiety and, when administered to the same individuals, shows the same efficacy and toxicity as that product, whose efficacy and safety has been established.

Definitions 1 and 2 are analogous to the FDA definitions. At an FIP Workshop in 1989, a more general definition for bioavailability was proposed. Consensus about it is not certain. For the time being, analogy with definitions in other guidance documents is considered to be more important. Definition 4 is analogous to that in the Dutch and the Australian recommendations.

Design, Conduct, and Evaluation of Studies

In paragraph 3, the need for knowledge about the pharmacokinetics of the active substance in question is stressed and refers to the EC document, *Pharmacokinetic Studies in Man* [17]. It goes into some detail in explaining the technical aspects of the studies required and their scientific background. The text reflects the existing consensus on technical aspects [18].

Following the usual practice, reinforced by Westlake [19], a bioequivalence range of 0.8-1.2 is taken within which the confidence interval of the relative bioavailability should lie. Smaller maximal deviations may be necessary (e.g., 0.9-1.1 for digoxin). Larger ranges may be allowed if technical limitations require them and if there are no objections concerning safety. Levy [20] has argued the appropriateness of larger deviations on clinical grounds. This, however, neglects the quality aspect of bioequivalence, which should be the first point to consider. This is still an unresolved issue.

For the chemical analysis, the applicant is referred to the EC recommendation *Analytical Validation* [21], especially to the paragraph on bioanalytical procedures. For the use of biotransformation products, instead of the active substance itself, the recommendation accepts the use of an active biotransformation product if the active substance cannot be determined for a sound reason. This is still in accordance with consensus. If active biotransformation products cannot be determined either, the use of inactive ones is acceptable.

In the selection of the reference product, the EC authorities will accept the innovator product from any member state as reference, if there is a guarantee of essential similarity with the corresponding products in other member states. This may cause problems, but only temporary ones, as the national markets are merging into one EC market.

Test products will often originate from test batches. This will be acceptable only if these are produced according to Good Manufacturing Practice (GMP) rules. After scale up, production batches must be compared with test batches in an appropriate in vitro test. The applicant should retain sufficient samples to allow repetition of bioequivalence studies, by an independent laboratory, at the request of the authority.

In the past two decades, major developments have taken place in the statistical evaluation of bioequivalence studies. Westlake [19] and Metzler [22] have stressed the difference between testing the null hypothesis and testing equivalence. Moreover, Westlake has proposed a useful method to test for equivalence. It has received much criticism, but it also has been the fruitful start of further developments. Bayesian approaches have been developed [12,13], and the automatic reliance on parametric methods has been changed by introduction of the approaches by Steinijans and Diletti [14]. All of these methods are based on existing foundations, but make the often forbidding statistics accessible for the nonspecialized, but intelligent, user. The FDA strongly recommends the use of two one-sided tests [23]. The EC recommendation is reticent in prescribing methods, because developments in this area are still advancing. However, a certain consensus is now being approached [24,25]. Computer programs that combine several tests in a package have been developed [e.g., 26,27] and are being developed further (Wijnand, 1990, personal communication). If used diligently, they are helpful in producing a comprehensive and balanced evaluation.

The text on reporting does not contain exceptional aspects. It enumerates in great detail the items to be reported. Strict and stern attention should be given to first, the identification of the reference product, and second, the proof or statement of identity of the test product and product submitted for marketing authorization. Sadly, quite a number of unreliable, if not fraudulent, studies have been submitted in the past years. Completeness of data should be proved, not be just implied. Changes in design, dropout of subjects, and other exceptions to protocol should be reported and justified.

Requirement for Studies In Vivo

1. *Applications for products containing new active substances*: In paragraph 4, dealing with new active substances, the emphasis is not placed on a substance's characteristics that imply bioavailability problems, but on the general requirement to produce a coherent picture of the pharmacokinetics of the substance in question, including systemic availability. Stress is also laid upon the bioequivalence requirement for experimental trial formulations and the formulation to be marketed. It is important for an innovator to produce one biopharmaceutically acceptable formulation for conducting clinical trials in an early phase, to avoid the need of multiple bioequivalence studies to validate the market formulation against several experimental formulations.

2. *Applications for products containing approved active substances*: Paragraph 5 of the old recommendation leaves much to be desired concerning clarity on when bioequivalence studies are or are not required. The new version intends to make this point clear: Patient risk is not the only reason for bioavailability studies. Primarily, bioavailability is a quality requirement [9], with, as background the general safety and efficacy requirement. This is especially true if the generic product in question is intended to substitute for the innovator product. Substitution implies the claim of bioequivalence. And claims have to be substantiated.

In paragraph 6 of the old version situations were mentioned in which there was no need for bioavailability studies: in some because it was irrelevant (e.g., formulations for intravenous administration) and in others as an exemption (e.g., minor modifications). These have been separated because their combination was illogical. The exemptions are now mentioned in paragraph 5.

"Open" and "Closed" Dossiers:

In the final version, no reference has been made to the new directive on protection to product information [28]. Applications for generic products containing approved active substances can be made only in the abbreviated form if the dossier of the substance is "open," i.e., if the innovator product containing that substance has received marketing authorization in the EC more than 10 years ago. If approval has been obtained fewer than 10 years ago the dossier is still "closed" and the applicant for the generic formulation has to submit all data, including pharmacologic, toxicologic and clinical.

Suprabioavailability

The point of suprabioavailability has been presented because it may happen that a well-designed generic product appears to be biopharmaceutically superior to an old innovator product. The competent generic manufacturer should not be punished by the verdict: "bioinequivalent." Similarly to the FDA, the EC regulatory authority intends to make biopharmaceutical improvement worthwhile for manufacturers. Adaptation of the strength may, however, be necessary to make the dosage unit therapeutically equivalent (equipotent) to existing ones. Confusion should be excluded by appropriate designation of the product. After obtaining marketing authorization, the suprabioavailable product may become a new reference product. So it must also be made clear to innovator firms that marketing a product is a process that regularly requires updating of the biopharmaceutical quality.

MODIFIED-RELEASE PRODUCTS

Products with modified release according to the *United States Pharmacopeia (USP)* are defined as:

> Dosage forms for which the drug-release characteristics of time-course and/or drug release location are chosen to accomplish therapeutic or convenience objectives not offered by conventional dosage forms [29].

In evaluating these products, attention is directed primarily to complete bioavailability and to the plasma concentration–time course in steady state. The differing manufacturing processes cause qualitative differences in plasma concentration–time courses of different products. As a consequence, substitution is generally not recommended, as will be discussed later. It will be clear that a claim of bioequivalence will require more human pharmacokinetic studies than are needed for a modified-release product per se.

Modified-release products can be divided into three subclasses with different properties, compared with conventional products (partly deduced from *USP XXII*):

1. Slow-release (SR) lower C_{max} $t_{1/2}$ not changed
   later t_{max}
2. Extended-release (ER) lower C_{max} apparent $t_{1/2}$ increased
   later t_{max}
3. Delayed-release (DR) same C_{max} $t_{1/2}$ not changed
   lag time

Slow-release products may be useful in decreasing the risk of concentration-dependent side effects. They do not allow an increase in dosage interval, because the apparent elimination half-life corresponds to the intrinsic half-life. Only if by decreasing the release rate in vivo the apparent half-life has been increased is it possible to increase the dosage interval: extended-release [30]. Delayed-release products are constructed to start the release of active substance later or more distally in the gastrointestinal tract (e.g. enteric-coated products).

Basic Evaluation Scheme

Extended-release (ER) products are designed to smooth, within the therapeutic window, the plasma concentration–time curves. It implies at least repeated administration over a longer course of time. This is reflected in the evaluation scheme (Table 2). At first, single-dose studies are needed to prove the extended-release characteristics of the product and to investigate the potential for interference by meals with the release in vivo. Variables to characterize ER character in a single-dose study are apparent elimination half-life [30], mean residence time (MRT) [31], half-value duration [32], and the period during which the drug plasma concentration is greater than 75% of C_{max} [33]. The latter two measures are very sensitive to random variations in C_{max}.

Next, studies in steady state are required to characterize the drug plasma concentration–time course in a situation mimicking practice. Variables used to this end are percentage fluctuation, percentage swing, difference area or AUC fluctuation according to Boxenbaum [30,34], and half-way AUC ratio [35]. Fluctuation, and especially swing, are sensitive to variations in C_{max} and especially in C_{min} [30,35]. The other variables are more robust because they are functions of AUC, a variable in which random variations in plasma concentration tend to cancel each other out. Depending on the extent of knowledge about the plasma concentration–effect relationship, clinical efficacy studies may be required.

Table 2 Basic Scheme for Evaluation of Modified-Release Products

Basic scheme for guidance on modified release	
Single dose	Steady state
MR characteristics and bioavailability →	Fluctuation of plasma concentration
↓	↓
Food interferences	Controlled clinical studies

National Modified-Release Guidance in European Community Member States

In the United Kingdom, general guideline on bioequivalence in vivo studies are required for MR products, no special requirements being mentioned. In a published commentary the Superintending Pharmacist of the United Kingdom regulatory authority has expressed views on in vitro and in vivo requirements that have been applied to regulatory practice [36]. These views are—as to be expected—fully compatible with concepts within the scientific community. Because of the increasing number of ER products that contain theophylline, a special guideline was issued in 1987. It includes a study of meal interference, which may not be surprising to those acquainted with—if not loving—the famous British breakfast.

The Superintending Pharmacist mentions another point of interest: substitution. Conventional products, if bioequivalent, may be substituted one for another. For ER products the situation is more complicated because of differences in release patterns in vivo between products. In his view, substitution should not now be encouraged [36]. The plasma concentration-time course of MR products with similar bioavailability may indeed be rather different in form without disqualifying any of the products. Bioequivalence, however, requires essentially similar plasma concentration-time courses [35].

The more recent MR guidance in the Netherlands has just been discussed with industry and will be published in 1990. It differs from others in that it discriminates between ER and SR products, on the grounds mentioned earlier. In the pharmaceutical paragraph the desirability of an in vitro-in vivo relationship is stressed. Release rate in vitro should be studied at *several* physiologically sensible pH values. Preferably the release rate should be independent of pH. Under the pharmacokinetic requirements, studies of meal interference by *appropriate* meals are mentioned. Circadian rhythms should be studied *if related* to claims or labeling. This guidance has attempted to account for new developments and experiences, without hampering procedures. The special guidance for ER products containing theophylline is also open for discussion. It is analogous to the corresponding British guidance.

European Community Guidance

This recommendation is now officially approved by the CPMP. The term *prolonged action* in the title puts emphasis on effects. The definition is more neutral:

> ... extended release [modified release] form is considered as a modified pharmaceutical form of which the release of the active ingredient and its subsequent absorption are prolonged in comparison with a conventional non-modified form.

After some dissection of the text one will recognize the basic structure shown earlier (see Table 2).

Biopharmaceutic Validation

The extended-release characteristics should be proved. The release rate in vivo of the active substance and its bioavailability, in comparison with the conventional form, should be determined. Inter- and intraindividual variability should not exceed that after the conventional product, especially at steady state. Different dose strengths should be compared in vivo. The influence on the performance of the ER product by nonformulation factors, such as meals, diurnal rhythms, or other, should be investigated, unless shown to be irrelevant.

Therapeutic Validation

Under this heading patient studies are mentioned: pharmacokinetic and clinical. Pharmacokinetic studies should concentrate on ER characteristics such as apparent elimination half-life, fluctuation, and so forth, and on the plasma concentration–time course relative to the therapeutic range. Only if the concentration–effect relationship is well known, and pharmacotherapeutic experience with the active substance is extensive and well described in the literature, may pharmacotherapeutic studies be waived.

If pharmacotherapeutic studies are necessary they should prove the efficacy in the dosage scheme recommended for the indications claimed and they should compare frequency and severity of side effects with standard conventional treatment or with a comparable approved ER product. Dosage range, dosage scheme, indications and conditions of use, definition of patient populations with special requirements should be justified. The advantages of the ER product over the conventional treatment should be shown by results of clinical studies.

Delayed-Release Products

Not only in the guidance discussed earlier, but also in FDA or Nordic guidance, little or no attention has been given to delayed-release products, although they are evidently included in several official definitions. The objective of this dosage form is protection of the gastric mucosa against the irritating or erosive effect of the active substance or, conversely, protection of the active substance against gastric conditions.

Both monolithic and disperse (microencapsulated) forms may satisfy this objective. However, gastric physiology may make the pyloric passage and, hence, the start of action of the monolithic form unpredictable [37,38]. An intact tablet pass the pylorus only after emptying of the stomach, carried on by the "housekeeper waves." Monolithic forms may be retained in the stomach for hours, days, or even weeks. Disperse products on the other hand, after disintegration behave like a liquid suspension and start passing the pylorus immediately. One may wonder if the monolithic form has not become obsolete if it can be replaced by an analogous disperse product. The authorities should give attention to this issue.

Comments on the EC Recommendation

The emphasis in the requirements in the EC guidance for MR products is on the clinical aspects. It is true that, in the past, too much weight has been attributed to pharmaceutical technology and to pharmacokinetic details of MR products. It is fortunate that in this guidance not only good pharmacokinetic sense is requested, but also more pharmacotherapeutic thought. It would have been desirable if the recommendation had also contained requirements concerning SR and DR products. This would have enabled a more distinct discrimination of SR products from ER products. Relationships between pharmaceutics and pharmacokinetics, pharmacotherapeutics are not stressed in the present draft.

International Coordination of Guidance on Modified-Release Products

At the moment in many parts of the world, guidance for MR products has been drafted. Definitive texts are in preparation in the United States, Canada, Australia, and the European Community. There is a rough consensus on the scientific aspects of MR requirements. It should be possible to produce a single document instead of a number of separate documents. It would be profitable for industry not to have to meet various similar, but different requirements. In addition, regulatory authorities would have a firmer stand, relying on worldwide guidance based upon consensus between academia, industry, and regulatory agencies.

VETERINARY MEDICINAL PRODUCTS

Medicinal products are developed and produced not only for humans, but also for animals. In several pharmacotherapeutic classes, the batch size of active substance produced for animals is measured in tons. The number of pigs yearly bred and slaughtered in the Netherlands approaches that of the population of the country, almost 15 million. Large-scale bred animals may be more intensively medicated than the pharmaceutical industry cares to imagine for human patients.

Veterinary pharmacotherapy differs from human pharmacotherapy in that it is predominantly aimed at groups instead of individuals, the pet animal group excepted. This influences the kind of formulations used: products for intramuscular administration, drenches, and medicated feed are most common.

During the last decade, awareness of biopharmaceutical aspects influencing bioavailability has grown and much research has been done in that area [39]. A glance in the veterinary journals shows also that increasing attention is being given to veterinary pharmacokinetics and to the effect of routes of administration on drug concentrations and effects in large animals.

However, in spite of EC registration requirements for veterinary medicinal products [40], relatively little attention has been given to problems of bioequivalence. This is amazing because not only pharmacotherapy may be influenced by differences in bioavailability between pharmaceutical equivalents or alternatives, but also the disappearance of residues. Especially for intramuscular (IM) or subcutaneous administration, slow absorption of dose from the injection site may turn a conventional IM product into a depot preparation. This will upset residue disappearance calculations and may give rise to residues where and when they are not expected.

This problem has been illustrated by pharmacokinetic simulations [41]. Nouws et al. [42] have shown the consequences of biopharmaceutical quality of ampicillin products on withdrawal time in calves. A rabbit model has been proposed recently to test intramuscular bioavailability and bioequivalence [43]. With some ampicillin products also studied by Nouws [42], results similar to those found in calves were found in the rabbit model. However, further validation of the model is necessary.

Indeed, in the EC Note for Guidance on pharmacokinetics of veterinary medicines, which is currently in preparation, bioavailability has been defined, but more in a sense of a pharmacokinetic than of a biopharmaceutic characteristic with consequences for bioequivalence. In the Directive 81/851/EEC on veterinary medicinal products in article 5, paragraph 10, the opportunity to submit an abridged application for marketing authorization is given, if the medicinal product in question is essentially similar to a registered product. A medicinal product—veterinary or other—is essentially similar to another product if it is pharmaceutically equivalent and if its bioequivalence with the other product has been implied or demonstrated [15].

In such a submission, the problem of demonstrating bioequivalence arises. Compared with the literature on bioequivalence of human medicinal products, that on veterinary products is scarce [44]. Sophisticated experimental designs and statistical evaluations are seldom used. Even if methods are developed and applied within a few years, it will be difficult to clean up a market flooded with products, the efficacy and equivalence of which have hardly been tested.

CONCLUDING REMARKS

In concluding this overview, it is pertinent to make some general comments.

As observed earlier, EC guidance is necessarily influenced by differences in attitude, administrative tradition, and medical and pharmaceutical training between member states. The difference reside not so much in official opinions and regulations, as in the way they are handled in practice. In the past years a trend toward a common practice has started, but differences are still too large to achieve mutual recognition. It will be of eminent importance for the future of the EC that especially the evaluators of all member states in a structured program are trained together so that they can interpret and apply EC directives and recommendations in the same spirit. Only in this way will reciprocal adjustment proceed in a timely manner.

Developments in the Eastern European countries in 1989 and 1990 have created a process leading to the closure of the gap between the EC countries and those in Eastern Europe. One may expect that regulatory cooperation on medicinal products will develop along with the other contacts. At present, cooperation on medicinal products between Eastern European countries is not an official Comecon activity, but a multilateral collaboration. This leaves much freedom in implementation of relevant guidance within each country (T. L. Paál, personal communication, 1990).

The underlying philosophy of requirements in Eastern Europe is analogous to that in the EC and elsewhere, but the practice shows differences. Thus, more weight is given to bioavailability and bioequivalence studies in animals. In the case of generics the level of requirements (in vitro, animals in vivo, or human studies in vivo) depend on the degree of differences between original products and generic products. In these countries pharmaceutical and medical training are on a high level. So cooperation on a scientific level will not present more problems than within the EC. Such cooperation has already existed for decades within the European regional organization of the WHO.

The bioequivalence issue in Europe is not as heavily contaminated with substitution politics as in the United States. This allows authorities to rely less on exhaustive regulation than in the United States. But by now the substitution debate has also started in Europe, and one should beware of simplifying science to serve political expediency.

Although consensus on definitions and technical details has not yet been reached, the larger problem resides in the demarcation of requirement for studies in vivo versus those only in vitro. Our ignorance, shared by academia, industry, and authorities alike, concentrates on the relation between efficacy limits and bioavailability limits. This ignorance compels us to keep "on the safe side," especially for products belonging to critical therapeutic categories [45]. Similar plasma concentration–time courses achieve similar therapeutic effects in the same patient. We still do not know which deviation from bioequivalence is still compatible with therapeutic equivalence. Interesting efforts to relate bioavailability by concentration–effect relations with efficacy have been undertaken by Olson et al. [46]. An organized research effort in this direction might answer many questions we now hardly dare ask.

However good the bioavailability and bioequivalence recommendations may be, and however well the authorities may maintain the regulations on marketing authorization, the quality of the medicinal products on the market and the trust one may put into substitution will still depend strongly on the efficacy of an EC system for pharmaceutical inspection after admission to the market. The evaluation of a product submitted for marketing authorization is just a snap-shot. The necessary maintenance of quality and bioequivalence can only be assured by a system of continuous and rigorous inspection supported by adequate sanctions.

REFERENCES

1. F. Sauer and R. Hankin. *J. Clin. Pharmacol.* 27:639 (1987).
2. Council Directive 65/65/EEC of 26 Jan. 1965. *Off. J. Eur. Commun.* No 22 (9 Feb. 1965).
3. Council Directive 75/318/EEC of 20 May 1975. *Off. J. Eur. Commun.* No L147 (9 June 1975).
4. Note for Guidance. *Investigation of Bioavailability. Off. J. Eur. Commun.* No L73. p. 27. (16 March 1987).
5. Nordic Guideline. *Bioavailability Studies in Man.* NLN Publication No 18, Nordic Council on Medicines, Uppsala (1987).
6. H. Junginger, U. Gundert-Remy, H. Möller, J. Pabst, and V. W. Steinijans. APV Guideline "Studies on Bioavailability and Bioequivalence." *Drugs Made in Germany* 30:161 (1987).
7. A. C. Cartwright. *Pharm. Int.* 4:196 (1984).
8. Medicines Act: Notes on Applications for Product Licences, Annex II to MAL 2, Department of Health and Social Security, London (1983).
9. D. D. Breimer. *Pharm. Weekbl.* 111:1121 (1976).
10. College ter Beoordeling van Geneesmiddelen (Committee for Evaluation of Medicines, Rijswijk, the Netherlands), Aanbeveling: "Onderzoek van Biologische Beschikbaarheid en Bioequivalentie. (Recommendation: Study of Bioavailability and Bioequivalence), Sept. 1985, revised Sept. 1987 (also available in English).
11. K. Schmitt-Rau. *J. Clin. Pharmacol.* 28:1064 (1988).
12. B. E. Rodda and R. L. Davis. *Clin. Pharmacol. Ther.* 28:247 (1980).
13. H. Fluehler, A. P. Grieve, D. Mandallaz, J. Mau, and H. A. Moser. *J. Pharm. Sci.* 72:1178 (1983).
14. V. W. Steinijans and E. Diletti. *Eur. J. Clin. Pharmacol.* 28:85 (1985).
15. *Approved Drug Products.* U.S. Department of Health and Human Services, Washington, D.C., p. 1-1 (1985).
16. Office of Technology Assessment. *J. Pharmacokinet. Biopharm.* 2:433 (1974).
17. Note for Guidance. Pharmacokinetic Studies in Man. *Off. J. Eur. Commun.* No L73 p. 32 (16 March 1987).
18. T. N. Tozer. In *Principles and Perspectives in Drug Bioavailability* (J. Blanchard, R. J. Sawchuck, and B. B. Brodie, eds.) S. Karger, Basel, p. 120 (1979).
19. W. J. Westlake. In *Principles and Perspectives in Drug Bioavailability* (J. Blanchard, R. J. Sawchuck, and B. B. Brodie, eds.) S. Karger, Basel, p. 192 (1979).
20. G. Levy. *Can. Med. Assoc. J.* 107:722 (1972).
21. Note for Guidance. *Analytical Validation.* Document No III/844/87 (1989).
22. C. M. Metzler. *Biometrics* 30:309 (1974).
23. D. J. Schuirman. *J. Pharmacokinet. Biopharm.* 15:657 (1987).
24. W. J. Westlake. In *Biopharmaceutical Statistics for Drug Development* (K. E. Peace, ed.) Marcel Dekker, New York, p. 329 (1988).
25. V. W. Steinijans and D. Hauschke. *Int. J. Clin. Pharmacol. Ther. Toxicol.* 28:105 (1990).
26. H. P. Wijnand and C. J. Timmer. *Comput. Progr. Biomed.* 17:73 (1983).
27. M. Olling and A. G. Rauws. *Method Find. Exp. Clin. Pharmacol.* 8:629 (1986).

28. Council Directive 87/21/EEC of 22 Dec. 1986, Official Journal No L15 (17 Jan. 1987).
29. *United States Pharmacopeia, XXII* ed. United States Pharmacopeial Convention, Rockville, Md., p. xliii (1989).
30. A. G. Rauws, and M. Olling. In *Oral Controlled Release Products* (U. Gundert-Remy and H. Möller, eds.) Wissensch. Verlagsges., Stuttgart, p. 195 (1990).
31. S. Riegelman and P. Collier. *J. Pharmacokinet. Biopharm.* 8:509 (1980).
32. J. Meier, E. Nüesch, and R. Schmidt. *Eur. J. Clin. Pharmacol.* 7:429 (1974).
33. J. H. G. Jonkman, W. C. Berg, N. Grimberg, K. de Vries, R. A. de Zeeuw, and R. Schoenmaker. *Eur. J. Clin. Pharmacol.* 21:39 (1981).
34. H. Boxenbaum. *Pharm. Res.* p. 82 (1984).
35. H. Blume, M. Siewert, V. W. Steinijans, and H. Stricker. *Pharm. Ind.* 51:1025 (1989).
36. A. C. Cartwright. *Manuf. Chem.* 58:(3)33 (1987).
37. K. A. Kelly. *Am. J. Physiol.* 239:G71 (1980).
38. C. Y. Lui, R. Oberle, D. Fleischer, and G. L. Amidon. *J. Pharm. Sci.* 75:469 (1986).
39. D. G. Pope. *J. Vet. Pharmacol. Ther.* 7:85 (1984).
40. Council Directive 81/851/EEC of 28 Sept. 1981. *Off. J. Eur. Commun.* No L317 (6 Nov. 1981).
41. A. G. Rauws. *Tijdschr. Diergeneesk.* 110:932 (1985).
42. J. F. M. Nouws, C. A. M. van Ginneken, P. Hekman, and G. Ziv. *Vet. Q.* 4:62 (1982).
43. M. Olling and A. G. Rauws. *Naunyn-Schmiedebergs Arch. Pharmacol.* 341:R106 (1990) (abstract).
44. G. D. Koritz. *J. Am. Vet. Med. Assoc.* 177:279 (1980).
45. J. L. Colaizzi and D. T. Lowenthal. *Clin. Therap.* 8:370 (1986).
46. S. C. Olson, M. A. Eldon, R. D. Toothaker, J. J. Ferry, and W. A. Colburn. *J. Clin. Pharmacol.* 27:342 (1987).

15
Bioavailability and Bioequivalence: An Australian Perspective

Susan Walters
Therapeutic Goods Administration
Canberra, Australia

Rodney Charles Hall
Merck Sharp & Dohme (Australia) Pty. Ltd.
Granville, New South Wales, Australia

INTRODUCTION

As in many countries, recognition of the teratogenic effects of thalidomide led to the development in Australia of legislation to require the premarket assessment of pharmaceuticals. Introduced in 1970, the legislation covered quality, safety, and efficacy. The first guidelines did not address the issues of bioavailability and bioequivalence.

Possible differences in absorption of active ingredients from different formulations were recognized as a potential health hazard when episodes of phenytoin toxicity were reported in an Australian city following changes to the excipients in a hard gelatin capsule [1]. The subsequent, well-publicized incident of clinically evident altered bioavailability of digoxin tablets that was associated with a change in manufacturing procedures [2] reinforced the need for rigorous testing of new or changed pharmaceuticals. The need to ensure bioequivalence between generic and innovator brands of the same drug product is critical in Australia because the government subsidy of pharmaceuticals is regulated through a national list of approved products [3] in which generic brands are listed alongside innovators.

Regardless of the brand specified by the prescriber, the dispenser will be remunerated according to the price of the one that is currently the cheapest. There is an incentive to supply the cheapest brand in that the patient must pay any additional cost. That different brands may be dispensed in hospitals because of separate generic tendering arrangements is a further source of brand switching as patients enter and leave a hospital.

The first Australian guidelines on bioavailability and bioequivalence were issued in 1975 [4]. These were followed, in 1980, by separate guidelines on slow-release oral formulations [5]. In the late 1980s, it was recognized in Australia that data on bioequivalence generated by a contract laboratory on behalf of two generic pharmaceutical companies had been unreliable. As a result, the agency began to require sufficient detail in study reports to permit evaluators to conduct more elaborate cross-checks. Subsequently, a number of bioequivalence studies for which such detail had been sought were found unacceptable. Consequently, the industry suggested that the guidelines be quite detailed as to how studies should be conducted and reported. The current guidelines were published in 1989 [6] after extensive review and are in two parts: the first component provides in general terms *guidelines* for the design, conduct, analysis, and reporting of bioavailability and bioequivalence studies. The second component describes regulatory *requirements* for various types of application, such as to market a new controlled-release product or to alter the formulation of an existing product.

Both documents were drafted by the Pharmaceutical Subcommittee of the Australian Drug Evaluation Committee, with input from clinicians and pharmacists workin in the bioavailability field, and from the Australian Pharmaceutical Manufacturers Association. The Australian Drug Evaluation Committee is an independent statutory committee of eminent physicians to which the Agency refers technical aspects of applications to market new drug products, and whose advice on these applications and on technical policy issues is rarely rejected.

As copies of the new guidelines are readily available [6], their contents are not reproduced here. A review and discussion of the major points follows.

DEFINITIONS OF BIOAVAILABILITY AND BIOEQUIVALENCE AND THEIR IMPLICATIONS

Bioavailability: The Australian guidelines define bioavailability as ". . . a measure of the rate and extent of absorption of the active form or forms of a drug from its formulation as reflected by the time concentration curve of the administered drug in the systemic circulation. An active form may be a metabolite."

Points to note here include the following:

Mention of *rate* as well as *extent*
Use of the term *active form*, rather than *parent drug*

Recognition that more than one chemical species may need to be assayed
Use of the term *systemic circulation* rather than *site of action*

Bioequivalence: "Two formulations of a drug are said to be bioequivalent if the rates and extents to which the drug reaches the systemic circulation after administration of the formulations are so closely comparable that their therapeutic effect with respect to both efficacy and safety will be essentially the same."

Note that the critical factor is therapeutic effect Although the guidelines go on to discuss an acceptable confidence interval width of ±20% in the general case for differences in area under the curve (AUC), mention is made of the possibility that, when close dosage control is critical, ±20% may be too wide, or that in other cases a wider confidence interval may be acceptable. In relation to rate of absorption, there have been examples of studies comparing a proposed new generic with an innovator in which the applicant has successfully argued to the Australian agency that an observed statistically significant difference in rate of absorption was not clinically significant. Other applications have been rejected because an observed difference in rate was considered clinically significant for that drug.

Whether differences in bioavailability between different dosage forms, generic copies, or reformulations of a product will result in significant differences in clinical effects depends on the nature of the drug concerned and the mode of its use. For example, the problems referred to earlier relating to phenytoin and digoxin are clear situations in which small differences in bioavailability can have serious complications. For some other drugs, such as the benzodiazepines, differences in bioavailability must be greater before clear evidence of inefficacy or undesirable clinical effects emerges. The Australian agency recognizes that it is not possible to formulate universally applicable rules, and that each product must be considered individually as to what constitutes bioequivalence.

It is noteworthy that the Australian definitions assume that if equivalent plasma levels of a drug or its metabolites, or both, are achieved, then this will result in equivalent efficacy and safety. No reference is made to the amount of drug in other body compartments, as might be measured by either assay or, for example, "quantitative pharmacoelectroencephalography" [7,8]. In relation to safety, adverse effects that may be associated with excipients are a matter for separate consideration and evaluation [9,10].

This view of bioequivalence permits flexibility in interpreting study results. For example, if a set of data suggest that the mean AUC or C_{max} for a generic is, with 90% confidence, within say 78–119% of the innovator mean, rather than rejecting the generic on the basis of a rigidly defined confidence interval of 80–120%, the agency will consider company arguments on whether or not the difference is likely to be clinically significant for that drug. However, it would be wrong to interpret this approach as suggesting that the agency is a "pushover" for soft data. The flexibility possible in Australia may reflect the fact that the industry is less litigation-minded than in some countries in which frequent resort to the courts pressures the agency into being more rigid. Perhaps this is a conscious policy on the part of the industry, stemming from an enlightened self-interest.

IN WHICH SITUATIONS SHOULD DATA ON BIOAVAILABILITY BE PROVIDED?

In general, the Australian agency now adopts the view that data on bioavailability are required for any application in the following groups, unless the applicant can demonstrate that such information is unnecessary:

New pharmaceutical products, including new chemical entities, new dosage forms, new generics, and new strengths of existing brands.
New routes of administration.
Changes in formulation, site or method of manufacture, manufacturing equipment, or source of raw materials.

This reflects not so much a change in the agency's views as to when data are required but, rather, a change in the onus as to who should argue the case. Formerly, when confronted with a new application, the agency would weigh up the arguments for whether or not a bioequivalence study was required on the basis of its own knowledge and experience. Now the onus is on the applicant to mount an argument as to why such data are not necessary.

The thrust of the applicants argument should in general be directed towards showing that:

Bioinequivalence or variable bioavailability would be unlikely to lead to adverse clinical consequences.
A bioavailability–bioequivalence study is not possible.
Formulation-related bioinequivalence is unlikely. The guidelines give the example that bioequivalence studies would not normally be required for drugs in simple solution that are intended for intravenous administration only.

It is helpful that the guidelines provide a list of the factors to consider when preparing a case for not conducting a study. These include the chemical and physicochemical properties of the drug and the dosage form, pharmacokinetic properties, any special claims made in labeling or prescribing information, and the clinical profile of the drug, including the margin between its effective and toxic plasma concentrations and the likely consequences of inequivalence or variable bioavailability.

TRIAL DESIGN

The Australian guidelines stress the importance of pilot studies and prior knowledge of a drug's pharmacokinetics in the design of bioavailability studies and the interpretation of results.

In general, it would be difficult to design a successful bioavailability study without prior estimates of the key variables associated with the drug and the dosage form, particularly the peak plasma concentration, the time to peak, and the persistence of the drug in plasma. The other key piece of information required is the variability to be expected between subjects for these parameters. Information on the properties of the drug will, in general, be available from either the literature or from data held by the company, depending on whether or not the company is the drug's innovator. For the specific dosage form under test, a pilot study should be considered and would also provide a basis for validating the assay method.

THE NUMBER OF SUBJECTS REQUIRED IN A STUDY

Generally, the number of subjects should be sufficient to provide the necessary discriminatory power. The key pieces of information needed to estimate the appropriate number are the variability to be expected between subjects and a knowledge of the clinically tolerable differences between formulations for each of the targeted parameters. If the intended statistical analysis of the study's results is in terms of the power of an analysis of variance, this calculation is easy. It is much more difficult when the statistically more acceptable confidence interval analysis is intended. The Australian guidelines suggest methods of estimating an appropriate number in the confidence interval case, but the calculation has the limitation that an *a priori* estimate is needed of the anticipated difference or ratio of the means for each pair of treatments. Metzler has published simulation curves that graphically present the probability of rejecting bioequivalence for various mean ratios [11], allowing a company a clearer assessment of the level of risk.

Over and above the statistical calculations, the Australian guidelines specify a minimum acceptable number of 12 and a maximum, on ethical grounds, of 24. However, although this is not stated, we suspect it is unlikely that the agency would reject studies using more than 24 subjects, particularly when conducted overseas where views on this ethical issue may be different. The stated maximum probably implies that studies using more than 24 subjects are not a requirement.

When calculations estimate that more than 24 subjects would be necessary, the guidelines suggest the following alternatives:

Cold-labeling techniques or studies in which treatments are replicated
Clinical efficacy or safety studies, or both

One may observe at this point that clinical efficacy or safety studies would almost always have a lower discriminatory power than any study involving plasma assays, whatever the intersubject variability. Perhaps the rationale is that the former would use patients and, although demanding more subjects, would not expose a large number of healthy volunteers to the drug. Separate statistical criteria, for example, in terms of the width of a confidence interval, are not specified for efficacy or safety studies.

Fortunately, a once commonly held belief that a sufficient number of subjects must be studied to look for random abnormal results in some individuals no longer has general acceptance. The objective of a bioequivalence study is to determine the relative properties of two formulations, not to examine the possible heterogeneity of the human race. Although there are situations in which two products may not be bioequivalent in all patients, such as when one product has acid-sensitive dissolution rate and may be given in the presence of hypochlorhydria [12] or during concomitant treatment with an H_2 receptor-blocker, these possibilities should be investigated in separate studies in which subjects are deliberately selected for chosen characteristics.

ANALYTICAL METHODS AND THEIR VALIDATION

It is now generally recognized that fully validated analytical methods are critical to the success of a study. Methods should be state of the art and should be specific and sensitive. Assay validation must be conducted in full and in the same laboratory that generates the study data and using the same technique. The Australian guidelines require provision in the report of full details of assay validation, including the shape of the calibration curve, specificity, accuracy, precision, sensitivity (minimum quantifiable concentration), recovery, and the stability of the measured species in plasma.

ASSAY OF ENANTIOMERS?

Although raised as an issue many years ago [13], the importance of stereospecific physiological handling of drugs has only recently received the attention that it deserves in regulatory circles. The Australian guidelines make only brief reference to the possible need to consider use of isomer-specific assays for drugs that are mixtures of enantiomers. Policy on data requirements in this area is now under development.

PRESENTATION OF DATA

The guidelines provide a checklist of items that should normally be included in the report of a study. Investigators would be well-advised to refer to this list when preparing reports. In particular, sponsoring companies should bear in mind that the Australian agency conducts its own independent assessment of bioavailability and bioequivalence data, including random checks of the kinetic and statistical calculations. Consequently, individual data must be provided, together with details such as the actual sampling times (for use in calculations) as well as the nominal times specified in the protocol.

In picking up a now well-accepted trend in ideas on ethics, the checklist seeks a statement of the means by which the study was monitored to confirm that it was carried out as proposed in the protocol. Monitoring should be in accordance with a recognized Code of Good Clinical Practice.

STATISTICAL ANALYSES

In reviewing the data, the Australian agency undertakes random recalculations of the statistical analyses. The statistical methods normally used by the agency are detailed in the guidelines. Sponsors may use other valid methods, but must justify them at the time of submission.

The question of outliers and their elimination from data sets is controversial, as less scrupulous sponsors have been known to select outliers on the basis of eliminating those data points that tend to reflect least favorably on the product under test. The Australian agency is preparing a set of criteria defining the circumstances under which outliers may be identified.

A MOVING TARGET?

Without a definitive and unchanging reference product against which other formulations may be compared, there is potential for both generics and innovators to change with time.

The Australian guidelines require that generics be shown to be bioequivalent to a formulation that is already marketed in Australia. The new brand should be compared with the leading Australian brand, which is normally the innovator. The batch of innovator used in the study must have been obtained on the Australian market because even transnational companies may market different formulations in different countries. If another product on the Australian market has significant usage, a three-way crossover trial may be desirable to show that the new product is bioequivalent to both frequently used products.

The logic of this requirement is fairly clear; namely, that the concern of the agency is that an Australian generic must be interchangeable with the leading brand in this country. But what if the benchmark changes?

Simplistically, generic A is compared with the innovator and is approved on the basis of this study. The innovator then undergoes an unauthorized formulation change as a result of a lack of communication within the company. Generic

B is compared against (unknowingly) the revised innovator formulation and is also approved for marketing. The agency then discovers the unauthorized formulation change. How does generic A compare with generic B? A very similar situation occurred recently within Australia. The agency was naturally reluctant to take action that would disadvantage either of the generic companies, as each had acted properly. But the public must be protected against inequivalent products.

A simple answer is to require a solution to be included in each bioavailability and bioequivalence study, as well as the formulations to be compared, whatever these are. A solution, whether administered orally or intravenously, can be reproduced exactly over time, providing an invariant benchmark. Not surprisingly, there is resistance to such a suggestion, as it increases costs and the exposure of volunteers to the drug.

In common with regulatory documents from elsewhere, the Australian guidelines do not address one of the most difficult problems in the bioavailability area, namely that of the moving benchmark.

CONCLUDING COMMENTS

Technical guidelines must be updated regularly as technology improves and ideas change. As examples, we have cited improvements in analytical methodology such that many enantiomers can now be separately measured when the racemate is present, and the more clinically oriented definition of bioequivalence. Nevertheless, it is reasonable for regulatory authorities to expect that the industry will keep abreast of developments in the field and will apply the latest technology (within reasonable cost limits), without there being a specific requirement to do so in published guidelines.

On the other hand, agencies are sometimes in the difficult position of having to assess data from studies that have been conducted to a lower standard than is now possible. Perhaps the study was conducted some years before submission, or perhaps the agency did not immediately evaluate the data when received. If the issue that arises is one of safety, the decision may be in favor of a new study. But if all that has happened is that new technology has provided an opportunity to generate "nice-to-know" information, the decision may go the other way. Of course, most real situations are less clear-cut. The agency has to bear in mind that to require a new bioavailability study will involve a further exposure of healthy volunteers, or in some instances patients, to the drug. Considerations of toxicity arise, and one might talk of a risk–benefit analysis of regulatory requirements. The ethics of demanding repeat studies using new technology require that there be real grounds for clinical concern that will be addressed by a new study.

It is our view that, although the Australian guidelines may be detailed, they do no more than set the scene for the conduct of scientifically and ethically sound studies that should be an integral part of any drug development program.

REFERENCES

1. J. H. Tyrer, M. J. Eadie, J. M. Sutherland, and W. D. Hooper. Outbreak of anticonvulsant toxicity in an Australian city. *Br. Med. J.* 4:271-273 (1970).
2. Bioavailability of digoxin [Editorial]. *Lancet* Vol. 2 no. 772:311-312 (1972).
3. Schedule of pharmaceutical benefits. Department of Community Services and Health, PO Box 9848, Canberra City Act 2601, Australia (Issued four monthly)
4. Guidelines for bioavailability studies. Australian Department of Health (1975).
5. Guidelines for slow release oral formulations. Australian Department of Health (1980).
6. Guidelines for bioavailability and bioequivalence studies; and Requirements for bioavailability and bioequivalence studies. Drug Evaluation Branch, Therapeutic Goods Administration, PO Box 100, Canberra City Act 2601, Australia (1989).
7. *Pink Sheets* pp. 3-4 (4 March 1985).
8. *Pink Sheets* T&G. pp. 2-3 (15 July 1985).
9. J. M. Smith and T. R. P. Dodd. Adverse reactions to pharmaceutical excipients. *Adverse Drug. React. Acute Poisoning Rev.* 1:93-142 (1982).
10. E. Napke and D. G. H. Stevens. Excipients and additives: Hidden hazards in drug products and in product substitution. *Can. Med. Assoc. J.* 131:1449-1452 (1984).
11. C. M. Metzler. Sample sizes for bioequivalence studies. *Stat. Med.* (in press).
12. H. Ogata, N. Aoyagi, N. Kaniwa, M. Koibuchi, T. Shibazaki, and A. Ejima. The bioavailability of diazepam from uncoated tablets in humans—effect of gastric fluid acidity. *Int. J. Clin. Pharm. Ther. Toxicol.* 20:166-170 (1982).
13. P. A. Lehmann, J. F. Rodriguez de Miranda, and E. J. Ariens. Stereoselectivity and affinity in molecular pharmacology. *Progr. Drug Res.* 20:101-142 (1976).

16

Bioequivalence: A Nordic Perspective

Tomas Salmonson and Hans Melander
Medical Products Agency
Uppsala, Sweden

Anders Rane
University Hospital and Medical Products Agency
Uppsala, Sweden

INTRODUCTION

The Nordic Council of Medicine is a joint Nordic organization with the objection to promote concurrence of legislation and administrative procedures related to pharmaceuticals in the Nordic countries. In cooperation with the drug regulatory authorities in Denmark, Finland, Iceland, Norway, and Sweden the council has prepared Nordic guidelines on bioavailability studies in humans, NLN 18 [1]. The guidelines are intended as an outline for the required studies that are considered necessary to document the rate and extent of bioavailability for new chemical entities, generic drugs, new dosage forms, and drug delivery systems.

By necessity, these guidelines may express only general views and suggestions on the required documentation. In this chapter, we will discuss how the Swedish Medical Products Agency applies these guidelines in its evaluation work. Our views represent only the views of the Medical Products Agency and the guidelines may be interpreted differently in other Nordic countries.

THE SWEDISH GENERIC DRUG MARKET

There are relatively few generic drugs on the Swedish market, compared with other countries. Several reasons may be identified, the major ones being

A limited market, since Sweden has only 9 million inhabitants.

A price-insensitive market, since the government reimburses almost the entire cost of a prescription. The prescribing doctor has the full formal right to choose the brand name of the drug, but is usually under "information pressure" from drug committees.

Generic substitution is not allowed at the pharmacies.

Table 1 summarizes the number of applications for general marketing of generic drugs, new dosage forms, and drug delivery systems that the Swedish Medical Products Agency has received during the last 5 years.

Even though the guidelines discussed in the following were published in 1987, the rejection rate seems to increase over the years. A possible reason for this is that the guidelines are not appropriately interpreted by the industry.

FUNDAMENTAL CONCEPTS IN NLN 18

The Nordic guidelines on bioavailability studies in humans covers the required documentation for new chemical entities, generic drugs, new dosage forms, and drug delivery systems. A generic product is defined as one that *contains the*

Table 1 Number of Applications for General Marketing in Sweden 1985–1989

	Generic drugs	New dosage forms	Drug delivery systems	Total	(%)
1985					
Accepted	10	14	2	26	
Rejected	2	0	0	2	(7)
1986					
Accepted	20	8	2	30	
Rejected	3	0	2	5	(14)
1987					
Accepted	28	8	6	42	
Rejected	6	1	5	12	(22)
1988					
Accepted	11	3	8	22	
Rejected	6	7	1	14	(39)
1989					
Accepted	13	13	3	29	
Rejected	5	1	5	11	(28)

same dose of the active ingredient in the same dosage form as a previously marketed drug product. Generic products should be bioequivalent to those already marketed. This definition is unfortunately unclear, since bioequivalence *between two products is achieved when the absorption (extent and rate) does not differ in any clinically important degree.* It is conceived that when bioequivalence exists, therapeutic equivalence also exists. However, sometimes therapeutic equivalence has to be demonstrated in comparative clinical or pharmacodynamic studies. This is obvious when considering an application for a generic topical ointment. Here, bioavailability studies may be of value for the safety assessment, but its value for the assessment of therapeutic equivalence is doubtful. Thus, a preferable expression in NLN 18 would be that generic products should be therapeutically equivalent to those already on the market.

The principles for bioavailability testing are the same for new dosage forms as for generic products. For drug delivery systems, data should be provided comparing the bioavailability for the new drug delivery system with the dosage form for which it is intended as a substitute. This shall be done both after a single dose and at steady state. In most cases, studies of factors suspected to influence the bioavailability (e.g., food intake) and clinical studies are also required. If clinical data are deemed necessary, they should be generated in comparison with the conventional dosage form.

Experimental Design

The type of documentation needed to prove that a product is bioequivalent to a marketed reference drug is not specified in NLN 18.

The following variables are traditionally used to determine the relative bioavailability:

The area under the concentration–time curve (AUC) as a measure of the extent of bioavailability
The time to the maximum concentration (t_{max}) describing the rate of absorption
The maximum concentration (C_{max}), which reflects both the extent of bioavailability and the rate of absorption

In addition, several other parameters are sometimes used to support the claims of bioequivalence, such as the mean residence time of a drug molecule in the body (MRT), absorption rate constant (k_a), and the elimination half-life ($t_{1/2}$).

The relative extent of bioavailability is, in many cases, demonstrated by comparing the total AUC for the products. This is done with the assumption that the elimination is the same, regardless of the dosage form. However, occasionally, the intraindividual variability in clearance capacity is large, requiring many subjects. If this is the case, the use of total urinary excretion to determine the relative bioavailability may be preferable. This comparison does not require that the total clearance is the same, but it is assumed that the renal/total clearance ratio is constant. For drugs that are excreted unchanged, to a large extent this ratio often varies less than the total clearance, since renal clearance contributes substantially to the total clearance. For drugs known to be completely eliminated in unchanged form by the kidneys, the absolute bioavailability can be calculated. It is our impression that the usefulness of urinary data to determine the extent of bioavailability is often underestimated.

The design of bioequivalence studies is often too standardized. This applies in particular to the sampling schedule. We all recognize the following standard sampling schedule:

Time after the dose was given: 0.25, 0.5, 0.75, 1, 2, 4, 6, 8, 12, and 24 hr.

For some drugs, this schedule may be very appropriate, but for others, it is not. In too many applications this schedule is used without considering the pharmacokientic properties of the drug and the pharmacokinetic variables that are intended to be determined. Usually, it is the possibility to accurately determine C_{max} and t_{max} that is lost. It should be obvious that the foregoing sampling schedule is not optimal for a drug that reaches its maximum concentration between 2 and 4 hours after the dose.

The guidelines recognize any appropriate design, but the parallel group and the crossover designs are explicitly mentioned. It is also stated in the guidelines that it is important to account for different sources of variability, such as subject and period effects, in the analysis. Apparently a crossover study is preferred as support for a bioequivalence claim. Nevertheless, in rare instances, applicants have relied on parallel group studies, and such applications have been approved.

The number of subjects is of crucial importance. According to the guidelines the sample size must be based on statistical considerations, and it is stated that it should be large enough to detect a $\pm 20\%$ difference with a type I error of 0.05 and type II error of 0.20. These explicit levels of significance and power should be regarded as recommendations, rather than as specific requirements. Here, there is a discrepancy in the guidelines. The sample size calculation is obviously supposed to be based on a conventional hypothesis test, whereas this method is considered inadequate for the analysis. The guidelines suggest a confidence interval (CI) approach for the establishment of bioequivalence. However, the sample size calculation should give only a rough estimate to be used in planning the trial, and a calculation based on confidence intervals should not differ much from the foregoing test-based criterion.

Evaluation of the Data

Since a generic drug, by definition, contains the same dose as a previously marketed drug product, the relative bioavailability can usually be determined by comparing the AUC and C_{max} without dose correction. In some cases, dose correction may be justified if the drug contents in the two dosage forms are different, but within acceptable limits. However, this will be accepted by the agency only if the correction was planned and stated in the study protocol.

As mentioned earlier, it is assumed that the clearance remains the same in the two study periods. In practice, however, the elimination capacity for many drugs varies with time, resulting in increased intraindividual variability. The variability in elimination capacity may be corrected for in several ways, for example, by the "half-life correction" method suggested by Wagner [2].

This method assumes that a change in $t_{1/2}$ solely reflects a corresponding change in elimination capacity without a concomitant change in the apparent volume of distribution (V_d). Such a correction would be acceptable if the applicant submits information to show that the elimination capacity varies more than the V_d, and if it is planned and described in the study protocol. The half-life correction method cannot be used if the rate of absorption is the rate-limiting step for the elimination ("flip-flop" phenomenon).

The advocacy of confidence intervals for the establishment of bioequivalence needs some clarification. First, should the confidence interval be calculated for differences of means or for the ratios of means (i.e., should the analysis be performed on observed data or on logarithmically transformed data)? The agency recognizes that a strong case can be made for the logarithmic transformation of at least AUC and C_{max}. Thus, analyses based on transformed data are accepted. It is important though that the decision to transform data was made independently of the data obtained in the actual study. Therefore, it should be decided a priori and stated in the protocol. An applicant may sometimes perform the analysis on both transformed and untransformed data and argue for the analysis that results in the shortest confidence interval. So far, we have not identified any approval that was dependent on the use of a logarithmic transformation.

What type of interval to use is a matter of discussion: A conventional confidence interval or an interval symmetric about the average of the reference. In the early 1980s, many of the applications were supported by symmetric confidence intervals according to Westlake [3]. If not, the data were reanalyzed in this manner by the agency. The symmetric intervals were later abandoned, since it works in favor of the applicant [see, e.g., Ref. 4]. From a regulatory perspective, conventional confidence intervals seem more appropriate.

Another issue concerning confidence intervals in bioequivalence studies is the level of confidence. The regulatory agency recommends and uses a confidence coefficient of 95%, irrespective of type of confidence interval.

Following Westlake [5] and Schuirmann [6] many applicants are arguing for 90% confidence intervals, which would increase their chance of demonstrating bioequivalence. The rationale behind this argument is that the 90% confidence interval is equivalent to a 5% significance test of the null hypothesis that the difference in bioavailability lies outside the acceptable range for bioequivalence (the "two one-sided test" procedure). Indeed, in efficacy studies of new drugs against placebo, the regulatory agencies accept a type I error of 5% in a conventional significance test of the null hypothesis of identical effect. Thus, it is argued that a 90% confidence interval is acceptable in bioequivalence studies. However, this analogy is not quite correct. The bioequivalence is usually assessed in only one study, whereas several independent studies are required for an approval of a claim of clinical efficacy. Hence, the overall type I error will be less than 5% in the clinical situation.

At present, we would not put forward the introduction of the two one-sided test procedure or the equivalent 90% confidence intervals.

Interpretation of the Results

The guidelines state that the confidence limits of the mean difference generally should be within ±20%. These limits may occasionally change, depending on the pharmacodynamic properties of the drug. It is important to realize that the intention with these requirements is that the limits may occasionally be narrower than ±20%.

The absorption rate is difficult to assess because it is not always well described by t_{max} and C_{max}. Since the rate of absorption is not always of importance for the clinical effect wider limits, or even differences in rate of absorption, may be acceptable. However, the NLN 18 gives no guidance when the rate of absorption can be considered clinically insignificant. It is the obligation of the applicant to convince the agency that the rate of absorption has negligible clinical relevance.

Recently, a company applied for general marketing of a generic nonsteroidal anti-inflammatory drug product. The indication included acute pain. To demonstrate bioequivalence the company submitted a study with the following results (Table 2, Fig. 1). The company argued that the difference in rate of absorption was clinically insignificant. This opinion was not shared by the agency. This example may seem clear-cut, but it illustrates the viewpoint of the agency.

In the previous example, the confidence interval for t_{max} was definitely too wide. However, the agency realizes that the ±20% rule cannot be applied strictly for t_{max} because then almost no drug that peaks early would be able to pass.

Table 2 Calculated Mean Parameters (± SD)

	Test	Ref	95% CI
AUC	96 ± 15	95 ± 16	96–105
t_{max}	2.2 ± 1.6	1.1 ± 0.8	135–267
C_{max}	18 ± 4	21 ± 4	78–94

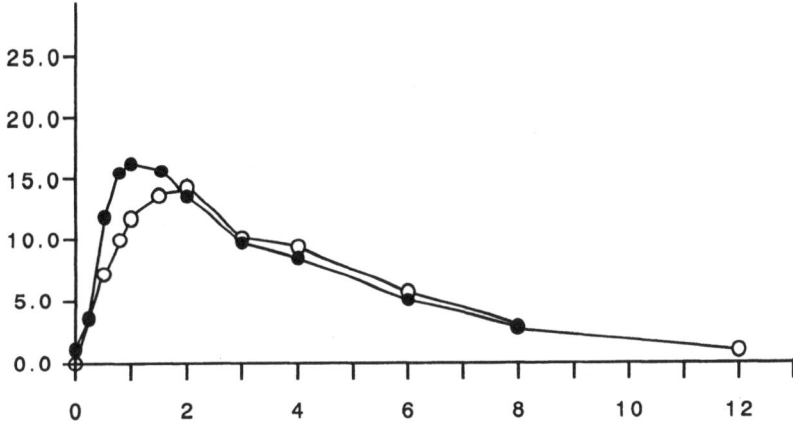

Figure 1 Mean concentration–time curves for the test (open circles) and the reference (closed circles) product.

When rate of absorption is relevant, the decision should be based on a clinical judgment of a confidence interval of the absolute differences expressed in, for example, minutes.

Presentation of the Results

A bioequivalence study submitted to support marketing of a generic drug is often very standardized. Therefore, the guidelines suggest a standardized way of summarizing the design and results of a bioequivalence study. This "standard protocol" has proved helpful in speeding up the regulatory review process. The protocol gives the reviewer a fast introduction to the documentation, but it also forms the basis for the evaluation report. The reviewer will append a cover with the results from his own statistical analysis and the review protocol is ready. A full report must be submitted with the standard protocol. In addition to description of the methods, results, discussion, and conclusion, the report should also contain

A detailed description of the validated analytical report
Individual concentration–time data, preferably also as figures, together with calculated pharmacokinetic variables
A statistical report
The study protocol

FUTURE PERSPECTIVE

Some inadequacies and problems in the current NLN 18 guidelines have been highlighted in the foregoing. The guidelines and their application are continuously discussed, and this may result in amendments to the future requirements.

The problems of finding the optimal sampling schedule is closely related to the problems with t_{max} and C_{max} when used to characterize the rate of absorption. These parameters are easy to assess without the need of model fitting. However, they are not determined solely by the rate of absorption, but also by the extent of bioavilability (C_{max}) and the rate of elimination (C_{max} and t_{max}). In view of the problems with the t_{max} variable (double peaks in the concentration-time curve or absence of sharp peaks with slow-release formulations), the agency would like to encourage the development of other measurements of the rate of absorption such as model-dependent techniques or determinations based on AUC—for example, time to a defined fraction of total AUC.

It seems logical to document the bioavailability/bioequivalence of the active chemical moiety. This implies that if a metabolite is responsible to a major extent for the clinical effect, the bioequivalence should be based on the concentration of the metabolite. Similarly, this has implications for documentation of racemic mixtures. This issue is currently debated at the agency and in the scientific community. The importance of documenting the kinetics of the active enantiomer(s) will undoubtedly be emphasized. The agency has not yet expressed specific requirements on chiral drugs. Should bioequivalence in the future be based on the active enantiomer(s) in a racemic mixture, instead of on the sum of the enantiomer concentrations? One might argue that since we are only interested in the biopharmaceutical qualities of two different products and, usually, it is achiral factors influencing the release rate from a tablet, the total concentration of the enantiomers adequately represents the biopharmaceutical quality of the formulations.

The current procedures to establish bioequivalence recognized by regulatory agencies are based solely on an analysis of average bioavailabilities. However, several authors [7-9] have questioned the adequacy of mean comparisons and, in some recent papers, alternative procedures are suggested. Anderson and Hauck [10] discuss in terms of within-subject bioequivalence and propose a method based on within-subject ratios of bioavailabilities. In two papers, Ekbohm and Melander [11,12] argue that bioequivalence should be interpreted as interchangeability. They suggest a criterion of interchangeability that is based on within-subject variability, subject-by-formulation interaction and also the average bioavailabilities. Their approach requires a design in which each subject is given each formulation at least twice, whereas an ordinary two-period crossover design is sufficient for the method of Anderson and Hauck.

Generic substitution has hitherto not been permitted in the Nordic countries.

Recently, however, an official report in Sweden discussed that issue. This report might have an impact on future regulations. If so, we will probably need a criterion of bioequivalence that takes interindividual responses into account.

REFERENCES

1. Bioavailability studies in man, Nordic guidelines. *NLN publication No 18*, Nordic Council on Medicines (1987).
2. J. G. Wagner. *J. Pharm. Sci.* 56:652 (1967).
3. W. J. Westlake. *Biometrics* 32:741 (1976).
4. T. B. L. Kirkwood. *Biometrics* 37:589 (1981).
5. W. J. Westlake. *Biometrics* 37:591 (1981).
6. D. J. Schuirmann. *J. Pharmacokin. Biopharm.* 15:657 (1987).
7. S. Hwang, P. B. Huber, M. Hesney, and K. C. Kwan. *J. Pharm. Sci.* 67:IV (1978).
8. W. J. Westlake. *Biometrics* 35:273 (1979).
9. J. D. Haynes. *J. Pharm. Sci.* 70:673 (1981).
10. S. Anderson and W. W. Hauck. *J. Pharmacokin. Biopharm.* 18:259 (1990).
11. G. Ekbohm and H. Melander. *Biometrics* 45:1249 (1989).
12. G. Ekbohm and H. Melander. *Report 14, Swedish Univ. of Agri. Sci., Dept. of Stat.* (1990).

Index

Abbreviated New Drug Application (ANDA), 3, 68, 170, 350
Absorption, 69
  animal models for, 235
  diseases and disease states affecting, 75
    cardiovascular, 88
    gastrointestinal, 75
    gastrointestinal infections, 85
    gastrointestinal motility, 79
    gastrointestinal surgery, 88
    hepatic, 93
    hyperthermia, 100
    hypothermia, 100
    large intestine, 85
    neurological, 100
    pulmonary, 99
    renal, 95
    rheumatoid arthritis, 100
    small intestine, 82
    stomach, 82

[Absorption]
  extent of, 5, 69
  factors affecting, 134
    antacids, 138
    blood flow, 134
    dissolution rate, 136
    drug metabolism in intestinal mucosa, 139
    fluid volume, 137
    food, 137
    membrane permeability, 134
    metabolic activity of the intestinal microflora, 141
    pH, 135
  intestinal, 160
    methods to study in animals, 160
    role in systemic elimination of drug, 161
  percutaneous, 129, 170, 192
  physiological basis of, 119
  rate of, 5, 69, 391

Allopurinol, 396
Analysis of variance, 38, 51
  uses in bioavailability studies, 53
Animal models, 235
  dog, 255
  monkey, 245
  rabbit, 242
  swine, 251
Antifungal products, 211
Austrialian regulatory perspectives, 443
  analytical methods, 448
  definitions of bioavailability and
    bioequivalence, 444
  enantiomers, 448
  number of subjects, 447
  presentation of data, 448
  statistical analysis, 449
  trial design, 447

Bioavailability, 36, 430, 444
  absolute, 18, 67
  assessment of, 17, 30
  design of studies, 19
  enantioselective, 102
  factors influencing, 117
    anesthesia, 102
    diseases and disease states, 67, 75
    pain, 102
    protein binding, 98
    surgery, 102
  metabolites, 20
  relative, 40, 67
    estimates of, 40, 44
  types of studies, 18
  variability, 37
Bioequivalence, 1, 36, 430, 445
  assessment of, 17, 117
  decision rules, 55
    Anderson-Hauck hypothesis test, 59
    Bayesian procedures, 60
    classic confidence intervals, 58
    symmetric confidence intervals, 59

[Bioequivalence]
  practices, criteria, and issues, 360
    accuracy, 365
    analytical procedures validation,
      364, 403, 448
    experimental design (see study
      design)
    linearity, 365
    range, 365
    reference product, 363, 402
    sampling times, 363, 402
    sensitivity limit, 366
    solution standards, 391
    specificity, 366
    study design, 19, 63, 361, 387,
      401, 430, 455
    subjects, 362, 400
    types of studies, 18
  regulatory perspectives (see
    individual Australian, Canadian,
    European Community, Nordic,
    and United States regulatory
    perspectives)
Blood concentration-pharmacologic
  response relationship, 22

Canadian regulatory perspectives, 381
  definition of bioavailability, 383
  dissolution and bioequivalence, 394
  dissolution limitations, 398
  drugs with complicated
    characteristics, 406
  Expert Advisory Committee, 383
  guidelines and standards, 399
  modified-release formulations, 409
  New Drug Submission (NDS), 381
  presentation of data, 404
  standards for bioequivalence, 405
  statistical analysis, 405
Clozapine, 28
Concentration-effect models (see
  pharmacodynamic models)
Confidence intervals, 46, 388
  as percentage, 48

Index

[Confidence intervals]
   classical t-based, 46
   nonparametric, 50
   Westlake's symmetric, 47
Controlled-release dosage forms, 21

Disease, 68
Dosage-form proportionality, 18, 28
Dose proportionality, 18, 29
Dose-response studies, 64
Drug-drug interaction, 163
Drug effect, 10
Drug transport, 132
   active transport, 134
   electrochemical diffusion, 134
   facilitated diffusion, 133
   ionic diffusion (*see* electrochemical diffusion)
   nonionic diffusion (*see* passive diffusion)
   passive diffusion, 132
   pinocytosis, 134

Enzyme systems:
   bacterial metabolism, 155
   colon mucosa, 155
   luminal enzymes, 150
   mucosal enzymes in small intestine, 153
   stomach mucosa, 153
Equivalent time, 294
European Community Regulatory Perspectives, 419
   bioavailability guidance, 421
   definitions, 430
   design, conduct, and evaluation of studies, 430
   Germany, Federal Republic of, 426
   in vivo studies, 432
   modified-release products, 433
   Netherlands, 424
   "open" and "closed" dossiers, 432
   Revised European Community Recommendation, 427

[European Community]
   suprabioavailability, 433
   United Kingdom, 423
   veterinary medicinal products, 437

Food, 26

Gastric acid secretion, 125
   phases of, 126
      cephalic, 126
      gastric, 126
      intestinal, 126
   regulation of, 126
Gastric motility, 124
Gastric mucosa, 121
Gastrointestinal tract, 119
   immunology of, 123

Hypothesis testing, 388

Ibuprofen, 398
Immediate-release dosage form, 26
In vitro–in vivo correlation, 223
   comparison of environments, 224
   guidelines for tests to determine, 226
   parameters used in, 225
Integrated pharmacokinetic-pharmacodynamic models, 313
   (*see also* Pharmacodynamic models)
   complexities in pharmacokinetic-pharmacodynamic assessment, 321
   effect compartment models, 317
   objectives, 313
   potential in bioavailability-bioequivalence studies, 323
   sampled matrix, 314
   simulations, 330
   steady-state measurements, 317
   use in predicting consequences of altered bioavailability, 328

Index

Interdigestive migrating motility complex, 241
Interspecies scaling, 267, 269
  absorption, 289
    animal models of, 289
    bioavailability, 291
  allometry, 271
  biological half-life, 292
  clearance, 273
  distribution, 284
    protein binding, 285
    volume of, 286
  dosing regimens, 292
  hepatic metabolic clearance
    in animals, 275
    in human, 278
    polymorphism, 280
    stereoselectivity, 280
  hepatobiliary clearance, 281
  renal clearance, 282
  total systemic clearance, 283
Intestine, 121
Intra/intersubject variability, 18

Kefauver–Harris Amendment, 2, 349

Lung capacity, 129
  assessment of, 129

Metabolism:
  bacterial, 155
  cutaneous, 130
  first-pass, 9, 140
  gut wall, 139
  intestinal, 149
    cannulated mesenteric vein, 157
    cannulated peripheral collateral veins, 158
    cannulated portal vein, 157
    changes in intestinal site of absorption, 159

[Metabolism, intestinal]
    comparison of drug and metabolite, 159
    dual isotope labeling, 159
    experimental evidence in humans, 157
    sampling of intestinal contents, 159
Michaelis–Menten kinetics, 20
Migrating myoelectric complex, 124
Minoxidil, 214
Multiple dose, 22, 30

New Drug Application (NDA), 3, 170, 349
Nordic Regulatory Perspectives, 453
  evaluation of data, 456
  experimental design, 455
  interpretation of results, 458
  NLN 18, 454
  presentation of results, 459
  Swedish generic drug market, 454

Pharmaceutical equivalents, 430
Pharmacodynamic models, 10, 301, 305 (*see also* Integrated pharmacokinetic-pharmacodynamic models)
  baseline compensation, 311
  E_{max} models, 308
  inhibitory E_{max} models, 311
  linear relationships, 305
  objectives, 303
  study design, 303
  terminology 303
  threshold effects, 312
Pharmacokinetic phases:
  absorption, 69
  distribution, 70
  excretion, 72
  liberation (*see* release)
  metabolism, 72
  release, 69
Phenylbutazone, 386, 394

Index

Physiological flow models, 268
Power analysis, 6
Protein binding, 98

Radiopharmaceuticals, 101
Routes of drug administration, 118
  buccal, 127
  inhalation, 128
  intranasal, 132
  oral, 118
  parenteral, 131
    intradermal, 131
    intramuscular, 131
    intravenous, 131
    subcutaneous, 131
  rectal, 132
  sublingual, 127
  transdermal, 129

Saturated first-pass metabolism, 9
Single dose, 22, 30
Skin:
  blanching assay, 203
    attenuated total reflectance infrared spectroscopy, 203
    laser doppler velocimetry, 205
    photopulse plethysmography, 205
    tristimulus reflectance meter, 206
    xenon clearance, 206
  characteristics of, 171
    age, 171
    barrier properties, 171
    hydration, 171
    race, 171
    site of application, 176
    skin condition, 176
  metabolism by, 177
    Phase I reactions, 177
    Phase II reactions, 177
  permeation, 192
Statistical criteria 35
Stomach, 121
Sustained-release dosage form, 26

Tetracycline, 395
Therapeutic equivalence, 1, 430
Thioridazine, 25
Topical dosage forms, 169, 170, 188
  animal models, 190
  clinical trials, 210
  human testing, 196
    biopsies, 198
    pharmacodynamic effects, 199
    skin stripping, 197
  in vitro methods, 191
  systemic availability of, 208
Transdermal delivery systems, 178
  in vitro testing, 187
  in vivo animal studies, 185
  in vivo human studies, 179
Transdermal dosage forms, 169, 170
Transformations of data, 65
  logarithmic, 65, 370, 387
Tretinoin, 212

United States Regulatory Perspectives, 347
  Abbreviated New Drug Application (ANDA), 350, 373
  bioequivalence practices, criteria, and issues, 360
  bioequivalence testing laboratories and compliance, 374
  DESI drugs, 351
  dissolution testing, 372
  historical perspective, 348
  Kefauver-Harris Amendments, 349
  New Drug Application (NDA), 349
  Regulations of 1977, 352
  statistical requirements, 367
  Waxman-Hatch Amendments, 352, 356

Variation, sources of, 51

Warfarin, 391
Waxman-Hatch Amendments, 189, 352